Peptide Immunotherapy

COLOSTRUM

A Physician's Reference Guide

Peptide Immunotherapy

COLOSTRUM

A Physician's Reference Guide

Andrew M Keech, PhD

Peptide Immunotherapy

Colostrum—A Physician's Reference Guide

Cover and book design by Atara Heiss

Edited by John Buhmeyer

Published by AKS Publishing

Second hardcover edition April 2010

Printed in China

Description: Macrophage engulfing bacteria. Computer artwork of a macrophage white blood cell (green) engulfing bacteria (gold). This process is called phagocytosis. Macrophages are immune system cells that phagocytose and destroy pathogens, dead cells and cellular debris. After phagocytosis they display fragments of a pathogen's proteins on surface receptors to direct other cells to attack the pathogen.

For additional copies of this book email Dr Keech directly at dr_keech@msn.com.

Library of Congress Cataloging-in-Publication data has been applied for.

ISBN: 978-0-692-00242-1

pep·tide

Pronunciation [pep-tahyd]

–*noun,* a compound containing two or more amino acids in which the carboxyl group of one acid is linked to the amino group of the other.

■ ■ ■ ■

im·mu·no·ther·a·py

Pronunciation [im-yuh-noh-ther-uh-pee]

–*noun*, treatment designed to produce immunity to a disease or enhance the resistance of the immune system to an active disease process, as cancer.

TABLE OF CONTENTS

PREFACE

I was born and raised on a dairy farm in New Zealand. Like many young dairy families in New Zealand, raising cows and children simultaneously was a challenge in a climate that would often experience four seasons in one day. We were somewhat isolated on a dairy farm, or maybe it was a good thing to be protected from the big city life challenges. Once a year, as kids, we would be driven by our parents about an hour to the big city (New Plymouth, about 40,000 people) to dine on Kentucky Fried Chicken. Well, that was a treat for a youngster who for 364 days a year was reared on potatoes, vegetables and red meat.

Growing up on a farm taught us kids the value of a good day's work. There was always something to do, whether we wanted to do it or not. Cows, pigs, sheep, horses, and chickens all had to be fed, lawns had to be mown, vegetables had to be grown, fences had to be mended, stock had to be moved, cows had to be milked, weeds had to be controlled, tracks and buildings had to be maintained, fertilizer had to be spread on the pasture, water lines and electric fences had to work, trees and riverbanks had to be maintained, swamps and pastures had to be drained, machinery had to operate, everything dirty had to be cleaned, firewood for the winter had to be cut and stored for drying, hay had to be collected and stored, rodents and pests had to be killed—I could go on and on, but you get the idea.

As a young boy on a dairy farm in New Zealand, one of my chores in springtime was to feed the young female calves my parents kept to one day become milkers, just like their mothers. Twice a day, before and after school, I would collect buckets of yellow milk that my dad milked from the new cows coming into the milk shed. My father would feed the boy calves with this yellow milk, and I would carry five gallon buckets of this yellow milk down to the female calf shed. After the boy calves were fed, a truck would come and take them away; they were of little use on a dairy farm as they did not produce milk, and no milk equals no money for the farm. The female calves were always excited about their twice daily feeding. They loved this yellow milk. In fact, we would have to ration it to them because they would drink it until they exploded if we gave them too much.

As I grew older and the farm got bigger and as my parents purchased neighboring farms, they hired staff to take care of these daily farm tasks. Fortunately, spelling and doing math problems were easy for me, so I got good grades at school. I left the farm at age eighteen and went to college for the next eight years to study science and engineering. After finishing my PhD on a Friday, I started work on Monday to help pay for my student loan. I began work as a Research Engineer for New Zealand Dairy Research Institute in Palmerston North. There I worked on projects to figure out ways to fractionate, or split apart, dairy proteins, oils, and other stuff.

After visiting my older sister, her husband and their three daughters, Bailey, Sienna, and Mikayla, in Palm Springs, California, I saw a bigger world in America, so I moved 6,000 miles to the land of the free, home of the brave. In 1997, I started work for Dairy Farmers of America, the largest dairy cooperative in the US, as their Whey Protein Technical Manager. One of my areas of interest was to develop colostrum extraction technologies. Over the next three years the focus moved from added-value ingredients back to commodities, so they shelved a lot of these projects. I asked if I could continue my work on colostrum during my own time, and I was given the green light.

In 2003 I teamed up with three individuals from the California dairy industry and built a new dedicated colostrum processing facility in Phoenix, Arizona. Having access to their new state-of-the-art facility has provided me with the opportunity to continue my work with colostrum.

There are a handful of publications on colostrum that present its benefits to human and animal health, but they are incomplete in context. In this publication

I have tryed to take the presentation of the quite remarkable benefits of colostrum and its constituents to a new level. Although clinical in nature and useful as a reference manual for those consumers and professionals seeking a greater understanding of colostrum, all will benefit in our constant struggle against the numerous challenges we face today in a world that is toxic and foreign to human body biochemistry.

I hope that this publication offers some enlightenment or knowledge for everyone who reads it so all can be aware of the wonderful healing and nutritional benefits that colostrum can give us. The true gem in the colostrum are the Proline-rich Polypeptides (PRPs). These peptides modulate, balance, regulate or initiate indirectly most of the biochemical processes in the mammalian body. They are probably the most significant natural substances in the human body relating to the immune system.

These are so important that God intended for us to have these peptides as soon as we enter this world.

They also happen to be found in abundance in colostrum—life's first food. Taking these peptides as we age, we redirect our bodies to function in homeostasis. Read on for more information about these healthful peptides.

■ **Andrew Keech PhD**

INTRODUCTION

Immunity has become a subject of interest to everyone at the dawn of the third millennium. Our confidence in Western medicine, and particularly in pharmacologic drugs, has been shaken by the appearance of drug-resistant strains of pathogenic (disease-causing) microorganisms and diseases, such as tuberculosis and staphylococcus, and entirely new and dangerous diseases that were unknown until recent years, such as AIDS, Ebola, SARS, and bird flu, all of which are resistant to all known antibiotics. Also, the drug industry is facing the dangers of new drug interactions and side effects of test-tube created alipathic medicines, ultimately keeping trial lawyers employed due to fully unproven new medications released by the Food and Drug Administration (FDA) or other government officials.

Fortunately, a new interest in an old remedy has emerged. It is a remedy that is as old as mankind itself, nay, older, as old as mammals. There are several natural products that have shown promise in empowering the body to treat itself. In this treatise we will deal with one that is probably the most successful natural product we have been leased to have. It is called colostrum, and it is the first food that all mammals taste in this life, the first milk that emerges from the mother's breast following the birth of the newborn. It is a fascinating mixture of immune and growth factors and basic nutrients all designed to give the newborn the best chance of surviving in its cold, new world. The process of birth is indeed a physical process. It is not until the newborn receives the colostrum that the immune system is truly activated. Newborns that do not receive the gift of colostrum do not thrive and typically face more health challenges than newborns that are given colostrum.

But the ancients also discovered that colostrum was good for people of all ages, not just newborns. It provided health maintenance long before the appearance of medicine as we know it and helped mankind weather the long years before the birth of civilization. Furthermore, up until the twentieth century it was our main source of immune protection against the many infectious diseases that regularly took their toll on humanity.

Over the last fifty years or so, scientists have begun to untangle the complicated web that is colostrum, teasing out the many different components that make it up. It has become clear that many of the substances in colostrum function as signal transducers that turn on or off different cell functions, particular those of the immune system. Signal transducers are one way the body regulates itself by "talking" to the trillions of cells that make up the body. These signaling molecules are usually small peptides,[1] polypeptides,[2] or proteins[3] that have corresponding receptors on the outer membranes of their target cells. When the signaling molecules are released, they travel through the blood to their target cells where they bind to the receptors, setting off a chain of events that result in a certain action taking place, such as the production of a specific protein, an immunoglobulin, for example. This is one of the principal ways that the body is able to function as a unit even though composed of many individual cells. The growth factors in colostrum function as signal transducers as do many other components of colostrum.

One family of components in colostrum consists of very short peptides or polypeptides. This family of peptides is characterized by having a greater frequency of the amino acid proline in their makeup than is normally found in peptides and proteins, hence the name Proline-rich Polypeptides, or PRPs.

For years scientists had known that there was an unidentified substance in colostrum of very low molecular weight that could be filtered out and used to transfer immunity from one individual to another. It was called "transfer factor," among other names, but for many years the identity of this substance was unknown. Then scientists in Poland found a complex of peptides in colostrum that had the

1 Short chains of amino acids
2 Longer chains of amino acids with no tertiary structure
3 Very long chains of amino acids that have a tertiary, or three-dimensional, structure that is often very complex

unique ability to modulate the immune response by activating the immune system when needed to fight an infection or inhibiting the immune response when the infection had been contained to avoid damaging healthy tissue. They termed these polypeptides colostrinin after the colostrum in which they were discovered. Another team of scientists in the United States found a similar substance in a dialyzable extract from leukocytes[4] that could also transfer immunity. Over the years it has become clear that all these were in fact PRPs.

Taking colostrum as a nutritional supplement helps maintain your health, particularly your gut health, which is critical to your overall health. Whole colostrum includes PRPs as well as a number of other immune factors, such as immunoglobulins, lactoferrin, and others, so you will receive significant immune benefit from taking whole colostrum. However, when you experience an infectious illness, such as a cold or flu, or if you experience an autoimmune condition, which indicates an overactive immune system that is attacking your own cells, then you need something stronger. PRPs are now available in a concentrated spray form that delivers maximum amounts of the immunomodulatory peptides to help modulate your immune system.

The purpose of this book is to introduce you to PRPs and how they can help you maintain your health. First we will start with an overview of colostrum, its history, and its components. Then we will examine PRPs in more depth, how they work, what they do, and what health conditions they may help. Our hope is to give you the information you need to use colostrum and PRPs wisely to maintain your health and the health of your family.

DISCLAIMER:
The statements contained herein have not been evaluated by the Food And Drug Administration. It is not intended to diagnose, treat, cure or prevent disease. The statements are for informational purposes only and is it not meant to replace the services or recommendations of a physician or qualified health care practitioner. Those with health problems or pregnancy are specifically advised that they should consult their physician before taking colostrum or any nutritional supplement.

4 White blood cells, also known as polymorphonuclear leukocytes.

PART I

COLOSTRUM

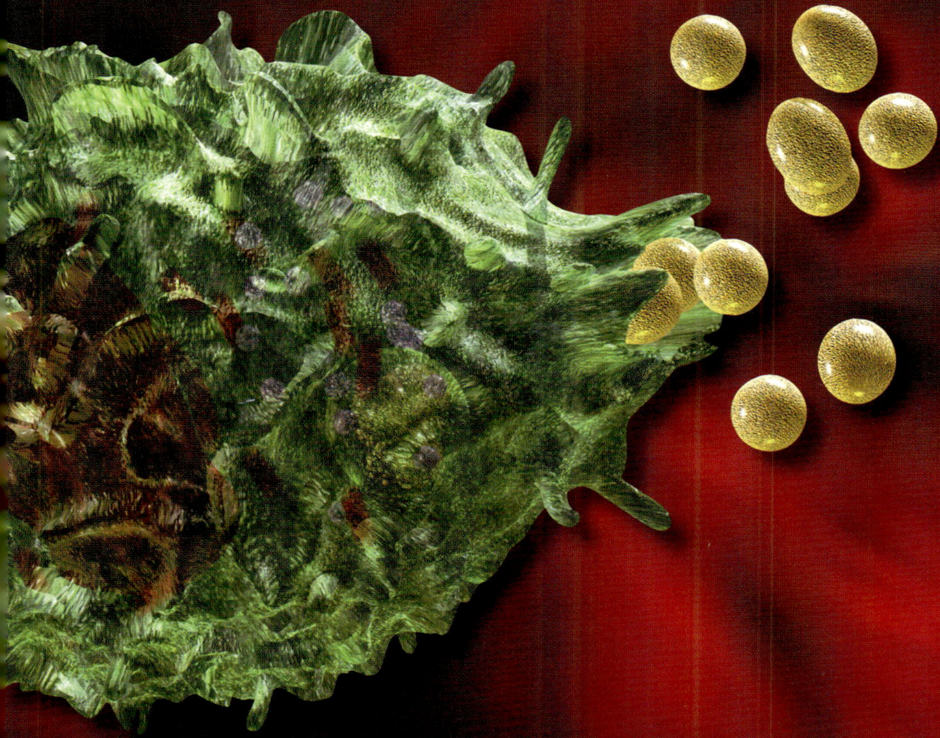

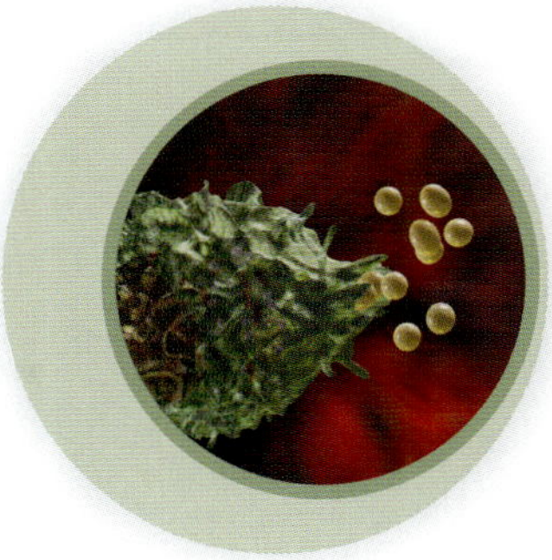

CHAPTER 1

WHAT'S IN COLOSTRUM?

Colostrum is the first pre-milk substance that is produced by the mammary gland of female mammals, including humans, following the birth of the newborn. It is the first food tasted in this life by all mammals. It is a special substance that is very unlike other foods, even milk. It is loaded with immune factors, growth factors, and protective proteins as well as all the nutrients the newborn needs to survive. The immune factors in colostrum provide the immunity necessary to ward off potentially fatal infections until the newborn's own immune system can get up to speed, and the growth factors help complete the development of the gut, which is not fully developed at the time of birth.

Mankind has known for thousands of years the benefits of colostrum to both the newborn as well as people of all ages. We will discuss the history of colostrum use in the next chapter, but it is important to understand that colostrum holds many benefits for all people. Strangely enough, however, it is not human colostrum that holds the greatest benefit for humans beyond the newborn stage but bovine (cow) colostrum. This is due to a difference in the placentas of cows and humans.

The human placenta allows the passage of immunoglobulin G (IgG), which is responsible for establishing systemic immunity, from mother to fetus. This means that a human baby is born with an immune system that is already primed and ready to begin its work defending the newborn against infection. The placenta of the cow, however, does not allow the passage of IgG from mother to fetus. Therefore when the calf is born it is completely unprotected from infection and needs the IgG in the mother's colostrum to survive. Thus bovine colostrum contains predominantly IgG (over 85% of total immunoglobulin) while human colostrum contains predominantly immunoglobulin A (IgA), which is designed for local immunity and is intended to help the newborn's immune system handle infections locally in the gut rather than establish systemic immunity. IgG, because it can pass immunity to a specific pathogen (disease-causing microorganism) from one individual to another, is therefore of much more benefit to humans past the stage of infancy. It is also produced in great quantities by the mother cow far exceeding the needs of the calf.

For the consumer seeking a nutritional supplement that will help maintain his or her health, it is important to remember that colostrum is a multifunctional complex of bioactive ingredients produced by mammals for mammals (which means you). If you walk into a natural foods store and examine the products on the shelves, nearly all are derived from plants, and generally speaking, most have only one function. It is also important to remember that most plant-derived supplements or herbs have little if any scientific research to back up their health claims, while many thousands of scientific studies from all around the world and virtually every leading research institution have been done on the health benefits of colostrum and its many ingredients.

Colostrum is so complex that we are only beginning to understand how it all works together. New components are still being identified, and the mechanisms of action of known components are still being worked out. The one thing that can be said with certainty is that there is no simple replacement for colostrum. It does a multitude of tasks, and the individual components work together in a synergy that no combination of plant-derived components could ever simulate.

What Are the Legal vs Actual Definitions of Colostrum?

It is well known that colostrum is the first pre-milk substance that is produced by the mammary gland of female mammals, following the birth of the newborn. However, the legal definition differs from the actual definition.

The legal definition: In the California Food and Agricultural Code, section 35602, ***"Milk shall be obtained by the complete milking of healthy cows or goats which are properly fed and kept. Milk shall not be obtained or used for human consumption within 15 days prior to or 5 days after parturition."***

Defining colostrum as milk that is collected up to five days is more of a legal definition rather than an actual definition.

Colostrum is more commonly defined as "milk that is in the mammary glands at the time of birth." Milk that is manufactured after the birth is characterized as "transitional milk"; actually, the third and fourth milking is transitional milk. By the time of the fifth milking, analytical methods indicate that the milk has essentially the same chemistry as that of mature milk.

One of the main reasons why this five-day period was implemented initially is because most cows, especially older cows, received antibiotic treatments to protect their udders from infection during their dry period, which is typically 45–60 days. After that period the cow could birth another calf. These older antibiotic treatments have a 72-hour withholding period, so, previously one should not have consumed the colostrum within 72 hours of birth.

With the advent of modern veterinary dry-cow therapies (beta-lactam drugs or preservatives), these typically have a 28-day withholding period. Thus the residual antibiotics have been removed well before the calf is born (45–60-day non-milking or dry period). So colostrum is safe to consume for animals and humans.

A consumer should seek colostrum powder in the market that is labeled "First Milking." This can also include the second milking because the second is actually the remaining first milk that was not removed on first milking. See Figure 1, page 64, HPLC graphs of colostrum showing IgG peak at 8 minutes for the first eight milkings after giving birth. A consumer should also look for colostrum peptide (PRPs) content not less than 3% by weight.

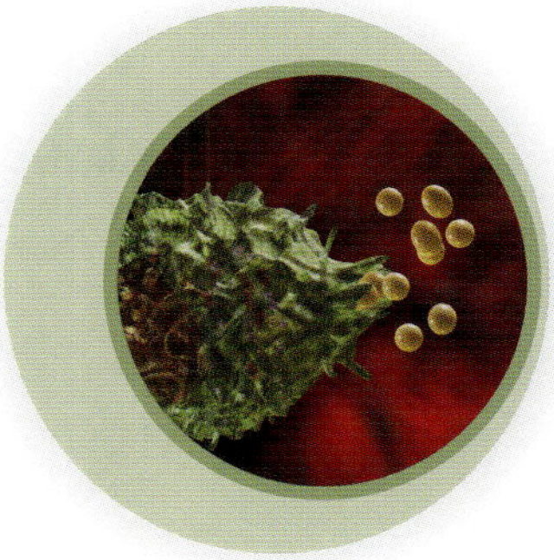

CHAPTER 2

A BRIEF HISTORY OF COLOSTRUM

The history of colostrum use, chiefly bovine colostrum, is as old as history itself. Cow and man have enjoyed a symbiotic relationship since before the last ice age. The cow served both as a source of food and a beast of burden. The cow was at the center of the primitive agricultural economies that were the foundation of civilization. The ancient ***auroch***, an extinct species of cattle from which modern cattle are descended, play a prominent role in the 17,000 year old cave paintings found in Lascaux, France—the oldest human art known. Selective breeding of cattle was practiced in Mesopotamia as early as 5,000 BCE.

In Europe, cows and men have lived intimately for centuries. Cows often shared the farmer's home in cold times. In England and Scandinavia, colostrum is a traditional tonic and folk remedy given to the entire family in the spring to keep them healthy for the entire year. The first milking of a cow following a calving is traditionally made into a pudding called ***beestings*** to celebrate the birth and promote good health.[1]

Ayurvedic medicine has used colostrum for thousands of years in India where it continues to be widely used today. Cows are considered to be gods in India.[2] Hieroglyphic texts show that colostrum was used by the Ancient Egyptians as well. On one stele in a temple dedicated to Hathor, the cow goddess and symbol of rebirth, the goddess is depicted suckling the Pharaoh, offering her colostrum as the elixir of metamorphosis to confer immortality upon the king.[3]

Masai tribesmen in Kenya drink bovine colostrum by the liter because they know how good it is for them. They are well-known for their toughness under extreme conditions and their healthy constitutions. Cows are considered their most important form of wealth, and they even sing songs of praise to colostrum in recognition of the health it gives them.[4]

However, taboos against the use of colostrum during breastfeeding are found worldwide. Delaying breastfeeding until the fifth day and using a combination of honey and clarified butter (ghee) to evacuate the meconium was practiced in India by the second century BC. In the Bible, a reference is made to giving curds and honey to the son born of a virgin "until he knows how to reject the evil and choose the good."[5] This taboo, derived from ancient Greek and Roman sources, carried through to seventeenth century England and France.[6] The taboo against colostrum persists in many cultures even today.[7]

When Antony van Leeuwenhoek—Dutch inventor of the microscope and discoverer of bacteria, red blood cells and protozoa—first peered through his new invention, he was looking at milk. This was in 1674.[8] Both Paul Ehrlich, the "Father of Immunology," and Elie Metchnikoff, another great nineteenth century immunologist, studied the immunologic properties of colostrum.[9,10,11,12] When Albert Sabin, inventor of the oral polio vaccine, made his first polio vaccine, he used antibodies from bovine colostrum.[13,14]

Prior to 1950, colostrum was intensively studied and used for its immune boosting powers and as a treatment for rheumatoid arthritis, for which it showed great promise. Unfortunately, with the advent of sulfa drugs, cheap antibiotics and other synthetic drugs, interest waned in natural remedies. The benefits of colostrum were largely lost for over forty years.

Prior to 1980 colostrum was harvested in North America from buffalo and goats. Post-1980s, colostrum was then sourced from bovine or cows owing to the abundant availability of this raw material.

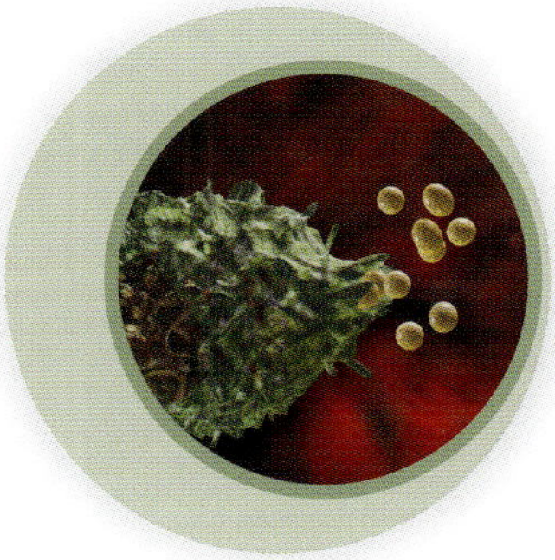

CHAPTER 3

THE REDISCOVERY OF COLOSTRUM

Doug and Kaye Wyatt's Story

Colostrum remained largely forgotten until 1994 when a man in Utah rediscovered its amazing qualities in his search for relief from his wife's intolerable suffering. That man was Doug Wyatt, and it was his efforts to find relief for his wife Kaye that opened the door to the rediscovery of the many health benefits of colostrum and began the nutraceutical revolution that continues today. Here is Doug and Kaye's story in Doug's own words:

> *The beginning of the story of colostrum begins for us in 1994. In 1994, my wife, Kaye, came to me and asked me to help her find a way to die. It was the most shocking experience, the most emotional experience, that I had ever had up until had that point. I'm a Vietnam veteran. I'm a Marine pilot, and I flew helicopters in Vietnam. That process, that emotional process for me was nothing compared to what happened that day when Kaye came to me with this startling request.*
>
> *I have to be very honest with you about this. At that point in time we had tried everything that the medical community had to offer, everything that the alternative community had to offer, every natural healing supplement, Chinese medicine, herbal products, homeopathic products, acupuncture…everything that you could imagine that was available up until that point in time, and nothing worked. The problem*

was that Kaye, when she was an infant, had had her thymus gland irradiated by a medical doctor. The thymus produces T cells, and if any of you have read any literature on AIDS, you understand what T cells are. They are the thing that we measure as a component to see how well the immune system is functioning during the process of an onset of AIDS and other immune diseases, like Hepatitis C, etc. If you can't produce T cells, in essence, you cannot ward off infection because they are the backbone of this, the very cornerstone of our immune system and how well it functions. So [it was] Kaye's inability to produce [T cells], with her thymus gland mostly destroyed through this treatment process, that, by the way, happened to about a half a million Americans, most of which are not alive today, and it was one of the big medical mistakes that took place in the '50s.

So the only thing that we had left at that time was prayer, and that prayer was in earnest. I have to tell you that we were honestly blessed out of that process because the very next morning I was working with a friend of mine who happened to have a couple of PhDs, and I didn't know about one. We were working on a financial issue for the State of Wyoming, and I found out during that process that he was also an MD, a naturopathic doctor, who had been trained in Europe. We got into this because he said, "Doug, you're not here with me this morning. We're not going anyplace, and I want you to talk about it. I know that might be difficult, but something is really going on."

So we started talking about the history of Kaye's process. Kaye's a very private person, and we'd never shared this. We hadn't shared this with her family, so I had no reason to share it with anybody outside of our relationship other than the medical professionals we were working with to try and find a process to deal with it. During that conversation he asked me if I had looked into bovine colostrum. This was really not all that long of a conversation. It was one of the first things that he actually went to, and it was something that I'd missed because it wasn't sitting on the shelf of the health food stores and none of the practitioners in the United States at that time thought about it, and of course, most of them are vegans, so you couldn't possibly get well from something that came from a cow.

It clicked with me, and I went, wait a minute, we're a mammal, we're not a plant. Plant phytochemicals are basically what we continue to look for. We look for those with drugs. We're down in the Brazilian rainforest and we're hunting for everything in the world and we create plant phytochemicals and that's what becomes our pharmaceuticals, but wait a minute, these are single action substances, and we're talking about an immune system here that isn't working, and I don't believe there's any one single substance on the planet that is going to replace Kaye's immune system. And I guarantee you there is not one single substance on the planet that will replace or provide a modulation for a human or a mammal's immune system except one thing and that is the immune system's components itself.

So when I was given this reward the next morning, which I felt was heaven sent, I immediately thought back to the time when I was a child when I worked on my grandfather's ranch in Southern Idaho. Every summer that was my summer experience. I got sabbatical out to put up the hay and milk the cows and brand the cows and cut the cows and go combine wheat, and I knew the calves, the horses, the foals, that this baby calf would die if it didn't get colostrum within 8 hours after birth. That was the end of it. That was how the immune system was passed on. So colostrum was the immune system, and it came to me at that point in time.

I bought a quarter pound of dried colostrum from this guy. He was actually drying it in his kitchen, of all places. He was getting it from a local dairy farmer. You have to dry it, or you don't have any shelf life. You don't want to throw colostrum away in two weeks because you only get it for one or two days out of the cow after birth, right after birth. So I took this home, and Kaye said, "You paid what for what? You take it back!"

I had a couple of abstracts that I'd been able to get out of him. He had a little bit of information on anti-inflammatory action and pain relief in colostrum, gastrointestinal, immune support, etc., and the fact that it imparts immunity to everything that the mother had been exposed to in her life. So this made sense, and I hid it and kept leaving these abstracts out. It was like a day or two later that Kaye sprained her knee very, very badly, and she came home barely able to make it. We go to the emergency room, she comes back, and it was a bad sprain, not a break, and she had a wrap-on cast on her leg, and she said, "OK, I'll take some of your dang stuff." "Your dang medicine," she called it. Of course, it isn't medicine, its natural food, but she took a couple of teaspoons of colostrum and went to bed in a lot of pain. Of course, trying to roll over in the middle of the night, this thing gets in the way, so she unstrapped it and threw it off by the side of the bed.

The next morning I'm up having coffee and reading the paper, and she walked in the kitchen. I went, "Kaye!" And she goes, "What!" It's early—no coffee yet. "Kaye!" She says, "What?" I said, "Your leg!" And she pulled up her nightgown and was like, "Huh?" All of the black and blue, all of the swelling, everything had gone virtually overnight. We couldn't believe it.

It was amazing, and it was so amazing that we were sitting back and saying, OK, maybe some of this other information that we were reading about colostrum is true too. So she kept taking colostrum, and within a couple of days—Kaye had had an ongoing, low-grade fever because of her inability to rid her body of constant infectious processes, so she constantly had infections going on, growing into this or growing into that—colostrum for the first time in about 8–10 years broke that low-grade fever, and it was the most startling event that had happened in all the time that I'd known Kaye, 15 years. And it changed her life.

I can honestly say this made the biggest and most important change in her life, in our lives, and in my life, in our family life, in giving us an ability to have hope for the future, to have an idea that maybe this request that she made to me could be set aside, that maybe we could think about having a life. That change worked and worked and worked, and it was so startling. What happened with her is that she didn't need antibiotics every 3 months. She didn't get every cold and flu that came along. In fact, if they came along, they were gone in an hour or two or overnight. That never happened with Kaye. Every time she got a cold it turned into flu, it turned into pneumonia; every time!

We were so startled by this that we were desperate to find out why. Now, at this time there was no web research for the public, in fact there was no internet except for those affiliated with Universities or the military. I knew some people that had talked about this internet and research data that was available but I was not allowed to get into this because it was not allowed expect for authorized personnel, and certainly not to the public. We lived at that time in Salt Lake City and we desperately needed to get on Pub Med (the medical researchers online research web that was only available to medical researchers and medical students). We found a friend through another divine intervention, another act of prayer and another gift the next day. I met this lady while working out and took her home and introduced her to Kaye. She became very good friends. But, what was interesting, and I don't know why she was inclined, was that she was a stranger who came to me out of the blue and said tearfully, "What can I do? My husband has been home and in bed for 2½, 3 weeks. He's on massive antihistamines, every drug that the doctors can find. He has massive allergies. He has hives all over his body, down his esophagus, inside and out, clear throughout him. He can't even stand to have a sheet touch him, can't stand to have his clothes touch him, can't eat because his whole mouth and all his insides are full of hives, and they itch and they're painful and they're killing him. They're driving him crazy." So I gave her some colostrum, Kaye and I did, and she took it home. Within a day, day and a half, she came back and said they'd all disappeared. All of these hives had disappeared that quickly.

We found out she was a medical researcher, so she got us into the University of Utah Medical School. We went online there, and we filled four file drawers full of research on colostrum that cost us thousands of dollars for. We did this, and I have the receipts for it,

> *and I can prove it. We did this, Kaye and I, and we wrote a book out of this. We wrote it with Dr. Daniel Clark out of Florida, who is a cancer and internal medicine specialist. We felt that the information that we found was the most astounding information that we could possibly put together. There weren't any MDs, there were no health-care specialists in our field, there were no wellness people that had ever seen any of this, it had not been published in the newspapers, it had not been published anyplace where the consumers could find it. We're talking thousands and thousands of clinical studies that had been published in peer review journals, and when I'm talking peer review, that means the kind of journals where the article is submitted and a group of doctors review the article for facts and for accuracy before it's ever published. We're talking over 10,000 articles that were published, clinical work that had been done on colostrum, bovine colostrum, its components (when you research colostrum you have to research its components not just whole colostrum), and the information was absolutely startling. That information gave us a basis in compiling that to go out and start educating people about what colostrum would do colostrum's overall benefits to a whole bunch of things besides Kaye's immune system.*
>
> *But I think it's important to understand really what happened in this. We were the pioneers of colostrum. There were no others.*

After discovering the amazing health benefits that colostrum provides, Doug decided he had to let others know about what he had discovered, and he had to find a way to mass produce the colostrum so that whoever needed it could get it. He soon discovered that there were no sources for colostrum anywhere in the US that met the stringent standards set by the USDA for the handling of milk for human consumption. Colostrum was considered a waste product by most dairy farmers. What colostrum was sent to the processors was usually set aside in a can by the side of the road until someone came to collect it. The only commercial sources for colostrum were animal feed companies who sold dehydrated colostrum in bags to dairy farmers who gave it to calves who needed more than their mothers could provide to survive.

Doug decided he needed to figure out a way to improve the collection, processing, and distribution of colostrum to meet standards for human consumption, and he needed to figure out a way to process the colostrum to give it a shelf life longer than two weeks, which is the approximate shelf life for whole liquid colostrum. Initially he used colostrum from dairy farms where he talked the farmers into using a freezer to store the colostrum until it could be picked up rather than leaving it by the side of the road. Then he worked on finding dairy companies who could process the colostrum using the same quality standards they employed for producing milk for human consumption. The FDA approves all dairies where milk is processed for humans, but colostrum processing at the time was only regulated by the USDA, and they regulated it as animal feed, which has much lower standards than human food. But Doug persisted, and he got a few dairies to start using sterilized equipment for processing.

Then he worked on the drying process. The traditional way of drying colostrum was spray drying. The colostrum would be sprayed through hot air coming off a gas flame. This worked to dry the colostrum, but the problem was the natural gas used for the heat. Natural gas produces nitrates as a combustion product, so the colostrum would pick up nitrates in the drying process. Nitrates can act as carcinogens, so a way had to be found to dry the colostrum without exposing it to natural gas.

Then Doug discovered New Zealand colostrum produced by the New Zealand Dairy Board. Here colostrum was produced to human standards in a country well-known for the pristine state of its environment. They have very strict environmental laws and no big pollution producing industry. At the time, New Zealand was producing the highest quality colostrum available, so Doug entered into an agreement with them to produce colostrum for sale in the US and throughout the world through the company he started, Symbiotics. When colostrum became popular as a nutritional supplement in the US, however, conditions began to improve. The demand for high quality colostrum gave dairy farmers an incentive to improve collection and handling techniques for colostrum. In 2003, the only processing plant exclusively dedicated to colostrum was built in Phoenix, Arizona. It draws colostrum from organic-like dairy farms located throughout the Southwest and produces the highest quality colostrum available anywhere. We will discuss the process of colostrum production in the next chapter

Doug Wyatt is now focused on giving back to society as the Managing Research Director for the Center for Nutritional Research (CNR) a non-profit research organization involved in disease prevention research focusing on bovine colostrum and complimentary natural prevention and remedies.

© Doug's story is offered here with copyright permission from the Center for Nutritional Research.

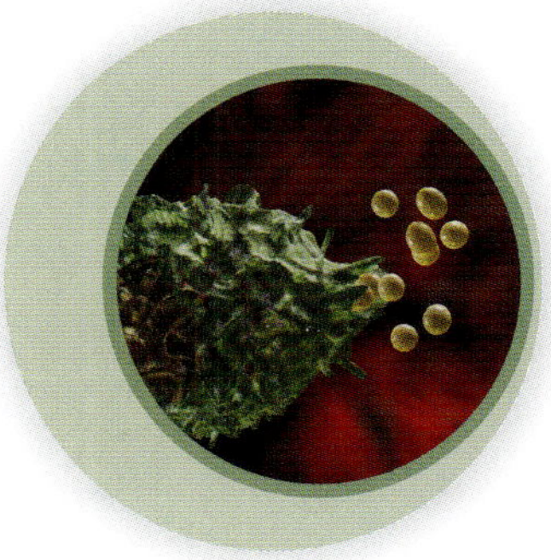

CHAPTER 4

WHAT IS COLOSTRUM GOOD FOR?

The first and foremost thing that must be understood about colostrum is what it ***isn't***, namely that colostrum is ***not*** a medication. Colostrum is designed to maintain health and prevent disease rather than cure a disease that you already may have. To make an analogy, it's better to close the barn door before the horse runs out than after it already has.

So what does it do for us as adults or for children older than babies?

Gut Health

Colostrum is an amazing cornucopia of everything we need to maintain a healthy, functional gastrointestinal tract, which is a key to good health in general since many diseases have their origins in the gut, and the proper absorption of nutrients is key to maintaining the body in top running condition. One of the primary functions of colostrum is gut health. The condition of our gastrointestinal tract— the mouth, the esophagus, the stomach, and the large and small intestines—is an important health concern due to the amount of potentially harmful material that passes through it and the fact that many, if not most, diseases originate in the gut in one way or another. Yet gut health is mostly ignored unless we're suffering from diarrhea, indigestion, or other GI problems. We don't like to think about our digestive processes. Improving our sex lifes or removing wrinkles on our skin is much more interesting.

When the proportion of beneficial bacteria in our intestines outnumbers the harmful bacteria, our intestines are said to be in a state of ***orthobiosis***, a term meaning "in balance" coined by Elie Metchnikoff, who was mentioned in Chapter 2. When that proportion gets off for some reason and the harmful bacteria predominate, we are in a state of ***dysbiosis***, or imbalance. Dysbiosis has a number of harmful consequences, including ***leaky gut syndrome*** where the permeability of the gut lining is increased so that toxins and pathogens normally excluded from passing through the gut lining now move freely into the body, which can cause or contribute to a multitude of diseases. Many autoimmune conditions, such as Crohn's disease and rheumatoid arthritis, and most food allergies can be traced to leaky gut syndrome. There are many other causes of leaky gut in addition to dysbiosis, including alcoholism, taking non-steroidal anti-inflammatory drugs (NSAIDs), aging, and excessive amounts of toxins in the gut. Whatever the cause, leaky gut can have serious, even life-threatening consequences.

Colostrum is the best remedy known for all-around gut health. Colostrum restores leaky gut to normal permeability levels.[15,16] It contains growth factors and hormones to help repair damage to the intestinal lining, including damage caused by NSAIDs and other medications, and restore gut integrity.[17,18,19] It contains massive doses of immunoglobulins which help control harmful bacteria and fungi, such as Candida, in order to restore orthobiosis. It has been clinically proven to control such harmful bacteria as ***H. pylori,***[20,21] which cause ulcers, and many other bacteria. Colostrum has also been shown to increase the surface area of the intestinal lining, improving the absorption of nutrients.[22,23,24] And there are no known side effects from using colostrum.

Intestinal Permeability

High intestinal permeability is a normal feature of newborn gut ecology. Colostrum functions to reduce inflammation protect against irritation from toxins, and check any potential infection, while promoting epithelial growth and repair. This combination of effects quickly reduces permeability, preventing toxins, irritants, allergens and infectious agents from entering body tissues.

A number of serious health syndromes are now known to be associated with an abnormally increased gut permeability. These include Crohn's disease, cholera, Salmonella and E. coli infection, HIV, arthritis, chronic fatigue syndrome, hepatitis, cystic fibrosis, alcoholism, muscular dystrophy, fibromyalgia, and scleroderma. Research shows that colostrum can correct this leaky gut syndrome with its unique combination of immune factors and growth stimulators, which includes epithelial growth factors.

In fact, research has shown that colostrum is the singlemost effective agent for correcting leaky gut syndrome. Of course, other factors can help, too. These include friendly bacterial flora, folic acid, vitamin B_{12}, and aloe. In addition, optimal nutrition should be ensured with a potent, broad-spectrum multi-vitamin and mineral supplementation program, high fiber intake, and lots of steamed vegetables and greens in the diet. Avoiding refined foods, sugar, alcohol, caffeine, chemical additives, and tobacco is also crucial.

Colostrum also promotes re-colonization of the bowel by friendly flora. These beneficial organisms help digest our food so that more nutritional value is available from the same diet and supplements. They also enhance nutrient absorption, feed epithelial tissue, produce bulk for healthier elimination of wastes, produce B vitamins, and prevent infection and disease. When colostrum normalizes this gut ecology, assimilation of nutrients is also enhanced. This means that other dietary, nutritional, herbal, homeopathic, and lifestyle interventions work better, too.

Leaky Gut Syndrome (LGS)

Leaky gut syndrome is the name given to a very common health disorder in which the intestinal lining is more permeable than normal. The abnormally large spaces present between the cells of the gut wall allow the entry of viruses, bacteria, fungi and other toxic material into the bloodstream. Leaky gut syndrome is at least as common as all the immune system diseases put together. Basically, it is caused by inflammation of the gut lining. This inflammation can be brought about by any of the following:

- Antibiotic use—leads to the overgrowth of abnormal bacteria in the gastrointestinal tract
- Alcohol and caffeine—these can irritate the gut wall
- Foods contaminated by parasites
- Foods contaminated by bacteria, such as E. coli
- Chemicals (including dyes and preservatives) in fermented and processed foods
- Prescription corticosteroids
- An abundance of highly refined sugars and other carbohydrates in your diet (e.g., candy bars, cookies, soft drinks, white bread)

LGS damages the protective coating of antibodies of the IgA family normally present in a healthy gut.[25] Since IgA helps us ward off infections, leaky gut problems make us less resistant to viruses, bacteria, parasites and Candida.[26,27] These microbes are then able to invade the bloodstream and colonize almost any body tissue or organ, thereby causing disease.

LGS also creates a long list of mineral deficiencies because the various carrier proteins needed to transport minerals from the intestine to the blood are damaged by the inflammation process.[28] For example, magnesium deficiency is a very common finding in conditions like fibromyalgia, despite high magnesium intake through diet and supplementation. If the carrier protein for magnesium is damaged, it doesn't matter how much of the mineral you take; it will not get into the body where it is needed. Similarly, the body can be deprived of zinc because of poor intestinal absorption, often resulting in hair loss. Copper deficiency can occur in an identical way, leading to high blood cholesterol levels and osteoarthritis. In addition, when calcium, boron, silicon and manganese are not absorbed into the bloodstream, bone problems develop. Bloating, cramps, and gas are common ailments associated with a leaky gut. Eventually, however, nutritional deficiencies can also lead to systemic complaints like fatigue, headaches, memory loss, poor concentration or irritability.[29]

Immune Health

Colostrum is unmatched as an immune system stimulant and modulator. There are numerous "one note" products lining the shelves of natural food stores that claim to stimulate the immune system. Only colostrum, however, plays the whole symphony. It is not only able to stimulate the immune system in a multitude of ways but also has the ability to modulate the immune response, turning it up or down as needed. No other health food product can claim that.

Colostrum can pass immunity to a wide variety of disease-causing pathogens to you. No shots required! Colostrum can protect you not only from dangerous bacteria, like Salmonella or Streptococcus, but it can also protect you against a number of viruses, from to HIV, fungi like Candida, and even protozoan parasites like giardia. Not even antibiotics can deliver that broad protection.

Our ability to survive in a world full of dangerous pathogens and toxins is dependent upon the ability of our immune system to neutralize and destroy these potential dangers. To accomplish this, our bodies have developed many strategies that attack or neutralize dangers in a wide variety of ways. Many of these are included in colostrum as well since one of the main routes of infection or toxin entry into the body is through the gut. In fact, no other supplement can come close to colostrum in the variety and effectiveness of its immune support.

Colostrum also provides a potent array of immune factors including immunoglobins, cytokines, interferon, lactoferrin and PRPs. Supplementation of these factors can dramatically restore immunity, prevent infection and speed healing and recovery from illness.

Bovine colostrum, in particular, is up to forty times higher than human colostrum in these immune factors. Plus, only bovine colostrum contains certain glycoproteins and protease inhibitors that naturally protect these immune factors from being digested in the intestinal tract.

Even so, prolonged exposure to stomach acid would decrease colostrum's immune effects. Swallowing colostrum in a capsule with a large glass of alkaline, antioxidant water (coral water or electrolysis water) between meals (or at the very start of a meal) should be optimum for immune benefits.

Colostrum is also one of the most potent known sources of methylsulfonylmethane (MSM), which relieves pain, aids in healing of scar tissue, deters parasites, supports liver detoxification and helps elimination of mercury, among its many other functions. MSM, or organic sulfur, is considered the number three mineral in the body.

Colostrum even contains powerful, soil-based organisms, which have been found to provide tremendous health benefits to human health.

According to the Centers for Disease Control, anywhere from 30% to 80% of commercial chickens are seriously contaminated with salmonella bacteria.[30] ABC TV quoted a government source that reported as many as 33 million Americans suffer food poisoning every year, and that over 5,000 die.[31] Colostrum has been shown to kill Salmonella, along with other disease-causing bacteria such as Campylobacter, ***E. coli*** (which can kill people when present in contaminated meat supplies), ***Helicobacter pylori*** (the main cause of stomach ulcers), Listeria, and multiple Streptococcus species and Staphylococcus.[70,163,313] This is good news in light of the increasing appearance of antibiotic resistant super strains, such as vancomycin-resistant ***Staphylococcus aureu***s. Colostrum has also been found to be effective against ***Candida albicans.***[32]

Research shows that colostrum prevents and controls infection in multiple ways. First, according to clinical studies, colostrum has been shown to inhibit attachment of bacteria to the body's epithelial (surface) tissue. This is a necessary first step for any infection to take hold. Secondly the lactoferrin and colostrum acts as a natural antimicrobial and antiviral.[533,539] Colostrum also imparts passive immunity to many high-risk organisms, including the leading intestinal killers ***E. coli*** and rotavirus. At the same time, immune factors enhance the body's natural defense against virtually all pathogenic bacteria and viruses.

Infections, such as intestinal infections that cause diarrhea, can be a real killer. Rotavirus, a major cause of diarrhea, is the world's leading killer in areas with poor sanitation and contaminated water, but it is also spreading rapidly due to increased travel and immigration. Clostridium and Shigella are two other major killers linked to diarrhea. Colostrum neutralizes the toxins produced by Clostridium, the organism linked to botulism.[33] Colostrum showed similar results against shigellosis.[34] Taking colostrum, along with friendly bacterial flora, whenever you travel abroad can be a lifesaver.

Infection is becoming increasingly important as a cause of chronic degenerative disease as we understand more about etiology. ***Chlamydia pneumoniae*** (an intracellular parasite), for example, may be a triggering factor in atherosclerosis.[35] Researchers now believe that this factor may account for up to 50% of all heart disease.

The best-known immune components of colostrum, of course, are the immunoglobulins, also known as antibodies.[36,37,38] Immunoglobulins, part of the adaptive immune system [see Appendix A for a brief review of the immune system], are special proteins produced by the body that can specifically bind virtually any bacteria, virus, protein, peptide, carbohydrate or cell that the body recognizes as "foreign." Once the immunoglobulins attach themselves to the foreign substance (called opsonization), scavenger cells of the immune system can attack and destroy or neutralize it.

The immunoglobulins in colostrum contribute to its ability to neutralize or kill many bacteria, viruses, fungi and even protozoan parasites. The list of pathogens against which colostrum has been shown to be effective is impressive,[39] including such dangerous bacteria as ***H. pylori***[40] (implicated in ulcer formation in the stomach), ***E. coli***[41,42] (a natural inhabitant of the GI tract that has a number of very dangerous strains that can cause severe diarrhea or intestinal bleeding), pertussis,[43] cholera,[44] and bacterial causes of severe diarrhea,[45,46,47] which can be lethal in those suffering from AIDS and which kill thousands of infants worldwide every year. It has also been shown to be effective against a number of viruses,[48] and even protozoan parasites, such as amoebas,[49] which cause dysentery and other GI diseases.

But immunoglobulins are only one weapon in colostrum's great arsenal. It has many other ways of providing protection and modulating our immune response. Three proteins found in colostrum—lactoferrin, lysozyme, and lactoperoxidase, part of the so-called innate immune system—provide non-specific protection against bacteria, viruses and fungi.[50]

Lactoferrin is one of the main proteins in colostrum, making up about 6% of the total protein. It is an iron-binding protein closely related to transferrin, which is a protein that transports free iron in the body. One of the ways lactoferrin destroys bacteria is by binding free iron, which many bacteria and fungi, such as ***Candida,***[51] need to reproduce. It can prevent the colonization of ***Haemophilus influenzae***, the primary cause of ear and respiratory infections in children, by inactivating its colonization factors.[52] Lactoferrin also has the ability to penetrate the cell walls of bacteria, which allows lysozyme to enter the bacterial cell, causing them to lyse, or burst.[53] It also acts in conjunction with lysozyme to destroy Candida.[54] Lactoferrin is a potent destroyer of viruses as well, including cytomegalovirus (can cause birth defects and death in fetuses),[55] HIV (AIDS virus),[56] hepatitis B[57] and C,[58] rotavirus (the main cause of diarrhea in infants),[59] influenza virus, respiratory syncytial virus (causes colds in adults[60] and severe bronchitis and pneumonia in children) and herpes simplex types 1 (cold sores) and 2 (genital herpes).[61,62]

In addition to its antimicrobial role, lactoferrin has other important immune functions. Lactoferrin from colostrum increases both motility and superoxide production by polymorphonuclear leukocytes (white blood cells), making them more effective in warding off infections.[63] It strongly augments natural killer cell and lymphokine-activated killer cell cytotoxic activity.[64] Lactoferrin is also a required growth factor for lymphocytes, the principal cell type of the immune system,[65] so it acts to stimulate increased activity of the immune system.

Lactoperoxidase combines with thiocyanate (a sulfur compound) and hydrogen peroxide to form a bactericidal compound that kills bacteria and viruses nonspecifically as well as degrades various carcinogens.[66,67]

Other components of the innate, or non-specific, immune system are also present in colostrum.[68] One important component of this system is the glycoconjugates found in colostrum and milk. Glycoconjugates are proteins, fats or complex sugars (polysaccharides) that have sugar molecules attached to them. These sugar molecules compete with pathogens for binding sites on the intestinal wall.[69,70] Complement,[71,72] part of the antigen-antibody system, is also found in colostrum. Complement proteins help to remove immune complexes, that is, immunoglobulin-antigen complexes, so that they do not accumulate in the tissues. In addition, there are a number of small proteins and peptides present that are also part of the innate immune system, such as defensins[73] (polypeptides that disrupt bacterial membranes, killing them), toll-like receptors[65,74,75] (pattern recognition detectors which help the immune system identify new pathogens), and cathelicidin-derived antimicrobial peptide[65] (another polypeptide that attacks the membranes of bacteria).

A unique feature of colostrum is its ability to modulate rather than just stimulate, compared to immune products from plants that only stimulate. Colostrum contains a substance known as PRPs or colostrinin, which has the ability to modulate the immune response by either turning up an underactive immune system or turning down an overactive one.[76] PRPs can also induce the growth and differentiation of resting B lymphocytes,[77] an important part of turning on the immune system in response to a threat.

Another way colostrum modulates the immune system is through controlling the production of interleukin-2 (IL-2), one of the cytokines—small, hormone-like proteins that regulate the intensity and duration of immune response. By controlling the production of IL-2, colostrum can increase or decrease the activity of natural killer cells[78]—specialized lymphocytes whose function is to attack and kill invading pathogens. Lactoferrin also stimulates the activity of natural killer and other immune cells.[79]

Diabetes

Both Type 1 and Type 2 diabetes can express autoimmune characteristics.[80,81,82,83] In a diabetic person, at some time in the body autoimmune antibodies against pancreatic beta-cells were created. These antibodies interfere with beta-cell production of insulin. This can cause an unstable production of insulin and the inability of the body to regulate blood sugars.[84]

Type 1, or juvenile onset diabetes, can also be considered an autoimmune disease.[85] Tests at UCLA and Stanford University showed that a protein called GAD, found in cow's milk, can trigger an allergic response that damages the insulin-producing cells of the pancreas.[86] Without insulin, the body is unable to use glucose for energy, so it is forced to burn fat instead. This severe metabolic imbalance can lead to a dangerous condition called diabetic coma.

This type of diabetes seems to occur most often in children who did not receive colostrum at birth or were not breast-fed for long. The immune factors in colostrum increased the tolerance for GAD, preventing the allergic response.[87]

Once an individual has developed Type 1 diabetes the treatment options are very few. Generally, the condition is controlled with a combination of dietary restrictions, and daily insulin injections. A 1990 study suggested that colostrum supplementation would be a very beneficial treatment for diabetics, based on the fact that a key growth factor, IGF-1, can stimulate glucose utilization. Researchers found that plasma levels of IGF-1 were lower in diabetic patients than in healthy individuals.[88] After administering IGF-1 to patients, the doctors noticed a two-fold increase in glucose transport to the muscles. The IGF-1 in colostrum could painlessly do the job of the daily insulin injections most diabetics now have to endure. Of course, any change in insulin medication should only be made under a doctor's supervision.

Autoimmune disease can be loosely defined as a condition where the body's immune defenses are turned on itself, or stated in another way, the body cannot distinguish ***self*** from ***non-self***. This state is usually characterized by the synthesis of specific antibodies to proteins that are normally found in bodily tissues and the mobilization of other aspects of the immune system (e.g., white blood cells and inflammatory cytokines), which in turn leads to wholesale tissue destruction.

In the specific case of diabetes, this situation is most readily observed in Type I diabetes (juvenile diabetes) where the immune system has attacked and killed the beta-cells that compose the Islets of Langerhans in the pancreas. These individuals lose the ability to produce insulin and must be augmented with insulin therapy for the remainder of their lives. Specific autoantibodies can be found in these individuals along with the activation of natural killer T cells that are normally targeted against invaders such as viruses. Even when people with Type I diabetes are treated with insulin, their autoimmune dysfunction still remains; more and more studies are being directed at the root cause of these issues in an effort to improve the overall prognosis of a complete treatment protocol. It is also true that patients with Type I diabetes are more likely to suffer from other autoimmune conditions such as rheumatoid arthritis or psoriasis. Therefore if progress is made on the autoimmune front for diabetes, there will surely be carryover to these other conditions.

More recently a great deal of attention has been paid to Type 2 diabetes, which is most often associated with obesity and inactivity. New work has shed light on the fact that there is much in common between Types I and 2 patients. One of these areas of commonality is the presence of autoantibodies. This fact alone suggests that on the many faces of diabetes (Types I, 1.5, 2, and now 3) there may be a common imprint of immune dysfunction. And with new revelations linking diabetes with Alzheimer's disease (so-called Type 3), there is even more at stake in deriving and understanding and, more importantly, developing new treatment protocols.

Autoimmune Conditions

Autoimmune conditions are serious diseases in which the body actually begins to make antibodies against itself, often for no clear reason. Colostrum, and PRPs specifically, have been shown to be of benefit in a number of autoimmune conditions,[89] such as multiple sclerosis,[90] rheumatoid arthritis,[91] asthma,[92] systemic lupus erythematosus,[93] several experimental autoimmune responses to red blood cells,[94] and hemolytic anemia.[95]

Chemokines (chemoattractants that attract immune cells to a site) and chemokine receptors have been implicated in a number of autoimmune conditions, such as rheumatoid arthritis, multiple sclerosis, allograft rejection, systemic lupus erythematosus, psoriasis, atopic dermatitis, lichen planus, and graft-vs-host disease. Expression of chemokines by endothelial cells of the blood vessels appears to be an important step in the development of these diseases. Antagonists of chemokine-chemokine receptor interactions alleviate the symptoms of many of these diseases in animal models.[96,97] This may suggest a role that PRPs play in the relief of autoimmune conditions.

Autism

Autism is an early-onset biological disorder that causes severe deficits of higher mental functions, as well as behavioral manifestations. There is no single, clear-cut cause and no complete cure for autism.[98] Causally speaking, immune factors, neurochemical factors, antibiotics,[99] genetic susceptibility factors and environmental factors (such as microbial infections and chemical toxicity) have been implicated. Autism is a very complex, multifactorial disorder that may include autoimmunity.[100] Immune therapies, such as PRPs and colostrum, have been of benefit in some cases, however.[101]

Heart Disease

We have heard so much in recent years about heart disease and what we can do to prevent it. Diet and exercise are some of the best weapons we can use to fight this killer, but for many, the immune and growth factors found in colostrum may be what are needed to win the war.

Altered immunity may be the hidden cause of atherosclerosis and cardiovascular disease. For example, the American College of Cardiology recently reported that a common type of Chlamydia bacteria has been associated with arterial plaque formation in over 79% of patients with heart disease.[102] Another recent study concluded that heart disease is the result of immune sensitization to cardiac antigens.[103] In other words, once heart tissue is damaged, the immune system begins creating antibodies which then cause more harm.

Because heart disease resembles an autoimmune response in this way, colostrum's PRPs can help limit the severity of the disease by toning down the immune system's attack on damaged heart tissue. In addition, the other immune factors found in colostrum can directly combat the Chlamydia bacteria. Finally, IGF-1 and GH in colostrum can lower LDL cholesterol while increasing HDL-cholesterol concentrations.[104,105,106] Colostrum growth factors promote the repair and regeneration of heart muscle and the regeneration of new blood vessels for collateral coronary circulation.[107] Both milk and colostrum contain hypotensive factors, called ACE inhibitory peptides (casokinins and lactokinins), which decrease blood pressure and lower the risk of heart attack and stroke.[108,109] The calcium found in milk and colostrum also contributes to lower blood pressure.[110]

Influenza

A recent study showed the efficacy of a two-month treatment with oral colostrum in the prevention of flu episodes compared with anti-influenza vaccination. After three months of follow-up, the number of days with flu was significantly higher in the non-colostrum subjects. The study showed that colostrum used by both healthy subjects and high-risk cardiovascular patients was three times more effective than vaccination in preventing flu and is very cost-effective. [111]

Cancer

Colostrum has also been shown to be of benefit against that most feared of diseases, cancer. Numerous research studies have shown that bovine colostrum has prevented the development of cancers, particularly cancers associated with the gastrointestinal tract, under experimental conditions.[683] More clinical research is needed to understand colostrum's role in preventing cancer ***in vivo***, which is, of course, much more difficult to study.

It has been estimated that one in three people living in Canada and the US will get some form of cancer during their lifetime. The causes of cancer (or cancers) are multiple. There are, of course, the well-known carcinogens like nitrates, hydrogenated oils, cigarette smoke, and radiation. Cancerous cells are continuously being formed and destroyed in almost every human body. The problem comes when a weakened immune system allows for the cancerous cells to spread and destroy other healthy tissues. Ironically, chemotherapy, the treatment of choice for many cancers, compromises the body's natural immune function, leaving patients susceptible to even more infection.

The benefits of natural immune boosters in the treatment of cancer was first popularized by the 1985 Steven Rosenberg book, ***Quiet Strides in the War on Cancer.***[112] Rosenberg had great success with cancer patients, including one complete cure, by using a treatment that flooded the body with killer immune cells, as well as chemical messengers called cytokines.[113,114] Since Rosenberg's time, the same cytokines found uniquely in colostrum (interleukins 1, 6, 10, interferon-γ, and lymphokines) have been the singlemost researched elements in the search for the cure for cancer.

Colostral lactalbumin has been found to cause the selective death of cancer cells, leaving the surrounding non-cancerous tissues unaffected. Lactoferrin has similarly been reported to possess anti-cancer activity. The incredible mix of immune and growth factors in colostrum can inhibit the spread of cancer cells. And if viruses are involved in either the initiation or the spread of cancer, colostrum could prove to be one of the best ways to prevent the disease in the first place.

PRPs have been shown to be a potent placental antiangiogenic hormone that prevents neovascularization[115] (see also: angiogenesis). Tumor cells engineered to express high levels of PRPs show markedly reduced growth rates as tumors in mice.[116] The protein also acts on human endothelial cells.[117]. It has been shown that the use of adenovirus vectors expressing PRPs can lead to complete tumor rejection and prolonged survival in a high proportion of animals bearing transplanted mouse B16F10 melanoma cells. [118,119,120,121]

A series of studies done in Japan on animal models of cancer showed in every case that lactoferrin either prevented the cancer from taking hold or prevented metastasis from established tumors.[122,123,124,125] Lactoferrin has also been shown to boost the cytotoxic activity of natural killer cells against blood and breast epithelial tumor cell lines[126,127] and to inhibit the growth of breast cancer cells.[128]

One study has shown that a number of human cancers become more sensitive to chemotherapy in the presence of epidermal growth factor, one of the growth factors present in colostrum.[129]

What colostrum does not do in regard to cancer is make it worse. There have been some stories put out that the growth factors in colostrum can cause cancers to grow faster, but these rumors are unfounded and not backed by research.[130]

AIDS (HIV)

Several unpleasant features make HIV frightening. First of all, the virus mutates so quickly that the body cannot produce an antibody to destroy it. Secondly, how can we fight off a virus that directly targets the body's main defense—the immune system? In fact, it is not finally HIV itself that poses the deadly threat associated with the AIDS disease. Rather, HIV attacks the immune system, rendering it extremely vulnerable to other invaders. In cases of severe immune damage, a simple cold or flu can be deadly.

In a 1995 article in ***Scientific American***, researchers concluded that "traditional" disease fighting methods (vaccines, for example) are just not effective in fighting HIV. Instead, they recommend reducing the viral level in the body and stimulating the body's natural immune response to have the best chance against the tricky virus.[131]

Another study[132] indicates that the colostral immune factor lactoferrin is one of the best ways to reduce viral levels in the body. For example, lactoferrin inhibited HIV infection of certain body cells. In addition, the immune factor was able to completely block Cytomegalovirus infection. This study also concluded that bovine lactoferrin was up to 2.5 times more potent than human lactoferrin.

Many of the immune factors in colostrum also help to stimulate or "jump-start" a weakened immune system. Lactoferrin, for example, is responsible for "turning on" the immune system in newborn babies and has been proven to do the same thing for adult AIDS patients. In addition, colostrum's growth factors also boost the body's immune function. Clinical studies have shown that HIV positive patients who are treated with certain growth factors (in particular growth hormone or IGF-1) were much less likely to develop full-blown AIDS than were patients who received different treatments.[133]

Growth factors also play an important role in preventing AIDS-associated wasting, or severe weight loss. Wasting occurs when the AIDS infected body begins using muscle for energy. Treatment with growth hormone and IGF-1 showed an increase in lean muscle mass among AIDS patients. This increase in muscle mass is one of the main keys to improving the quality of life of AIDS sufferers.

Mass wasting is most often brought about by severe, chronic diarrhea, one of the first symptoms of AIDS. Cryptosporidia and rotavirus take advantage of the weakened immune system, causing acute diarrhea. This results in a loss of vital nutrients and fluids and also depletes much of the supply of intestinal antibodies leaving the sufferer even more susceptible to dangerous pathogens.

Because it is one of the most serious, potentially fatal problems that AIDS sufferers face, much of the research thus far has focused on finding a way to prevent diarrhea. One study[134] showed that out of 37 immuno-deficient patients with chronic diarrhea, 72.4% experienced a significant improvement with the use of immunoglobulins from colostrum. Over half of the patients remained diarrhea free for at least four weeks after the treatment. A 1990 study stated that colostrum immunoglobulins have been able to treat opportunistic, diarrhea-causing infections in AIDS patients where no other treatment was effective.[135]

At the very least, colostrum will benefit the AIDS patient by prolonging and greatly improving the quality of life.

Athletic Use

But wait, that's not all. Athletes love colostrum because the growth factors in it help burn fat while building lean muscle. Colostrum builds strength and shortens recovery time. It also protects athletes from getting sick when at their most vulnerable following a vigorous workout when the immune system is temporarily disabled. Some athletes and trainers have even labeled colostrum as the "new creatine."

In the 2000 and 2004 Summer Olympics, Australian athletes stunned the world by earning more medals than China, a nation with over 100 times as many people and potential athletes. What was their secret? Colostrum!

Fitness

Studies are now showing significant gains in fitness with colostrum supplementation. A widely reported study in Australia found a 20% increase in strength, stamina and shortened recovery time for both soccer players and cyclists. Many body builders and fitness experts say colostrum works better than any other legal substance they ever experienced.

The growth factors found in colostrum are now known to enhance muscle tone, burn off body fat, promote skin elasticity, and increase bone density. TgF-alpha and -beta (transforming growth factors) stimulate production and repair of RNA and DNA, as well as repair of damaged muscle fibers in athletes. EGF (epithelial growth factor) stimulates enhanced skin healing. IGF-1 (insulin-like growth factor 1) is able to "promote muscle growth by itself," according to ***Muscle and Fitness*** associate editor Steve Schwade.

Bovine IGF-1 is effective in humans, differing in its structure by only 3 out of 67 amino acids, and bovine colostrum is found to be even higher in IGF-1 than human colostrum. The growth factors in colostrum stimulate protein synthesis and slow protein breakdown, resulting in increased lean muscle mass. At the same time, they shift the metabolism from burning carbohydrates to burning more fats.

Olympic skiers taking colostrum experienced less fatigue and improved their performance in a placebo-controlled study in Finland. They also showed only half the level of blood creatine-kinase, a marker of muscle injury, compared to placebo control. Another Finnish study confirmed that athletes taking colostrum during strength and speed training did in fact show increased blood serum concentrations of IGF-1[136].

Overall, colostrum is considered as powerful as steroids at generating increased muscle mass when used in conjunction with exercise, but without the risks and side effects.

Studies have shown that the growth factors present in colostrum increase between 2,500 to 4,000% (from 2–5 ng/mg to 50–200 ng/mg) with exposure to acidity. To gain the maximum fitness benefits from colostrum, take it in powder form (empty the capsule in your mouth or onto food) toward the end of a meal or 45 minutes before a physical workout session with a protein drink like One Step. Friendly flora, which naturally promote a healthy acidity level in the colon, may also enhance the benefits of colostrum.

Strenuous exercise associated with athletic training and competition places a tremendous strain on body systems, including the immune system. Studies on the effects of extreme exercise on the immune system have shown profound immune system changes following marathon runs or other forms of athletic performance that push the body to the limit. One study on marathon runners showed that white blood cell counts decreased dramatically after a three-hour run but returned to normal levels within 21 hours.[137] Another study on marathoners showed decreased natural killer cell activity after a race.[138] This would suggest that athletes who push themselves to their limits are much more susceptible to infectious diseases, such as upper respiratory infections, which is indeed borne out by research.[139] Colostrum, combined with proper nutrition and rest, helps prevent this. Colostrum, with its growth and immune factors, cuts recovery time and boosts immune function, reducing the susceptibility of athletes to infection after exercise,[140] and it can help heal "leaky gut" in athletes which can be caused by protein supplementation.[141] Colostrum also speeds the healing of muscle, tendon and ligament injuries.

Other studies on athletes have shown that colostrum can lower recovery times and increase anaerobic power.[142,143,144] Colostrum supplementation also builds lean muscle tissue and burns fat.[145]

In recognition of colostrum's natural ability to improve an athlete's health and physical condition, the IOC ruled that colostrum is an acceptable supplement. They based their decision on the fact that although colostrum supplementation stimulates the production of IGF-1 in the body, the IGF-1 in colostrum is not actually absorbed but digested.[146,147]

So colostrum emerges as an ideal supplement for athletes, whether they're Olympic or professional level athletes or weekend warriors. It builds lean muscle, burns fat, protects from disease and heals the leaky gut condition often associated with athletic training and performance.

Anti-Aging

Getting a little long in the tooth? Then colostrum is for you. Colostrum has many antioxidant and anti-aging components to keep you in top shape longer. It helps keep skin looking young and healthy. It removes dangerous free oxygen radicals, metabolic waste products that can cause you to age more rapidly. It supplies us with growth factors and other important substances that normally decline with age, leading to cell senescence and accelerated aging.

Oxidation is the normal metabolism of nutrients in the body. As we age, we are less able to remove the byproducts of metabolism resulting in high levels of reactive oxygen species (ROS) which results in oxidative stress in the tissues. What this means to us is rapid aging, damage to DNA, proteins, and lipids, and cancer and degenerative diseases, including arthritis.[148,149,150] Colostrum can help clean up these waste products and counteract their negative effects on the body. It contains a number of powerful antioxidants, including glutathione, the most powerful antioxidant known, and its chemical precursors.[151] Glutathione itself is not absorbed through the intestinal wall, but the glutathione in colostrum still plays a major role in maintaining gastrointestinal health. The precursors, cystine, glycine, and glutamic acid, are absorbed and contribute to glutathione production in the body.

Colostrum reduces respiratory burst output in white blood cells (polymorphonuclear leukocytes), which has both an antioxidant and an anti-inflammatory effect.[152,153] PRPs contribute to the antioxidant effect of colostrum by down regulating lipid peroxidation, inhibiting glutathione depletion and reducing intracellular levels of ROS (reactive oxygen species).[154] Lactoferrin also has antioxidant properties, preventing lipid peroxidation.[155] Haemopexin is a protein found in milk and colostrum[156] that strongly binds haem, a low molecular weight form of iron that takes part in oxidative reactions in tissues. Haemopexin can inhibit these reactions by up to 90%.[157]

Detoxification

Traditionally, detoxification means taking a powerful herbal concoction that causes the body to dump fluids, thus flushing the system of impurities and toxins. From the point of view of colostrum, however, this is a limited and potentially dangerous concept of detoxification that puts unneeded stress on the body and can do more harm than good. Colostrum detoxifies the body beginning in the gastrointestinal tract in a much healthier and efficacious manner. Colostrum inhibits or destroys harmful pathogens which can colonize the gut and cause major health problems, such as ***Helicobacter pylori***, the main cause of gastric and duodenal ulcers,[158,159,160,161] ***Candida albicans***, a fungus that can overgrow the intestines, forcing out beneficial bacteria,[162] and many other pathogens,[163,164] while promoting the growth of beneficial bacterial colonies. Colostrum also acts to heal the damage to the intestinal lining caused by the pathogens and toxins that can accumulate there. This prevents pathogens and toxins from entering the body and restores normal gut functioning. Colostrum also helps protect and heal both the liver and the pancreas from the effects of toxins in the body by helping to remove dangerous toxins and by stimulating these organs to replace damaged tissue.[165]

Weight Loss

Whole first milking colostrum contains leptin (approximately 50 ng/g). Leptin, discovered in 1994, derives its name from the Greek word ***leptos***, meaning thin. This is a polypeptide hormone produced in adipose and many other tissues with many different roles related to the inhibition of food intake and stimulation of energy expenditure.

In embryology, its levels are associated with fertility and reproductive maturity in many species. There are several additional hormonal roles in the adult including satiety, adiposity, and metabolism.

Higher levels of leptin as a neurotransmitter can accelerate the communication signals to stop eating sooner.

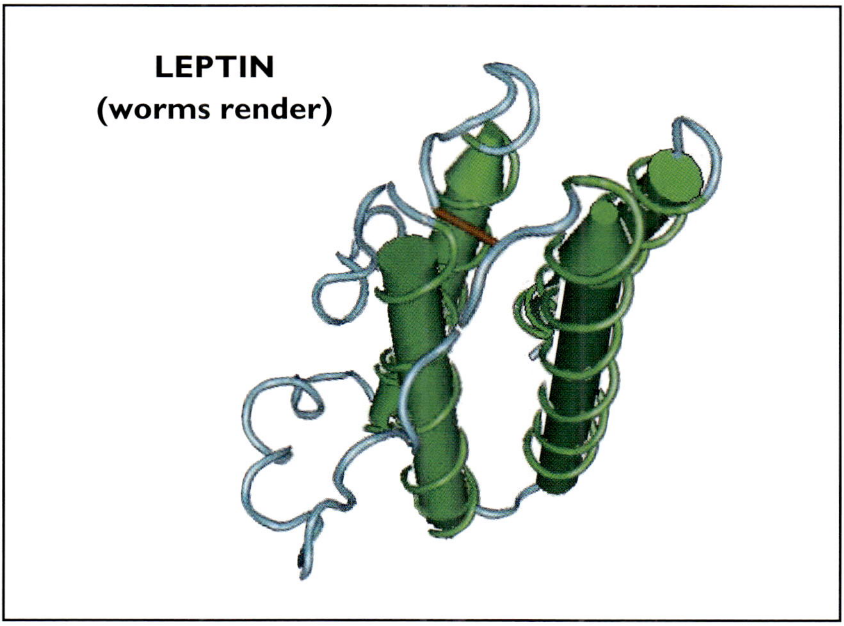

Healing, Tissue Repair and Recovery from Injury

Colostrum has been known for its healing abilities since earliest times, being mentioned in Egyptian hieroglyphic texts for its healing properties. Skin cells have receptors for growth hormone and IGF-1, showing that they have the ability to react directly to growth hormone stimulation.[166] IGF-II, also found in colostrum, plays a similar role.[167] Fibroblast growth factor (FGF) and epithelial growth factor (EGF), both found in colostrum, are important in healing skin wounds.[168,169] Burns suppress the levels of IGF-1 in the affected area,[170] which explains why colostrum, with its high concentration of IGF-1, is excellent for burn recovery.
The growth factors in colostrum also accelerate the healing of muscle, tendon and ligament injuries, such as are commonly experienced by athletes.[171,172,173,174]

Colostrum's growth factors stimulate regeneration and repair of muscle, bone, cartilage, skin, collagen and nerve tissues, as well as RNA and DNA. This not only means faster, more complete recovery from injury and illness. It is also how colostrum stimulates age-erasing effects.

With prolonged use, the skin becomes more youthful, while age-spots and liver spots disappear. Sexual function is enhanced and bone density increases. Research published in the ***New England Journal of Medicine***[175] has shown that transforming growth factor (TGF-β) found in colostrum is also produced by osteoblasts, the cells that build bone. TgF-β was found to dramatically increase cell apoptosis (programmed cell death) among osteoclasts, the cells responsible for breaking down and reabsorbing bone. In addition to colostrum, microcrystalline hydroxyapatite and DHEA are proven to increase bone density.

Colostrum also helps to balance blood sugar and replenish neurotransmitters, resulting in better alertness and concentration, while enhancing mood. Both serotonin and dopamine are released in greater quantities, while their re-uptake is prolonged, allowing each molecule to work longer and more efficiently. For this reason, it is generally best to take colostrum in the morning and again sometime before about 4 PM (e.g. around lunchtime or a couple hours after).

Topical Applications

Colostrum, mixed into a paste with water, helps the body heal injuries such as burns, cuts, abrasions, ulcers, acne and even surgical wounds with topical application.[168,176] Topical use in the mouth helps relieve gingivitis, canker sores, sensitive teeth and speeds recovery from dental work.

The Perfect Food

Colostrum is the perfect food, combining all the crucial immune and growth factors in the exact synergistic combination necessary to promote life. For many, it is considered the ideal alternative to hundreds of pharmaceutical drugs, from antibiotics to steroids.

Research on colostrum has documented benefits from dosages in the range of 2 to 60 grams per day with no known contraindications, side effects or allergic reactions reported over thousands of years of use. It is even safe for those with lactose intolerance. Some experts recommend taking it in a divided dose (at least 1 gram twice a day) with antioxidant water on an empty stomach for maximum benefits.

Here is a partial list of some of the benefits of colostrum:

Anabolic activity
Antiaging
Antifungal
Anti-Inflammatory
Antimicrobial
Assimilation
Athletic performance
Body building
Bone density
Cytokines
Digestion

Elimination
Friendly flora
Immunity
Intestinal permeability
Muscle tone
Prevention
Recovery time
Retinoic acids
Skin elasticity
Soil-based organisms
Sports performance
Stamina
Terrain
Weight loss
Wound healing

Following is a list of some of the major conditions that your body may be able to better heal or prevent with colostrum:

Alcoholism
ALS (Lou Gehrig's Disease)
Anemia
Arthritis
Atherosclerosis
Autoimmune conditions
Bacterial infection
Bone marrow transplant
Bullous Pemphigoid
Campylobacter
Cancer
Candida albicans
Chlamydia
Cholera
Chronic Fatigue Syndrome (CFIDS)

Crohn's disease
Clostridium
Cystic fibrosis
Diarrhea
Dysbiosis
Epstein Barr virus (EBV)
Fibromyalgia
Food poisoning
Fungal infection
Guillan-Barre Syndrome
Heart disease
Helicobacter pylori
Hepatitis
Herpes virus
HIV
Influenza
Intestinal parasites
Irritable Bowel Syndrome (IBS)
Kawasaki Syndrome
Listeria
Multiple Sclerosis
Muscular Dystrophy
Myasthenia gravis
Neutropenia
Osteoporosis
Overweight
Premature birth
Rheumatoid Arthritis (RA)
Rotavirus
Scleroderma
Shigella
Staphylococcus aureus
Systemic Lupus Erythematosus (SLE)
Thrombocytopenia

Ulcers
Viral infection
Yeast infection

Colostrum as Functional Food

Functional foods are defined as those foods that have potential healthful benefits beyond the traditional nutrients they may contain. As such, colostrum has great potential as a functional food that can be easily combined with other healthful food products. Whole colostrum or various components of colostrum show great promise as an additive to infant formulas, for example, as well as other dairy products, such as yogurt. It is used as an ingredient in nutritional supplements such as Nutriboost. By itself colostrum can be put in capsules or tableted for easy consumption.

In Summary

Mankind was never designed to eat processed foods, breath polluted air, drink polluted water, or lead sedentary lives. Colostrum can help us restore some of our lost balance. It has shown great promise to help each and every one of us to lead a happier and healthier life.

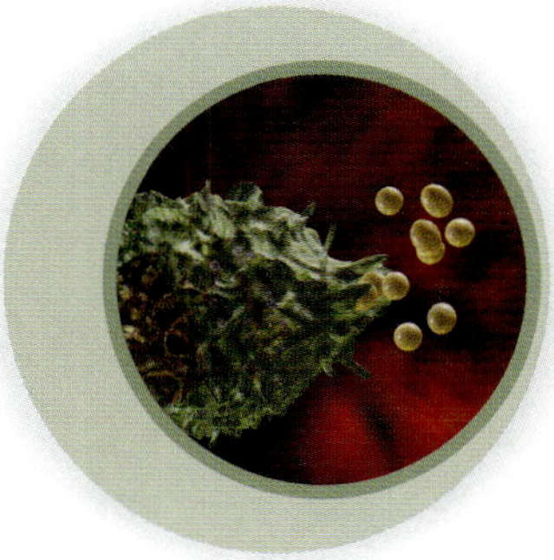

CHAPTER 5

COLLECTION AND PROCESSING

How colostrum is collected and processed matters. Care must be taken to preserve the bioavailability of the components of colostrum in order for it to be effective.

First and second milking colostrum are the richest in immunoglobulins, growth factors and peptides. These milkings should be done only after the calves have had their fill to ensure their survival. The graph below shows that first and second milking colostrum has a higher percentage of IgG than subsequent milkings.

While the concentrations of immunoglobulins and growth factors decrease over time, other factors, including lactose, increase. The amount of lactose is important for lactose-intolerant individuals as higher levels are more likely to produce an allergic response.

The Southwestern United States is ideal for colostrum production as cows give birth year round, rather than just in the spring as occurs in most locales. Grass used for feed is grown on DDT-free soil. The dry desert climate helps minimize insect populations without the need for pesticides. The cows should not be given hormones or antibiotics.

After collection, the colostrum should be frozen or cooled below 40°F to maintain freshness until it reaches the processing plant. At the plant, the frozen colostrum must be thawed and then homogenized to restore the casein micelles that protect

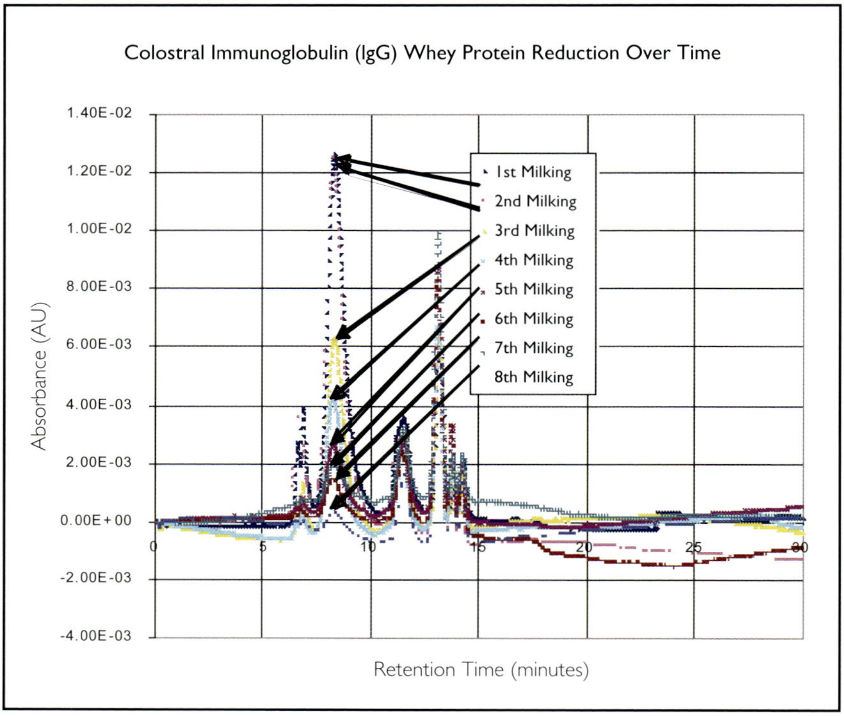

Figure 1. HPLC graphs of colostrum showing IgG peak at 8 minutes for the first eight milkings after giving birth.

the proteins. Freezing colostrum does not damage its proteins if done properly.[177] Processing should be done daily to ensure freshness and maximum quality.

Whole colostrum will quickly go rancid if not properly stabilized in the processing. If rancidity occured in the whole colostrum, it will deactivate many of the components of colostrum, such as vitamin A,[178] and makes it unpalatable. One hundred percent whole colostrum powder is preferred for human nutrition compared to a skim colostrum powder. There is no evidence that defatting the colostrum in any way affects the bioavailability of its components.

As with any dairy product, the colostrum must be pasteurized to guarantee safety. Many producers of colostrum use high heat pasteurization and drying processes that can denature the proteins in colostrum. They use this technique because

Time After Birth, hr	Total (i) Protein %	Casein %	Albumin %	Fat %	Lactose % (ii)	Ash %	Total Solids % (iii)
0	17.57	5.08	11.34	5.10	2.19	1.01	26.99
6	10	3.51	6.30	6.85	2.71	0.91	20.46
12	6.05	3.00	2.96	3.80	3.71	0.89	14.53
24	4.52	2.76	1.48	3.40	2.98	0.86	12.77
36	3.98	2.77	1.03	3.55	3.97	0.83	12.22
72	3.86	2.70	0.97	3.10	4.37	0.84	11.86

Source: Immuno Dynamics, Inc. ICN Biomedical, Inc. Costa Mesa, CA.

FIGURE 2. PROPORTIONS OF VARIOUS COMPONENTS OF COLOSTRUM AT DIFFERENT TIMES FOLLOWING BIRTH.

(i) Contains cytokines and other protein compounds of very low molecular weight that act as Biologic Response Modulators (BMRs), which intervene locally in most biological processes.
(ii) Lactose has a great influence on allergic-like responses experienced by some individuals due to the lack of lactase and β-galactosidase. Unlike immunoglobulin IgG, lactose rises in value from the first milking through subsequent several milkings.
(iii) Total solids are determined by the dried solids by the original quantity of liquid started with.

they process their colostrum in milk processing plants that use high heat pasteurization to pasteurize the milk. This batch pasteurization method can destroy up to 58% of the IgG in colostrum.[179,180] Ultra high temperature (UHT) sterilization of colostrum destroys all IgG and protein activity.[181,182] Unfortunately, most commercially available milk in the US is prepared using UHT, resulting in most milk in the grocery dairy section being biologically inactive. A preferable technique called high temperature short time (HTST) pasteurization, or flash pasteurization, preserves the bioactivity of the proteins while still ensuring that any pathogens are killed. Both temperature and time are important in maintaining bioactivity of IgG in colostrum. The higher the temperature, the shorter the time it takes for denaturation of IgG to take place.[183] Other components, such as growth factors, are similarly affected.[184] Lactoferrin subjected to UHT was not destroyed, but its ability to bind various bacterial species was decreased, and its ability to inhibit bacterial growth was destroyed.[185]

Following pasteurization, the colostrum is dried into a fine pale yellow powder. The preferable method is spray drying at temperatures less than 145°F using an indirect steam heating method. Many colostrum producers use direct heating from gas flames which introduces dangerous nitrogen oxide chemicals into the colostrum.

Following drying, the colostrum should then be agglomerated to produce consistently sized particles. This allows the colostrum to more readily dissolve in liquid. It is also important that the manufacturer follow Good Manufacturing Process (GMP), including microbiological analysis on each batch to ensure safety and the highest quality.

Immunoglobulins should be quantified using Ion Exchange HPLC-IX (Ion Exchange, not by Ion Exchange HPLC Protein G alone), or by Radial Immunodiffusion (RID). Calibrations of these columns should be done using Bovine IgG standards, most likely provided from Sigma Aldrich Company.

Coating the Colostrum Powder with Various Phospholipids

Most manufacturers stop here, but the highest quality colostrum will have a lipid coating that forms liposomes (lipid globules) around the proteins for protection and easy absorption in the gut. This replicates the globules in milk produced in the mammary gland and provides the best possible delivery system for the colostrum. The best liposomes are formed using the same phospholipids found in milk globules and which also make up the cell membranes of all cells in the body, phosphatidylethanolamine, phosphatidylcholine, phosphatidylserine, phosphatidylinositol, and sphingomyelin. Phospholipids are unique in that they are soluble in both water and oil, ensuring they remain in solution until they reach the gut lining where they fuse with the cell membranes of the cells lining the gut. Their contents then pass into the bloodstream for use within the body without being digested or degraded.

There are several types of phospholipids that can be used to produce the liposomes. One is extracted from the anhydrous milk fat in cream and may be referred to as Alpha-lipid, Beta-lipid or BIO-lipid™. These are terms for the same phospholipids found in milk. These milk lipids can be called milkfat globule membrane (MGM). Another type of phospholipid that is used for liposomal delivery systems is lechithin, which is usually composed of phosphatidylcholine, one of the major membrane phospholipids in the body. A new type of coating is made up of vegetable oils, usually derived from soybeans. Phospholipids tend to form liposomes spontaneously in solution. The basic makeup of a cell membrane is shown in Figure 1.

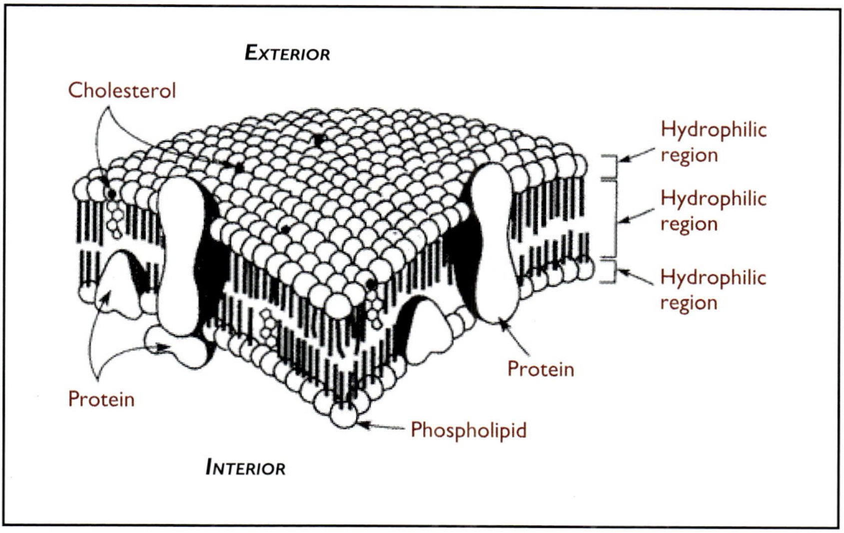

FIGURE 1. TYPICAL CELL MEMBRANE STRUCTURE WITH BILAMELLAR PHOSPHOLIPID ORGANIZATION.

Note that the hydrophilic ends of the phospholipids all point out, and the hydrophobic (lipophilic) ends all point in towards the other layer of the membrane. The benefit of using phospholipids to make the liposomes in the delivery system is that phospholipids themselves are beneficial to one's health, particularly brain and nervous system health, cell signaling pathways, and anti-aging benefits.

In addition to protecting the contents from digestion in the gastrointestinal tract, liposomes also aid in dispersion. The large proteins in colostrum tend to clump together and disperse poorly if just put into solution. Inside liposomes, they disperse evenly and thus are more likely to be absorbed in the gut. Freeze facture electron microscopy of phospholipid liposomes show that they can be produced in unilamellar or multilamellar forms for different applications.

Always check to make sure that any colostrum you purchase meets the criteria listed in this chapter. Only then will you receive any benefit from the colostrum. Colostrum is a biologically active product. The quality of a good colostrum is determined by the quantity of bioactive constituents of the colostrum product and not by marketing hype.

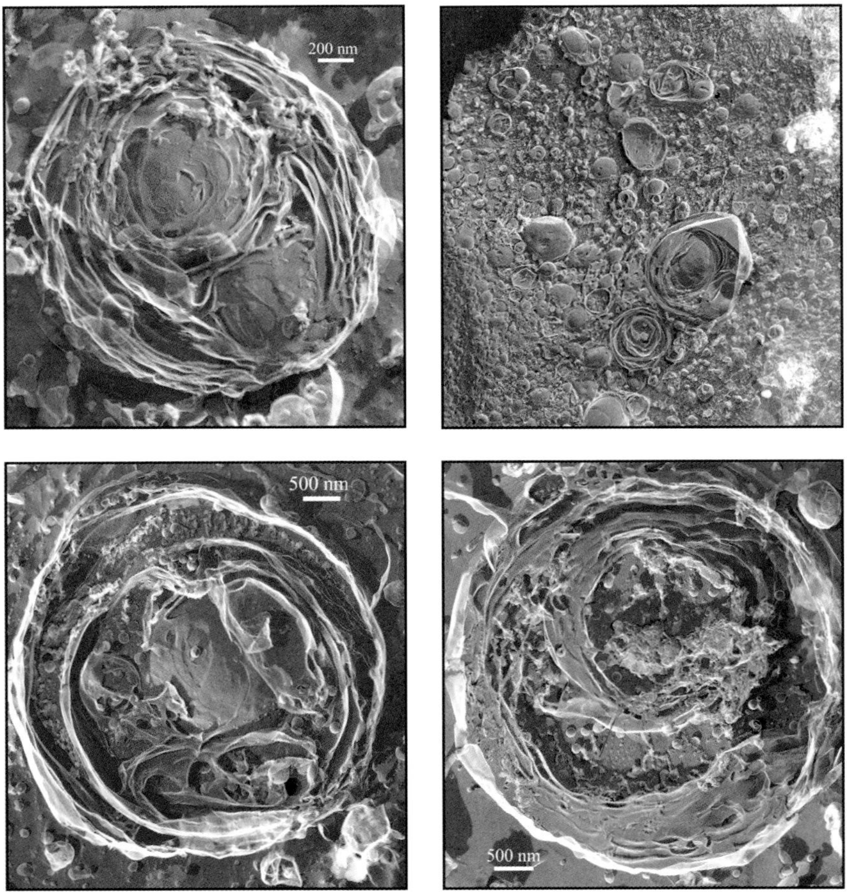

FIGURE 2. FREEZE FRACTURE ELECTRON MICROGRAPHS OF DIFFERENT MILKFAT GLOBULE MEMBRANE PREPARATIONS SHOWING BOTH UNILAMELLAR AND MULTIMLAMELLAR LIPOSOMES.

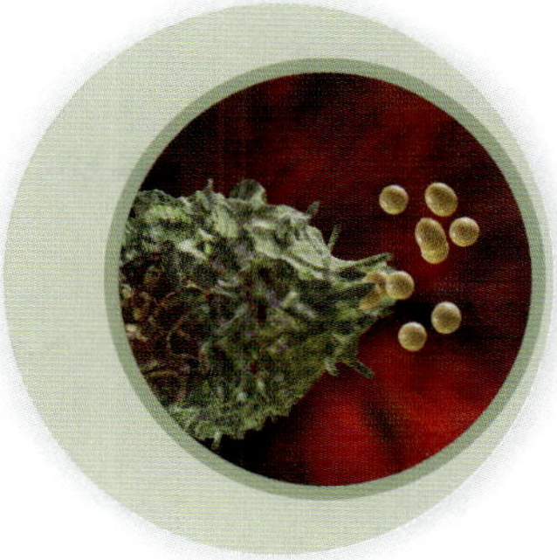

CHAPTER 6

WHAT'S IN COLOSTRUM?

Not an easy question to answer! Scientists are still unraveling the amazingly complex web we call colostrum. However, we have a good idea of the main ingredients and how they work. This list is not exhaustive but indicative of how complex this life-giving substance is.

IMMUNE COMPONENTS

Immunoglobulins

The natural environment contains a large variety of infectious microbial agents—bacteria, viruses, and fungi. If left unchecked and allowed to multiply, pathogenic species will eventually kill the host. In normal healthy animals most infections are of limited duration and cause little if any permanent damage. This is due to the immune system—a natural defense mechanism that helps ward off or combat infectious agents.

Immunoglobulins have an integral role in this defense system in that they function as ***antibodies***. There are five classes of immunoglobulin recognized in mammals: IgG, IgA, IgM, IgE, and IgD. While the most prevalent class in most mammals is IgG, the other immunoglobulins also have very important functions. The fact that in human milk and colostrum IgA is the predominant immunoglobulin should be noted. The main function of these molecules is to bind to invading organisms and to activate specific mechanisms that help rid the body of disease-causing agents.

In human and animal trials it has been demonstrated that specific antibodies exist in bovine colostrum which are effective against both enteropathogenic and enterotoxigenic organisms.

Immunoglobulins are also known as antibodies. They are the main component of the adaptive immune system (for a brief explanation of how the immune system works, see Appendix A). When an antigen (a foreign protein) is discovered in the body by immune scout cells, a chain of events is begun that results in antibodies specific to that antigen being produced by certain blood cells called B lymphocytes. The antigen might be a protein from a bacteria or virus, or it could be from a toxin. It could even be a protein produced by your own body, as happens in the case of autoimmune conditions. These specific antibodies fit the antigen like a key fits a lock. The disabled antigen can then be targeted for elimination by the immune system. There are different types of immunoglobulins found in the body, and these are also found in colostrum.

Immunoglobulins are glycoproteins and are present in serum and other tissue fluids, including the milk and colostrum, of all mammals. Antibodies are produced in response to the host being exposed to immunogenic foreign substances (antigens), such as infectious microbes. They are an important element in the adaptive immune response in that they are directed specifically to the antigen that induced their formation and that they impart memory. In this manner the body is effectively prepared to repel any later invasion by the same organism.

Antibodies are produced by activated B cell lymphocytes (plasma cells). Each plasma cell secretes one class of antibody, and all the antibody produced by a single plasma cell is of the same specificity. There are five classes of immunoglobulin that are recognized in mammals: IgG, IgA, IgM, IgE and IgD. The most prevalent class of immunoglobulin in all species of animals is IgG. However, in humans the IgA class is the predominant form found in breast milk and colostrum. The function of these molecules is to bind to invading organisms and to activate specific actions that help rid the body of disease-causing agents. They function in cell killing, inflammation, and prevention of bacterial and viral attachment.

IgG is the form in which antibodies occur most abundantly. In all species of mammals IgG is passed from the mother to its young, although the actual mechanism of transmission varies from species to species. In humans and apes it has been shown that IgG and its complement of antibodies pass across the placental barrier from mother to fetus during the second two-thirds of gestation. This passage appears to be selective in that IgG is transferred but not the other immunoglobulins. Albumin is also transferred, but to a lesser degree. Other plasma proteins are not transferred across the placental barrier. In cattle it appears that the same type of selection occurs in absorption of antibody through the gut in that there is a preferential passage of IgG but not IgA, IgM, IgD or IgE.

Immune factors in colostrum include immunoglobulins (A, D, E, G, M), cytokines, including interleukins 1, 3, 4, 5, 6, 8, 10, 12, 13, 16, 18, interferon-γ, and lymphokines, leukocytes, lactoferrin, Proline-rich Polypeptides (PRPs), protease inhibitors, trypsin inhibitors, antibodies, glycoproteins, Lactobacillus, Bifidus, Acidophilus, oligopolysaccharides, glycoconjugates, orotic acid, secretory IgA, IgA specific helper, β-lactoglobulin, lactalbumin, albumin, prealbumin, alpha-1 antitripsin, alpha-1 fetoprotein, alpha-2 macroglobulin, alpha-2 AP glycoprotein, C3 and C4 orosomucoids, lysozyme, lactoperoxidase, thiocyanate, peroxidase, xanthine oxidase, vitamins A, B_{12}, E, and sulfur.

Immunosupplementation of the Gut

Local protection in the form of immunosupplementation with bovine milk antibodies has been shown to be an effective means of providing local protection to the GI tract against disease. Bovine immunoglobulin in the form of specific antibody has been shown to be effective against various enteric diseases. In trials it has been successfully shown that specific antibodies in bovine colostrum are effective against both enteropathic and enterotoxic ***Escherichia coli***, ***Cryptosporidium parvum***, rotavirus, and ***Shigella flexneri.***[186,187,188,189,190,191,192]

Clinical research by Dr. David Tyrell in England in 1980[193] revealed that a high percentage of the antibodies and immunoglobulins present in colostrum are believed not to be absorbed but remain in the intestinal tract where they attack disease-causing organisms before they penetrate the body and cause disease. The remainder are believed to be absorbed and distributed to assist in our internal defense processes. It is this combination of actions that is believed to make colostrum so unique and effective as an oral supplement.

> "Studies with human volunteers found that the preservation of the biological activity of IgG (Immunoglobulin), in the digestive secretions of adults receiving bovine colostrum orally, indicates passive enteral (intestinal) immunization for the prevention and treatment of acute intestinal diseases..."
> – Dr. L.B. Khazenson, Journal of Microbial and Epidemiological Immunobiology[194]

Bovine Immunoglobulins

The cow is an ideal source of natural occurring antibodies. Though all species of mammals have antibodies to various pathogenic microbes, the established supply and volume of cow's milk available make this species an ideal candidate as a source of the natural antibodies. Further, as mentioned previously, a very important aspect of this local immune protection is that it is not species specific, so we as humans and all other animals can use bovine colostrum for its various health benefits.

The principal immunoglobulins that function as antibodies are IgG, IgA and IgM. Also present in bovine colostrum and other biological fluids are IgE and IgD, though only in small amounts. All these immunoglobulins function synergistically in such a way as to complement one another's ability to hunt down, fight and destroy invading pathogenic microbes. The immunoglobulin fraction in bovine colostrum is composed of approximately 70–80% IgG, 10–15% IgA, 10–15% IgM, while IgE and IgD are found in small amounts.

The function of these immunoglobulins (antibodies) is as follows:

IgG—predominant immunoglobulin in bovine milk colostrum; primary function is to identify and help destroy invading pathogenic microbes.
IgA—predominant immunoglobulin in human milk and colostrum; primary role

is as first line of defense, protects mucosal surfaces and prevents the attachment of pathogens to them.

IgM—primary role is "first to fight;" enhances phagocytosis by destroying invading pathogens.

IgE—involved with the allergic reaction and histamine-associated allergic reaction; also involved with active defense against enteric parasites.

IgD—attached to B cells; it stimulates lymphocytes to produce antibodies by presenting antigens to them.

Bovine immunoglobulins, once again, are a group of bioactive molecules, all of which work together to fight disease. IgG is simply a member of this mighty defense system. IgG measurement is typically used as the marker to designate the overall immune strength of colostrum, but this is only a small part of the immune defense system. The fact that IgG only constitutes approximately 80% of the overall total immunoglobulin present in colostrum should be noted. To illustrate the differences and functions of the three predominant immunoglobulins the following schematics may be of value:

BOVINE IMMUNOGLOBULIN G (IgG)

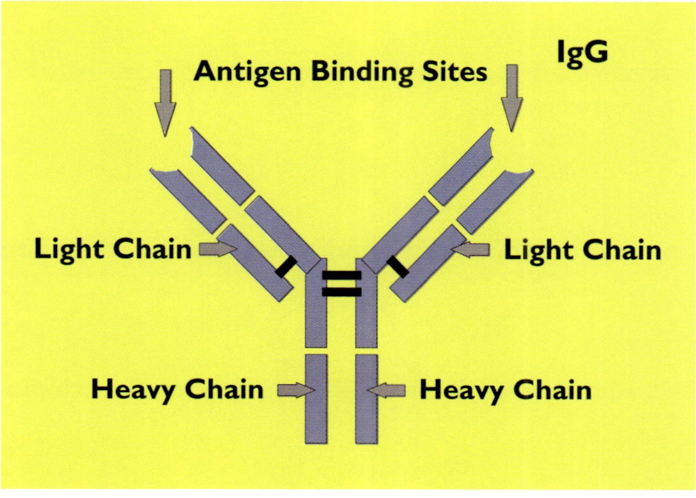

Note the basic immunoglobulin structure: the "Y" and the two antigen binding sites.

BOVINE IMMUNOGLOBULIN A (IgA)

In colostrum and milk IgA is present as secretory IgA

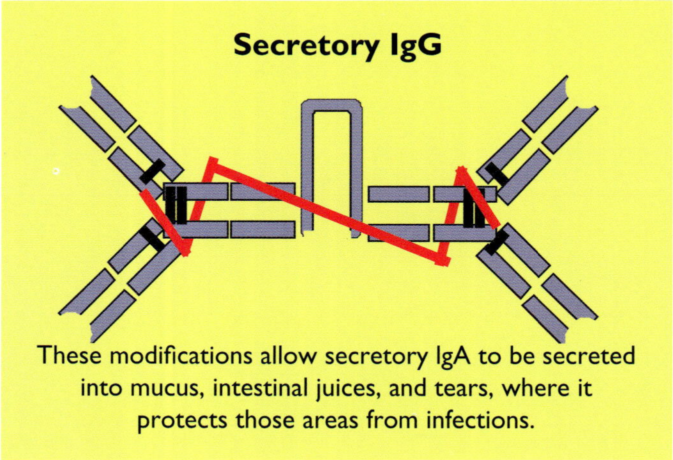

Note the presence of two "Y" elements and the presence of four antigen binding sites.

BOVINE IMMUNOGLOBULIN M (IgM)

In colostrum and milk IgM is present as secretory IgM

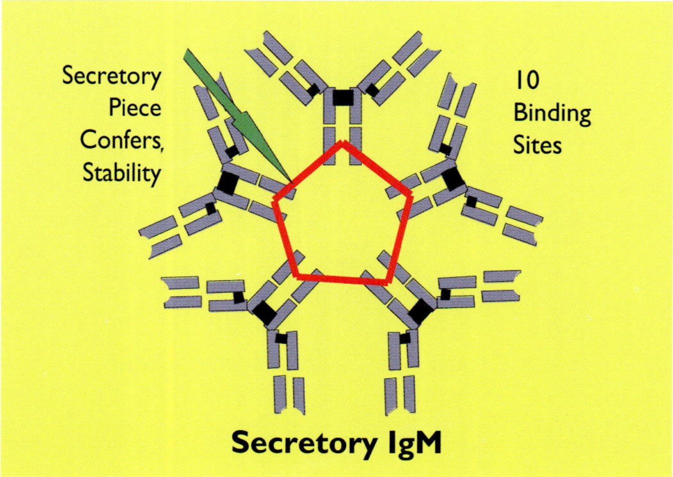

Note the presence of five "Y" elements and the presence of ten antigen binding sites.

COMPARISONS BETWEEN THE MAJOR IMMUNOGLOBULINS IN COLOSTRUM

IgG	sIgA	sIgM
▪ 45 mg/ml	▪ 5.5 mg/ml	▪ 6.9 mg/ml
▪ ~80%	▪ ~10–15%	▪ ~10–15%
▪ 150,000 Daltons	▪ 380,000 Daltons	▪ 980,000 Daltons
▪ 2 ABS	▪ 4 ABS	▪ 10 ABS
▪ Specific	▪ Specific & Non-specific	▪ Specific & Non-specific
▪ Blood, Tissue Fluids, Milk & Colostrum	▪ Mucous Fluids, Tissue Fluids, Milk & Colostrum	▪ Mucous Fluids, Tissue Fluids, Milk & Colostrum
▪ 90 ABP	▪ 22 ABP	▪ 69 ABP

Note how significant the Antigen Binding Potential (ABP) of sIgA and sIgM are in bovine colostrum.

Bovine Secretory Immunoglobulin A (sIgA)

The beneficial aspects of milk and colostrum in maintaining health and well-being are well established. In humans it has been shown that the incidence of common infections of the intestinal and respiratory systems is significantly reduced in breast-fed infants when compared to non-breast-fed infants. The protective effect of human milk has been attributed to its immunoglobulin content, primarily secretory IgA, whereas in most other animals it is primarily IgG. Other nonspecific factors have also been implicated, including lactoferrin and lysozyme. The pharmacological action of milk and colostrum lies in its ability to function as an antibacterial, anti-inflammatory, and antiviral agent. All these activities have been attributed to secretory IgA.

The IgA and IgM immunoglobulins present in bovine colostrum are of the secretory type—secretory IgA and secretory IgM. Though far more research has been conducted on secretory IgA because of its importance in human immunity, its counterpart, secretory IgM, most probably possesses similar bioactive properties.

Antibacterial/Antiviral Activity

In humans, secretory IgA is the predominant immunoglobulin in seromucosal secretions such as colostrum, milk, saliva, tears, nasal mucus, tracheobronchial secretions and genitourinary secretions. Structurally, secretory IgA consists of two monomeric IgA molecules linked by disulfide bonds to a joining chain (J-chain) and one molecule of secretory component. The main features distinguishing secretory IgA from the other immunoglobulins is that it functions predominantly in mucosal immunity and that the molecule is protected from proteolytic degradation by its association with secretory component. Secretory IgA can be regarded functionally as "antiseptic paint," providing a first line of defense that prevents infectious organisms from entering the body proper. It is probably most important early in life where it may limit the extent of infection and give the newborn's system time to mature.

Adherence to epithelial cells of mucous membranes is essential for viral infection and bacterial colonization. Secretory IgA functions to inhibit the adhesion of these pathogens, thus limiting disease. In addition, secretory IgA functions to neutralize the toxins and virulence factors from microbial pathogens by immunoagglutination. The leading cause of death for newborns in developing countries has been attributed to infantile diarrhea.[40] This is also true of domestic animals where scours (enteric dysentery) is the major cause of mortality in newborn calves.[41] The enterotoxic form of ***Escherichia coli*** is one of the pathogens most frequently associated with this disease state.[41,42,43,44] Secretory IgA has been shown to neutralize this toxin, as well as enterotoxins of ***Vibrio cholerae***, ***Shigella***, and ***Salmonella.***[45]

Anti-inflammatory Activity

Inflammation is a complex localized event in response to either injury, invasive foreign substance (pathogen) or in some instances to internally produced substances (such as in rheumatoid arthritis). This is a protective adaptation that serves to isolate, destroy, and rid the infected area of both the injurious agent and the injured tissue. Inflammation is characterized by an increase in vascular permeability and vasodilation with a subsequent migration of leukocytes into the inflamed area. Clinically, inflammation is associated with pain, swelling, tenderness, redness and general discomfort. Prostaglandins (PG) and leukotrines (LT) play an important role in mediating the process of inflammation by increasing histamine-mediated vascular permeability. It is predominantly this action that causes the discomfort associated with inflammation. The common anti-inflammatory analgesic and antipyretic drugs, such as corticosteroids, aspirin, and indomethacin, inhibit PG and or LT synthesis. In fact, most, if not all, of the anti-phlogistic actions of steroidal and non-steroidal anti-inflammatory drugs act by inhibiting prostaglandin synthesis. The anti-inflammatory effect of aspirin and indomethacin is inhibition of cyclooxygenase, whereas those of corticosteroids are thought to inhibit the release of fatty acids from phospholipids either by inhibition of phospholipase A2 or by interfering with the release of membrane phospholipids.

The adverse side effects associated with certain anti-inflammatory agents limit their use. In the case of natural and synthetic corticosteroids, the potential side effects include the elevation of blood pressure, water and salt retention, increased calcium and potassium excretion, gastric upset and possibly peptic ulceration. In addition, the use of these compounds may also aggravate diabetes mellitus. The non-steroidal anti-inflammatory compounds (salicylates) are synthetic biochemical substances, which can be toxic at high doses. The possible side effects associated with these substances include gastric upset and gastric bleeding, prolonged clotting time and liver damage. Though the number of various anti-inflammatory agents is great, so are the potential side effects and adverse reactions associated with these compounds. It has been shown by ***in vitro*** studies that the secretory component of secretory IgA inhibits phospholipase A2 activity and therefore prostaglandin and leukotrine synthesis by limiting the release of arachidonic acid.

This inhibition of prostaglandin and leukotrine synthesis thus gives supporting evidence that secretory component and secretory IgA possess anti-inflammatory properties. As was mentioned previously, it is most probable that secretory IgM possesses similar biological functions to secretory IgA.

Stability

An important consideration is the stability of antibodies in the digestive tract. In a study conducted to ascertain the stability of bovine immunoglobulins to proteolytic digestion, it was found that antibodies that possess specific activity can pass through the gastrointestinal tract of infants without being completely destroyed.[195] This indicates that the specific action of antibodies in the gastrointestinal tract is not adversely affected and that biological activity is retained. Secretory IgA and IgM have been shown to be more resistant to degradation and that the secretory piece is responsible for the added protection.

Immunoglobulin G (IgG)—The predominant antibody found in bovine colostrum, making up about 85% of the total immunoglobulins.[196] Human colostrum, as was mentioned, contains significantly less IgG and much more IgA due to the differences in human and cow placentas. IgG imparts systemic immunity. That is, it can induce immunity in one individual if taken from another individual who already has immunity to a certain pathogen. This is how a mother cow imparts her own immunity to her calf. It is also how the same immunity can be transferred from a cow to a human via colostrum.

There are four subclasses of IgG, known as IgG_1, IgG_2, IgG_3 and IgG_4.[197] While all function as antibodies, they differ in the types of antigens they protect against. IgG_1 and IgG_3 are predominantly antibodies against proteins found in bacterial toxins, such as those produced by diphtheria and tetanus bacteria, and viral proteins. IgG_2 is made up of antibodies against the polysaccharide (complex sugar) capsule of certain pathogenic bacteria, such as pneumococcus and ***Haemophilus influenzae***. IgG_4 is involved in repeated, long-term antigenic stimulation.[198]

A study by Borrisenko et al (page 291 of this book) exposed 19 different pathogenic bacteria and yeasts to a 15% IgG colostrum and were assayed using enzyme linked immunosorbent assay (ELISA). The Specific IgG Antibody Titers were then measured. The 19 bacteria were:

- ***Bacillus cereus***—food poisoning, mastitis
- ***Campylobacter jejuni***—food poisoning
- ***Candida albicans***—thrush, yeast infection
- ***Clostridium difficile***—food poisoning
- ***Escherichia coli***—commensal bacteria
- ***Escherichia coli* 0157:H7**—food poisoning
- ***Haemophilus influenzae***—bacterial meningitis, can be fatal
- ***Helicobacter pylori***—stomach ulcers
- ***Klebsiella pneumoniae***—pneumonia, urinary tract infection
- ***Listeria monocytogenes***—food poisoning, can be fatal
- ***Propionibacterium acnes***—acne
- ***Salmonella enteritidis***—food poisoning, can be fatal
- ***Salmonella typhimurium***—food poisoning, can be fatal
- ***Staphylococcus aureus***—pneumonia, osteomyelitis, carditis, meningitis, arthritis, toxic shock syndrome, antibiotic resistant—MRSA (methicillin-resistant *Staphylococcus aureus*)
- ***Staphylococcus epidermidis***—multiple antibiotic resistance (MAR)
- ***Streptococcus agalactiae***—mastitis, bacteremia, meningitis, pneumonia, can be fatal
- ***Streptococcus mutans***—periodontal disease, tooth decay, atherosclerosis, endocarditis
- ***Streptococcus pyogenes***—strep throat, flesh-eating bacteria, myositis, strep shock syndrome, rheumatic fever, kidney disease
- ***Yersinia enterocolitica***—food poisoning, septicemia, can be fatal

They found success in killing all 19 bacteria. It was also found that colostrum was better in killing these bacteria than milk hyperimmunized against the same 19 bacteria.

Immunoglobulin A (IgA)—This immunoglobulin is mainly involved with local immunity against pathogens. The type of IgA in colostrum is called secretory IgA (sIgA) because it has a protective protein attached to it to protect against digestive enzymes, to help the molecule pass through the intestinal lining, and to prevent the attachment of pathogens to mucosal surfaces in the gastrointestinal tract. Its main function in colostrum appears to be to prevent gastrointestinal infections.

Immunoglobulin M (IgM)—Basically five or six IgG molecules strung together in a circular arrangement, IgM is the first antibody produced in response to an antigen. While its function remains unclear, it is involved in aggregating antigens and reactions involving complement.[199,200,201]

Immunoglobulin E (IgE)—Involved in allergic responses to antigens. It binds to mast cells and basophils, specialized cells in the body that participate in allergic reactions. When an antigen comes into contact with IgE, the mast cell or basophil releases histamine and other chemicals which produce the allergic reaction.[202] Highly antiviral.

IgE Binding Factor (IgEbf)—This molecule binds to IgE to suppress its action and may provide the anti-allergic function of colostrum.[203]

Immunoglobulin D (IgD)—IgD acts as an antigen receptor on B cells. It is also highly antiviral.[204]

OTHER IMMUNE FACTORS

Complement

Technically part of the innate immune system, complement is triggered by the adaptive immune system to form part of the membrane attack complex that penetrates the cell membrane of pathogens and results in their destruction. Complement is composed of over twenty separate proteins and protein fragments.[205,206]

Lactoferrin

An antiviral, anti-bacterial, anti-inflammatory, iron-binding protein with therapeutic effects in cancer, HIV, Cytomegalovirus, herpes, chronic fatigue syndrome, ***Candida albicans***, and other infections. Lactoferrin helps deprive bacteria of the iron they require to reproduce and releases iron into the red blood cells enhancing oxygenation of tissues. Lactoferrin modulates cytokine release, and its receptors have been found on most immune cells including lymphocytes, monocytes, macrophages, and platelets.

Lactoferrin is a large iron-binding protein with a complex structure. It has a multitude of functions and is found in all mucus secretions of the body.[207] It is closely related to transferrin, a protein that transports iron in the body. It is an integral part of the innate immune system, a non-specific first line of defense against pathogens. Lactoferrin is a potent anti-microbial against bacteria, viruses,[208] fungi (such as ***Candida***),[209] and protozoan parasites (like ***giardia***).[210,211] It kills pathogens by withholding the iron they need to reproduce, blocking the attachment of pathogens to target cells,[212] binding to the outer membrane of microorganisms, causing them to lyse (burst), along with other effects. In addition, it is an essential growth factor for lymphocytes (immune blood cells),[213] stimulates the activity of polymorphonuclear leukocytes (white blood cells),[214] strongly promotes natural killer (NK) cell cytotoxic (cell killing) activity,[215,216] stimulates the production of various cytokines (chemicals that promote or inhibit the inflammatory response to infection)[217], and is a powerful antioxidant and anti-inflammatory[218]. It inhibits tryptase, an enzyme secreted by mast cells and which may be a causative agent for asthma[219]. In experimental animal models, lactoferrin has been shown to prevent cancer[220]. Lactoferrin has been shown to have an immunomodulatory effect on the immune system, controlling the release of cytokines and regulating the proliferation and differentiation of immune cells[221]. In addition, lactoferrin helps maintain iron homeostasis in the body, regulates bone metabolism, and is involved in reproductive function and embryonic development[222].

Lysozyme

An enzyme that is capable of degrading the outer membrane of gram-positive bacteria.[223] It also acts in concert with lactoferrin to kill gram-negative bacteria.[224] Lysozyme is also a hydrolyzing agent and immune system booster capable of destroying bacteria and viruses on contact.

Lactoperoxidase

Another enzyme which, in the presence of hydrogen peroxide (formed naturally in the body), catalyzes the oxidation of thiocyanate, a component of saliva, to form hypothiocyanate, which can kill both gram-positive[225] and gram-negative[226] bacteria.

Growth Factors

Colostrum, as might be expected, contains many growth factors.[227,228] Their presence in colostrum is primarily to complete the growth and development of the newborn gut, but in older children and adults they act to repair damage to the gut lining that might result in leaky gut syndrome as well as other health maintenance functions.[229,230] Their main function in the organism is to regulate the growth and development of cells.[231] They play a major role in wound healing and the repair of broken bones[232] as well as injured tendons and ligaments.[233] Growth factors, just like PRPs, are generally peptides that function as intercellular signaling molecules to turn on or turn off the production of specific proteins in the target cells.

The body's growth factors are capable of increasing T cell production, accelerating healing, balancing blood glucose, reducing insulin need, increasing growth, and repair of vital tissues while metabolizing fat for fuel. Medical studies have shown the vital growth factors IgF-1, TGF-α & β, and nucleotides from bovine colostrum to be identical to human in composition. They help provide the raw materials to repair vital DNA and RNA in the body's cells. By stimulating DNA formation, it has been shown that they can help stimulate normal cell and tissue growth, regeneration, and accelerated repair of aged or injured muscle, skin collagen, bone, cartilage, nerve tissues, heart muscle and new blood vessels for collateral coronary circulation. These growth factors facilitate the healing of tissues damaged by ulcers, trauma, burns, surgery, or inflammatory disease.

> "Transforming growth factors-α & β (TGF-α & β) in bovine colostrum were involved in normal cellular activities such as cell proliferation, and tissue repair. Also reported it promoted the synthesis and repair of DNA—the master code of the cell."
>
> – July 1992, New England Journal of Medicine

Colostrum provides a good source of IGF-1 as a complementary therapy for successful weight loss and building of lean muscle. IGF-1 is required by the body to metabolize fat for energy through the Krebs cycle, but with aging, less IGF-1 is produced in the body. It helps stimulate the body to burn fat for fuel instead of the body's own muscle tissue in times of diet and fasting.

> "High age is associated with reduced levels of growth hormones GH and IGF-1. Induction of GH and IGF-1 increase body weight through muscle growth of aged subjects"
>
> – Drs. Ullman, Sommerland and Skottner, Departments of Pathology and Pharmacology, University of Gothenburg, Sahlgren Hospital and HabiVitrum AB, Stockholm, Sweden

Human trials in 1990 reported that IGF-1 stimulates glucose utilization. It can help balance blood sugars (non-insulin diabetics and hypoglycemia). Inadequate levels of IGF-1 are associated with an increased incidence of Type 2 diabetes and difficulty in losing weight despite a proper nutritional intake and adequate exercise. Additionally, IGF-1 and GH in colostrum normalize LDL cholesterol while increasing HDL cholesterol concentrations (the good cholesterol).

Genetically engineered versions of IGF-1 and GH are now marketed, but they are found in high concentrations in colostrum. Biotechnology companies are currently selling IGF-1 for as much as $800 per 50 cc vial. GH is also very expensive. Even less expensive products marketed as growth hormone releasers (designed to help the body to manufacture their own hGH) are markedly more expensive than colostrum. None of these expensive products contain any of the vast array of immune factors in colostrum.

Colony-stimulating Factor-1 (macrophage colony-stimulating factor)—A growth factor that stimulates stem cells in the marrow to differentiate into macrophages, phagocytic ("eating") cells that enter the connective tissue in order to clean up dead pathogens and other debris from infections.[234]

Epidermal Growth Factor (EGF)—Stimulates the proliferation and differentiation of epidermal cells, including the lining cells of the gut that maintain the gut integrity and the proper permeability.[235,236] It exerts its effects by binding to the EGF receptor protein in the cell membrane of the target cell.[237] It has been used to promote wound healing by stimulating cell proliferation in the wound.[238]

Betacellulin—A member of the EGF family of growth factors, the function of betacellulin remains unclear, but it appears to play a role in the growth and development of the neonatal gastrointestinal tract.[239,240]

Fibroblast Growth Factor (FGF)—Fibroblasts are the cells in the connective tissue that help to promote wound healing by stimulating cell proliferation in the wound. It also helps maintain normal bone and repair fractures.[241,242] It also plays a role in the healing of ulcers.[243]

Granulocyte Colony-stimulating Factor (G-CSF)—Increases growth, differentiation and activation of granulocytes (eosinophils, basophils, neutrophils).[244]

Insulin-like Growth Factor 1 (IGF-1)[245]—Originally known as somatomedin C. It is very similar in structure to insulin. IGF-1 affects nearly every cell in the body, in particular muscle cells, cartilage, bone, liver, kidney, nerves, skin and lungs.[246] It regulates cell growth and development as well as cellular DNA synthesis. Studies have shown that both TGF-β and IGF-1 speed the healing of bones, which is particularly important in the elderly whose bones heal very slowly.[247] IGF-1 also is responsible for increasing muscle mass in response to muscle overloading.[248] Both IGF-1 and IGF-2 promote the growth of arterial cells, and disruption of the dynamic balance between IGF-1, IGF-2 and IGF binding proteins has been implicated in the formation of atherosclerotic plaques in the arteries and resulting restenosis (narrowing of the artery).[249] IGF-1 has also shown promise in peripheral nerve regeneration.[250] In the newborn, IGF-1 plays a critical role in the development of the newborn gut.[251]

Insulin-like Growth Factor (IGF-2)—Very similar in function to IGF-1. Its major function is to promote growth during fetal development.[252]

Insulin—Insulin is also present in bovine colostrum, starting out at high levels (327 µg/l in first milking colostrum) and tapering off thereafter.[253] While the exact role of insulin in colostrum is unclear, it is known that insulin receptors are found in the membranes of intestinal epithelial cells,[254] indicating it may act as a growth hormone.

Insulin-like Growth Factor Binding Proteins (IGFBP)—Proteins which bind to IGF-1 and IGF-2.[255] An important part of the IGF axis that forms a dynamic balance to regulate the activity of IGF in the body.[256] IGFBP-3 is the most common form of IGFBP in bovine colostrum and milk.

Platelet-derived Growth Factor[257]—Plays a role in bone metabolism as a mitogen (stimulator of cell division) for osteoblasts.[258] It is important in angiogenesis (the formation of blood vessels).[259] It also stimulates fibroblast division in wound healing[260] and the healing of ulcers.[261] Its role in tissue modeling involves both the stimulation of growth as well as apoptosis (programmed cell death).[262,263]

Transforming Growth Factor-alpha (TGF-α)—Induces epithelial development[264,265,266,267] and stimulates neural development in the injured brain.[268] It is closely related to EGF.

Transforming Growth Factor-beta (TGF-β)—Has three isoforms, TGF-β1, TGF-β2 and TGF-β3.[269,270,271,272] Only TGF-β1 and β2 are found in human and bovine milk and colostrum. TGF-β controls cellular proliferation and differentiation.[273] It stimulates the production of IgA by B lymphocytes.[274,275] It is particularly important in the development of cartilage and bone.[276,277]

Vascular Endothelial Growth Factor (VEGF)[278]—a member of the PGDF family, VEGF plays a role in the healing of injuries and wounds, such as ligament and tendon injuries, by providing blood supply to damaged areas.[279]

Lactalbumin

Research indicates that lactalbumins may be highly effective against numerous forms of cancer and viruses. Colostral lactalbumin has been found to be able to cause the selective death (apoptosis) of cancer cells, leaving the surrounding non-cancerous tissues unaffected.

Lactobacillus, Bifidus, Acidophilus

Friendly flora, which are necessary for the digestion of food and in the reduction of the growth of harmful bacterial in the digestive system. They have been shown to effectively combat ***Candida albicans***.

Vitamins and Minerals

Colostrum is not a supplement; it is whole food for the newborn. Its combination of vitamins and minerals are naturally occurring and in perfect combination. Vitamins A, B_{12}, and E are found in small amounts, while traces of all others are also present in colostrum.

Sulfur

A mineral with multiple uses in metabolism and as part of many structural body proteins.

Enzymes

Lactoperoxidase-thiocyanate, peroxidase and xanthine oxidase oxidize bacteria through their ability to release hydrogen peroxide.

Trypsin Inhibitors and Protease Inhibitors

Prevent the destruction of immune and growth factors in colostrum from being broken down in the GI tract. They also prevent ***H. pylori*** from attaching to the walls of the stomach and can have a beneficial role in the treatment of peptic ulcers.

Lymphokines

Hormone-like peptides produced by activated lymphocytes which mediate the immune response.

Oligopolysaccharides and Glycoconjugates

Attract and bind to pathogens, such as ***Streptococchus, E. coli, Salmonella, Cryptosporidia, Giardia, Entamoeba, Shigella, Clostridium difficile*** toxins A & B and cholera, preventing them from attaching or entering the mucous membranes.

Orotic Acid

Stops the formation of pyrimidine nucleotides and prevents hemolytic anemia.

Neurotransmitters

Endogenous signaling molecules such as leptin that alter the behavior of neurons or effector cells. Neurotransmitter is used here in its most general sense, including not only messengers that act directly to regulate ion channels, but also those that act through second messenger systems and those that act at a distance from their site of release. Included are neuromodulators, neuroregulators, neuromediators, and neurohumors, whether or not acting at synapses.

Cytokines

Cytokines are also small peptides that exert either a pro- or anti-inflammatory effect on the immune system. Colostrum is known to stimulate the production of cytokines in peripheral blood cells.[280] Cytokines found in colostrum include interleukin-1 (IL-1),[281] IL-1β,[282] IL-1ra,[283] IL-3, IL-4,[284] IL-5,[285] IL-6,[286] IL-8,[287] IL-10,[288] IL-12,[289] IL-13, IL-16, IL-18,[290] interferon-gamma (INF-γ),[291] tumor necrosis factor-alpha (TNF-α),[292] and TNF-α receptors.[293]

IL-1—pro-inflammatory, can induce fever in large amounts

IL-1β—pro-inflammatory, similar in action to IL-1

IL-1ra—IL-1 receptor antagonist, a protein that binds to IL-1, inhibiting its action and producing an anti-inflammatory effect

IL-2— was the first interleukin molecule to be discovered, that is instrmental in the body's natural response to microbial infection and in discriminating between foreign (non-self) and self.

IL-3—pro-inflammatory, growth and differentiation of granulocytes and red blood cells, growth of mast cells and release of histamine

IL-4—anti-inflammatory, proliferation and differentiation of B cells, proliferation of T cells, plays important role in allergic response with IgE

IL-5—production of eosinophils, differentiation of B cells and production of IgA by B cells

IL-6—differentiation of B cells into plasma cells, antibody secretion by plasma cells, differentiation and acute phase reaction of T cells, differentition of stem cells. Pro-inflammatory cytokine involved in the production of C-reactive protein (CRP).

IL-8—actually a chemokine, neutrophil chemotaxis (movement of neutrophils to site of inflammation)

IL-10—anti-inflammatory, activates B cells, cytokine production by ma-rophages, inhibits Th1 response, stimulates Th2 response (see Appendix 1)

IL-12—pro-inflammatory, differentiation into cytotoxic T cells, increased TNF-γ and INF-γ, decreased IL-10

IL-13—anti-inflammatory, stimulates growth and differentiation of B cells, inhibits Th1 and production of macrophage inflammatory cytokines, decreased IL-8, IL-10, IL-12

IL-16—anti-inflammatory, CD4+ lymphocyte chemoattractant

IL-18—pro-inflammatory, induces production of IFN-γ, increases NK cell activity

TNF-α—pro-inflammatory, the controlling cytokine for the entire inflammatory cascade

TNF-α receptors—anti-inflammatory, proteins which bind to TNF-α, inhibiting it

Osteopontin—a member of the tumor necrosis family of cytokines that is expressed at high levels in both human and bovine colostrum and milk;[294,295] vital to cell-mediated immunity[296] and may activate T lymphocytes

Osteoprotegerin—another member of the tumor necrosis family of cytokines, osteoprotegerin inhibits osteoclast ("bone-eating") differentiation, preventing bone destruction; also induces apoptosis (programmed cell death) in T lymphocytes to inhibit their proliferation; may help prevent immune and bone disorders in the newborn[297]

INF-γ—inhibits proliferation of certain cell types, immunomodulatory, required for the proliferation of IL-2 receptors on T lymphocytes, inhibits proliferation of B cells stimulated by IL-4

Cytokines are any of several regulatory proteins, such as the interleukins and lymphokines, that are released by cells of the immune system and act as intercellular mediators in the generation of an immune response. Cytokines are produced in the human body by the actions of PRPs. Two main cytokines that are produced by PRPs are IFN-α and IFN-β. The function and applications of just these two cytokines are described below. Cytokines IL-1, -6, interferon-γ, and lymphokines stimulate the lymph glands and are thought to be highly effective antiviral immune substances. Interleukins that regulate the duration and intensity of the immune response are responsible for cell-to-cell communication and boost T cell activity and the production of immunoglobulins. Interleukin-10 is strongly anti-inflammatory, especially in arthritic joints.

The benefits of cytokines in the treatment of cancer was first popularized by the 1985 Steven Rosenberg Book, ***Quiet Strides in the War on Cancer***. Since that time, the same cytokines found in colostrum (IL-1, 6, 10, interferon-γ, leukocytes, lymphokines, tumor necrosis factor) have been the most researched protocols in scientific research for the cure for cancer.

The term cytokine, or immunocytokines, was used initially to separate a group of immunomodulatory proteins, also called immunotransmitters, from other growth factors that modulate the proliferation and bioactivities of non-immune cells. However, this terminology suggesting a clear-cut distinction cannot be maintained and may not be altogether meaningful. Some cytokines are produced by a rather limited number of different cell types while others are produced by almost the entire spectrum of known cell types.

Today the term cytokine is used as a generic name for a diverse group of soluble proteins and peptides that act as humoral regulators at nano to picomolar concentrations and that, either under normal or pathological conditions, modulate the functional activities of individual cells and tissues. These proteins also mediate interactions between cells directly and regulate processes taking place in the extracellular environment (for some mechanistic concepts underlying cytokine actions see also: autocrine, paracrine, juxtacrine, retrocrine). Many growth factors and cytokines act as cellular survival factors by preventing programmed cell death.

Chemokines

Small pro-inflammatory cytokines that act primarily as chemoattractants to draw immune cells to the site of infection and activators of specific types of white blood cells. Chemokines found in milk and colostrum include CXLC 1-7 (chemokine ligands),[298] eotaxin (chemoattractant for eosinophils),[299] GRO-alpha (Growth-Related Oncogene, also called CXLC1; activates neutrophils, chemotactic for neutrophils),[300] IP-10 (may contribute to migration of intestinal T lymphocytes to enhance mucosal immunity),[301] MCP-1 (Monocyte Chemoattractant Protein; monocyte chemotaxis),[302] MIG (Monokine Induced by interferon Gamma, also called CXC chemokine ligand 9; chemotactic for tumor infiltrating lymphocytes),[303] and RANTES (Regulated upon Action, Normal T cell Expressed, also called CCL5; chemotaxis of T cells, eosinophils and monocytes).[304]

Proline-rich Polypeptides (PRPs)

Peptides are short chains of amino acids—the building blocks of proteins—without the complex tertiary structure of proteins. Proline-rich Polypeptides, so-called because they contain an unusually high proportion of the amino acid proline, are intercellular signaling molecules that have the unique ability to modulate the immune system, turning it up when needed to fight an infection, or turning it down when it is overactive, such as is the case in autoimmune disorders.

Proline-rich Polypeptides (PRPs) function as a hormone that regulates the thymus gland (the body's central command for the immune system, and the gland responsible for the normal development of immunologic function in the body), stimulating an underactive immune system or down regulating an overactive immune system as seen in autoimmune disease (MS, rheumatoid arthritis, lupus, scleroderma, chronic fatigue syndrome, allergies, etc.). They have been shown to improve or eliminate symptoms of both allergies and autoimmune conditions. PRPs inhibit the overproduction of lymphocytes and T cells and reduce the major symptoms of allergies and autoimmune disease: pain, swelling, and inflammation.

> "PRP, in bovine colostrum, has the same ability to regulate activity of the immune system as hormones of the thymus gland. It activates an underactive immune system, helping it move into action against disease-causing organisms. PRP also suppresses an overactive immune system, such as is often seen in the autoimmune conditions. PRP is highly anti-inflammatory and also appears to act on T-cell precursors to produce helper T cells and suppresser T cells"
>
> – Drs. Staroscik et al, Molecular Immunology[305]

> "PRP turns white blood cells into functionally active T cells. Results were shown in treatment of autoimmune disorders and cancer. An important immune modulator stimulates an underactive immune system and tones down an overactive one"
>
> – Drs. Janusz & Lisowsk,; Archives of Immunology[306]

We will explore PRPs in much greater detail later in this book.

Defensins

Polypeptides that disrupt bacterial cell membranes, such as pertussis,[307] killing them.[308]

Soluble CD14

CD14 is a membrane-bound pattern recognition protein found on monocytes and expressed mainly by macrophages and, to a lesser extent, neutrophil granules. It acts as a co-receptor with toll-like receptor 4 (TLR 4) to detect bacterial lipopolysaccharide in the presence of lipopolysaccharide-binding protein as well as other pathogen associated molecules. CD14 is found in a soluble form in colostrum and milk where it acts to directly induce B cell growth and differentiation, thus enhancing IgG secretion.[309]

Toll-like Receptors

Pattern recognition detectors that help the immune system recognize new pathogens.[310,311]

Cathelicidin-derived Antimicrobial Peptide

Certain peptides of the cathelicidin family of peptides found in milk and colostrum have antimicrobial activity against both gram-positive and gram-negative bacteria.[312] They have been found to be particularly effective against antibiotic resistant opportunistic pathogens found in AIDS and cystic fibrosis patients, including ***Pseudomonas aeruginosa, Burkholderia cepacia, Stentrophomonas maltophilia,*** and *Achromobacter xylosoxidans*.

Glycoproteins

Colostrum contains a number of complex carbohydrates, including glycoproteins, glycolipids, glycosaminoglycans, mucins, and oligosaccharides, which are basically complex sugars either alone or in combination with proteins or lipids (fats). They are known to inhibit pathogen binding to gut lining cells, preventing their entry into the bloodstream, usually by competing for binding sites on the cell membranes. One fucosyloligosaccharide inhibits ***E. coli*** toxin. Another inhibits ***Campylobacter jejuni***, which is a major cause of gastroenteritis and food poisoning. Oligosaccharides inhibit the binding of ***Streptococcus pneumoniae,*** which causes many infections such as pneumonia, meningitis, otitis, osteomyelitis, peritonitis and endocarditis, and enteropathogenic ***E. coli***, which causes diarrhea. A mannosylated (mannose is a type of sugar) glycopeptide inhibits the binding of enterohemorrhagic ***E. coli***, which causes bloody diarrhea. One of the glycosaminoglycans prevents the binding of HIV structural protein to CD4+ cells (T cells), which is the first step in HIV infection. Mucin, found in milk and colostrum, inhibits the binding of S-fimbriated ***E. coli*** (fimbriae are thread-like structures used by certain bacteria to adhere to cells). Ganglioside GM1, a membrane protein, reduces diarrhea due to cholera toxin and ***E. coli*** labile toxin. Glycosphingolipid Gb3, another membrane protein, binds to shiga toxin, a toxin produced by ***Shigella dysenteriae*** (cause of dysentery) and the shigatoxigenic group of ***E. coli***. Shiga toxin functions much like the deadly toxin ricin by inhibiting protein synthesis in target cells.[313]

Kappa-caseino Glycomacropeptide

This is a peptide from the casein fraction of milk and colostrum that interferes with the binding of viruses and bacteria in the intestine, binds cholera and ***E. coli*** toxins, promotes the growth of beneficial bacteria in the gut, and helps modulate the immune system.[314,315,316]

Fatty Acid Binding Protein

A member of the lipocalin family of secreted proteins, fatty acid binding protein regulates two molecular pathways in macrophages that coordinate inflammatory activity and cholesterol uptake.[317]

β-lactoglobulin

Another member of the lipocalin family of proteins, β-lactoglobulin has antimicrobial and antiviral activity.[318,319]

Orosomucoids

Increased levels of this glycoprotein are associated with inflammation. It acts as an anti-inflammatory mediator, particularly in the endothelium of capillaries where it inhibits the effect of histamine.[320,321]

Clusterin (Apolipoprotein J)

Clusterin plays an important role in cell-cell and cell-substratum interactions.[322] It also acts as an extracellular molecular "chaperone" that "steers" proteins into cells.[323]

Haemopexin

A transporter and binder of free haeme (iron) molecules.[324] It has an antioxidant function by preventing the participation of haeme in oxygen radical reactions in tissues.[325,326] It also plays a key role in the homeostasis of nitric oxide. It is also known to suppress tumor growth. The haeme-haemopexin complex supports and stimulates the proliferation of T lymphoblasts (lymphocyte stem cells).[327] It has an anti-inflammatory effect by suppressing neutrophil accumulation and phagocytosis[328] and by inhibiting the magnesium-dependent adhesion of polymorphonuclear leukocytes (white blood cells).[329] Its anti-inflammatory activity could be of use in autoimmune disorders.

Haptoglobin

A protein binder of free hemoglobin. Binding free hemoglobin prevents hemoglobin-induced oxidative damage to healthy tissue, so haptoglobin is in effect an antioxidant. Levels of haptoglobin are increased in acute phase inflammation where they act to selectively suppress monocyte production of pro-inflammatory cytokines TNF-α, IL-10, and IL-12 while not inhibiting IL-6, IL-8, or IL-1 receptor antagonist. This is thought to selectively dampen the inflammatory effects of lipopolysaccharide (a component of bacterial cell walls that acts as an endotoxin), probably to modulate cytokine release and protect against endotoxin damage to tissues.[330]

Sporozite Inhibitory Lipid (SIL)

A new addition to the list of immune components in bovine colostrum is sporozite inhibitory lipid (SIL). This is a lipid that inhibits the adhesion of ***Cryptosporidium parvum*** sporozites to host cells, preventing infection. SIL has been identified as oleic acid, a monosaturated fatty acid likely released from colostrum triglycerides and phospholipids by digestion in the small intestine. A related lipid, linolenic acid, also displays potent inhibitory activity.[331]

Nucleotides

Dietary nucleotides, the building blocks of DNA and RNA, enhance dietary growth and maturation as well as humoral and cellular immunity.[332] Infants who receive human milk with nucleotides have higher antibody levels, lower rates of diarrhea, and higher natural killer cell activity.[333,334]

Hormones

Colostrum includes a number of hormones. Their presence in colostrum is somewhat problematic as it is often unclear if they act upon the infant or are artifacts of lactation. Hormones identified in colostrum include:

EPO (Erythropoietin)—stimulates red blood cell production.[335]

Estrogen—The "female" hormone is found in bovine milk. It appears to be an artifact of maternal serum.[336]

Gonadotropin-releasing Hormone (GnRH)—A hypothalamic hormone that stimulates the release of gonadotropin, a hormone that promotes gonadal growth and development.[337,338] It is believed that GnRH is an artifact from maternal serum.

Growth Hormone—Also known as somatotropin. A pituitary hormone that promotes body growth, fat mobilization and inhibition of glucose utilization.[339]

Insulin—In addition to the activity already mentioned above, insulin promotes glucose utilization, protein synthesis and storage.[340]

Leptin—Secreted by fatty tissues, acts to curb appetite and increase energy expenditure as body fat stores increase.[341]

Luteinizing Hormone-releasing Hormone (LHRH)—a hypothalamic hormone that stimulates the release of luteinizing hormone.[342] Another artifact from maternal serum.

Melatonin—Produced by the pineal gland, controls circadian rhythms.[343]

Procalcitonin/Calcitonin/Thyrotropin—Produced by the parathyroid, thyroid and thymus glands. Increases the deposit of calcium and phosphate in bone and lowers their levels in blood.[344]

Progesterone—The "pregnancy hormone" that prepares the corpus luteum of the uterus and the placenta for pregnancy[345]. An artifact of maternal serum.

Prolactin—Pituitary hormone that stimulates the production of milk in the mother. Artifact of maternal serum.[346]

Relaxin—A peptide hormone that aids delivery.[347] Artifact of maternal serum.

Somatostatin—Inhibits the release of somatotropin and the release of insulin and gastrin.[348]

Thyrotropin-releasing Hormone (TRH)—hypothalamic hormone that stimulates the release of luteinizing hormone.[349] Artifact of maternal serum.

Cardiovascular Health

A number of components of colostrum are important to cardiovascular health, including ACE inhibitors that help regulate blood pressure, and clotting factors.

ACE (Angiotensin-I Converting Enzyme) Inhibitors and Competitive Substrates

Bradykinin—vasodilatory peptide activated by ACE[350]
Enkephalins—endorphin-like peptides found throughout the body, natural pain killer, antidepressant, and immune modulator
Substance P—a neurotransmitter and potent vasodilator and secretagogue (agent that promotes secretion)
Casokinins—casein-derived ACE-inhibitors[351]
Lactokinins—whey-derived ACE inhibitors[352]
α-lactorphin[353]—antihypertensive milk peptide

Thrombospondin—Extracellular proteins involved in cell-to-cell and cell-to-matrix communication, including cell adhesion, platelet aggregation, cell proliferation, and tissue repair; potent inhibitors of angiogenesis and tumor growth; interact with coagulation and anticoagulant factors in blood.[354,355,356]

Kappa-caseino glycomacropeptide—In addition to the functions given above, this component of colostrum helps prevent the formation of arterial thrombi (blood clots), a leading cause of heart attack and stroke.[357]

κ-caseinoglycopeptide—A peptide produced by digestion of kappa-casein, found in both bovine and human colostrum and milk, which is absorbed into the blood serum and which has antithrombic properties, preventing platelet aggregation.[358,359]

α_2-macroglobulin—Inhibits thrombin and other proteases.[360,361]

α_2-antiplasmin—Thrombin inhibitor, fibrinolysis inhibitor.[362,363]

Antithrombin III—Inhibits thrombin (coagulation protein).[364,365]

Apelin—First identified as a ligand for the APJ-receptor;[366] functions as a mediator of cardiovascular control, including blood pressure and blood flow; the most potent stimulator of cardiac contractility known;[367] important in maintaining fluid homeostasis.[368]

Digestive Enzymes and Proteins

Colostrum contains proteins that inhibit the action of digestive enzymes, allowing the contents of colostrum to reach their targets without significant degradation.[369] Protease inhibitors also facilitate the passage of macromolecules through the gut lining, which is important in the newborn.[370] Colostrum also contains various enzymes that help the components of colostrum do their job. Enzymes basically function to facilitate chemical reactions in the body.

Protease Inhibitors[371]

C1-inhibitor—inhibits C1 protease, a digestive enzyme
Chymotrypsin inhibitor—inhibits chymotrypsin, a digestive enzyme[372,373]
Elastase inhibitor—inhibits elastase, a digestive enzyme[374]
Inter-α-trypsin inhibitor—inhibits inter-α-trypsin, a digestive enzyme
Trypsin inhibitor—inhibits α_1-trypsin, a digestive enzyme[375,376,377]

Of the enzymes found in colostrum, some of the more interesting are matrix metalloproteinases, which are zinc-dependent endopeptidases.[378] There are two found in human colostrum, matrix metalloproteinase-2 (MMP-2) and tissue inhibitor of metalloproteinase-4 (TIMP-1). Matrix metalloproteinases degrade extracellular matrix proteins and are important in tissue remodeling, cell proliferation, migration and differentiation, angiogenesis, apoptosis and host defense. They are widespread in both the animal and plant kingdoms. A good example of their function is the metamorphosis of a tadpole (with a tail) to a mature frog (no tail).

Fats

Although normally defatted when converted into a powder, whole colostrum also contains fats, including phospholipids, fatty acids (linoleic acid, dihomo-gamma-linoleic acid, alpha-linoleic acid, octadecatetraenoic acid, eicosatrienoic acid, docosahexaenoic acid, docosapentaenoic acid, and arachidonic acid), saposins (A, B, C, D), prosaposin, tocopherols, and cholesterol.[379,380,381] These are necessary nutrients for the newborn, while in the adult, milk fat in whole milk is believed to be beneficial to the regulation of blood sugar levels and appetite.[382]

This is only a partial listing of the components of colostrum, as was stated. There are also abundant nutritional components as colostrum supplies all of the newborn's nutritional needs until transitional and mature milk begin to flow. These include vitamins, minerals, essential fats, and bulk proteins, such as albumin. There are also components that aid the digestion and absorption of the nutrients as well as contribute to the maturation of the gastrointestinal tract of the newborn. Additionally, there are beneficial bacteria that help seed the newborn's gastrointestinal tract with the flora that will help keep it healthy.

Another thing that may be noted from reading through these components is that very often one finds both stimulatory and inhibitory components, for example, MMP and TIMP, which inhibits MMP. This illustrates the fact that the processes of the body are always in a state of dynamic balance. As soon as the balance is disrupted, the body acts to bring it back into equilibrium. Most enzymes, such as MMP-2 and TIMP-1, as well as other proteins exist in a "turned off" state until activated.

Drug manufacturers have tried to copy (genetically engineer) and market several of the individual components of colostrum, most notably interferon, gammaglobulin, growth hormone, IGF-1, and protease inhibitors. Some of the following colostrum components may very well be next on the list of major breakthroughs by the pharmaceutical/ nutraceutical industry: Immunoglobulins (A, D, E, G, and M) are the most abundant of the immune factors found in colostrum. IgG neutralizes toxins and microbes in the lymph and circulatory system, IgM destroys bacteria, while IgE and IgD are highly antiviral.

It is important to note that some of the components listed have thus far only been identified in human colostrum and milk, or that of other species than cows. They are included on the assumption that the colostrum from different mammalian species is essentially the same. This has generally proven to be the case. Bovine colostrum has been shown to be essentially bioidentical to human colostrum, the major difference being in the relative amounts of some components, such as IgG and IgA.

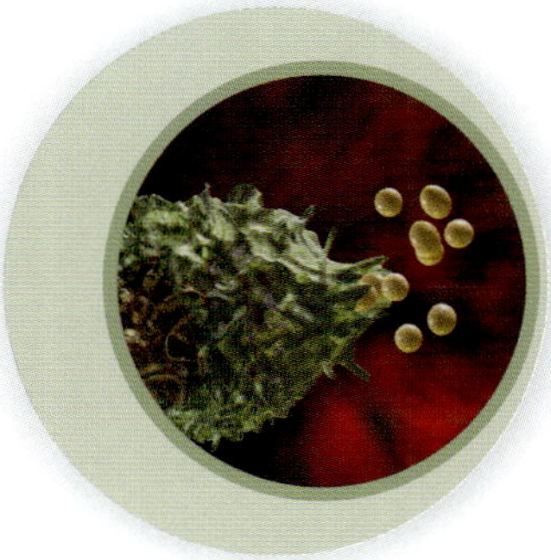

CHAPTER 7

YES, BUT DOES IT WORK?

Colostrum does indeed contain many amazing components, but the bottom line is, does it actually work? Let's look at what actual users and professionals have to say about colostrum.

GUT HEALTH

Colitis

I was diagnosed with colitis 1½ years ago. None of the medications helped me. Several made me worse. High doses of prednisone helped, but symptoms would worsen when trying to reduce dosage. I took 6–8 Imodium daily, and water ran straight through me. I could barely eat for almost a year. I began searching for help on the Internet when none of the medications would work. I read about colostrum and decided to try it. I saw immediate results when I started taking it. It made me feel bad, so I dropped the dosage to two pills every other day for several months. I wouldn't stop taking it even though it made me feel bad because it was drastically reducing my diarrhea. I still had to watch my diet for about 6 months, and I gradually got better. I eventually also started taking multi-enzyme pills that really helped with my stomach cramps. I can't say that I know it cured me, but it definitely helped. I also completely changed my lifestyle and reduced stress in my life by working at home. I really had no choice. I couldn't leave the house too long at a time and sure couldn't eat. I feel that a combination of things has completely cured me: the power of God, stress reduction, my diet and colostrum. I would definitely recommend anyone trying it that has colitis or any other illness. I eat a full normal diet—even pizza and milk! I am fat and sassy once again!

– Dianne B., Houston, Texas

Ulcerative Colitis

Approximately two years ago my then eleven-year-old son was diagnosed and then hospitalized with severe ulcerative colitis. His weight dropped dramatically down to 56 pounds (he was then 4'10") and nothing helped until, after a month and only days away from losing his entire colon, they tried a very powerful experimental drug on him, one that shut down his immune system. That, along with prednisone (a steroid), allowed him to be released from the hospital and begin to recover and lead a fairly normal life. However, after six months, now off the prednisone and on a milder version of the immune suppressant drug, he stopped gaining weight, was still 4'10" and some of his symptoms had returned. Afraid that we were going to have to go back on the steroids (which gave him a big, puffy face—tough for a middle schooler) and higher doses of Purinethol (mercaptopurine), we began to search for more natural, alternative cures.

We discovered colostrum through a doctor friend in the Midwest. He advised Sean to take two capsules before breakfast and two at bedtime. Within weeks we saw an amazing change in our son. He began gaining weight, getting stronger, and he even seemed to be growing faster! He has now been taking colostrum for about a year now. He weighs 100 pounds, is 5'4" and is the pitcher on his baseball team. In other words, he is the picture of health! He leads a totally normal life and amazes his doctor here at UCLA who calls his recovery nothing short of a "miracle." We know that colostrum has made all the difference—and given us back a happy, healthy now thirteen-year-old son. We are forever grateful for your product.

– Jean L., Westlake Village, California

Irritable Bowel Syndrome

Two years ago I received massive antibiotic treatments for **H. pylori** *(ulcers), which cured my stomach pain but devastated my intestinal tract! I had chronic intestinal pain, cramping, diarrhea, indigestion and could no longer tolerate many of the foods*

I used to enjoy. Eventually I was diagnosed with Irritable Bowel Syndrome after losing 20 pounds, and I was miserable. Four months ago I began taking colostrum with probiotics and began to exercise. I now feel better than I've felt in years. I have regained 15 pounds (mostly muscle), and my IBS symptoms have improved dramatically! I wholeheartedly recommend colostrum for IBS sufferers.

– John Q., Lodi, California

IMMUNE SYSTEM

Colds and Flu

Last winter I think I had every flu bug and virus that came around. I was on one after another type of antibiotics, trying to shake what was bound to get the best of me. I had acute sinus problems, the inside of my mouth broke out in blisters, as did my throat. My ears ached and popped constantly. The worst part was the chronic fatigue and general feeling that I was going downhill fast and nothing seemed to help. I also had a serious case of acid reflux and terrible heartburn. Wow, I was a mess! I went to the local health supplement store to purchase another supplement and brought home some literature on colostrum. After reading the literature, I decided to try it...what the heck, nothing to lose, right?

That was about three weeks ago. I started taking the colostrum faithfully. My sinus problems, blisters in the mouth and throat and ear popping and aching have stopped. The acid reflux and heartburn have stopped, and the intestinal problems have stopped. What can I say except thank God I read that literature and started taking colostrum!

– Shari R., Libby, Montana

Staph Infection

It was July 4th of 2002 when a friend called me, and during the conversation she began talking as if she was drunk. Because I know of her commitment to a health lifestyle, I knew this was out of character. She told me that she hadn't been drinking or taken any medication but that she did have a staph infection. This lady is the victim of mercury poisoning which severely compromises her immune system and means that any sign of infection must be met with aggressive measures. However, her adherence to natural health principles and her experience has led her to be adamantly opposed to antibiotic therapy. She didn't respond adequately and immediately to the presence of the staph infection and instead kept her appointment for an out-of-town trip. By the time she returned home, the staph infection had gone out of control. An alternative-minded medical doctor told her that the symptoms warranted an immediate trip to the emergency room and intravenous antibiotics. She refused!

Had I known the danger of staph infection or that her "drunkenness" was evidence of blood poisoning that had reached the nervous system and brain, I probably would not have had the courage to do what I did next. (Ignorance truly is bliss!) I told her I would be right over with the intention of trying to persuade her to go to the emergency room even though I too can't tolerate antibiotic therapy. The cure is never worth the suffering that ensues. Before leaving the house I asked God what I should do. As clearly as you would speak to me, I heard, "take your colostrum," so I grabbed it and ran out the door. Upon arriving, her drunken state had increased, but initial appeals to go to the emergency room were rejected. I went to her kitchen and began mixing five heaping tablespoons of powdered colostrum, which may have equaled closer to ten tablespoons if measured accurately. I sat with her anxiously waiting to see if there was any improvement and using the time to negotiate "Plan B" with her, watching for signs of progress or deterioration. One hour and forty-five minutes later she turned the corner and slowly began to come out of the drunkenness. Two hours later she had returned to normal, and I was able to go home. I strongly encouraged her to go to an alternative doctor in town the next day for an intravenous ultraviolet light treatment, which is beyond conventional antibiotics in effectiveness without the harmful side effects, and she agreed.

From that moment on, if I read any information that attempts to question the health benefits of colostrum, I just have to laugh. There's no way I would believe that a product that can pull a person out of a septic condition could also be responsible for producing harm. Several RNs have responded in awe when I've told them this story and shared the horror of what it means to be septic. Again, I say that I'm thankful I didn't know so I would have the courage to see this miraculous event.

Thank you for making such a wonderful product!

– Kathy B., Austin, Texas

Fever of Unknown Origin

For approximately two years we had been taking our daughter to Children's Hospital to find out what was wrong with her. She was coming down with a fever of 102.8–103.6°F every 4–5 weeks without fail! No doctor could find out what was wrong. She would get so ill at times that she had to take antibiotics to get over the infection. She missed so much school because of her illness that the school spoke to us about it, but thank goodness that she is a superb student because she still did very well with all her subjects. She would feel horrible when it would hit. She was bedridden 5–6 days each time it happened!

We felt helpless. Children's Hospital infectious disease doctors knew us on a first name basis because we were there so often. They were puzzled and had us bring her in every time she was sick to draw blood and examine her.

We were at our wits' end until a friend gave us a bottle of colostrum and said it helped him recover from an illness that forced him to retire from veterinary practice prematurely. He said it couldn't hurt her and it might help! I thought we had nothing to lose. She was beginning an infection right when we were given the first bottle. We gave the colostrum to her 2 tablets 4–5 times a day. After one day on the colostrum the lymph node swelling went down completely! The next day she was completely normal, feeling totally well. From that point onward, she has not gotten sick ***at all****! It has been 1 ½ years and she has been around numerous people that were sick but hasn't gotten sick at all. Thank you, from the bottom of our heart!*

– William S., San Diego, California

Herpes and Hashimoto's Disease

I have suffered from herpes encephalitis Type A severely for approximately ten years. My symptoms have been weakness, breathlessness and seizures. I have also had drop attacks and intense pressure in my head. Of course, I've had eruptions of herpes on the skin as well. I also suffer with Hashimoto's disease, a lupus disease which attacks the thyroid, since having my thyroid gland irradiated in 1984. This radiation process was the medically prescribed treatment of Grave's disease—an inherited disease in my family.

Since taking colostrum (two pills twice daily) I've noticed less weakness, much milder seizures, less pressure occurring in my head and an added bonus of mood elevation. My menstrual cycles are even easier. I've felt a definite surge of immune function…I noticed a difference in about one week. With the help of colostrum I look forward to complete recovery—I believe it is possible.

Also, my dog, Traveler, has severe allergies to grass and certain weeds that appear in the spring. He can scratch himself to the point of bleeding. In the past I had to resort to cortisone treatments. With the usage of colostrum (one pill a day), it is a remarkable change. He hardly appears to itch at all—ever, even when he's directly exposed to allergens!

– S.N., Woodacres, California

Mononucleosis

I received a positive blood test for mono last spring while trying to work and go to college and just before I was scheduled to house-sit for my employers while they were on vacation. They loaded me down with everything in their Health Food store that might help me fight the disease, including colostrum. I pretty much forgot to take everything else, but I faithfully took the colostrum. The first week I went to school full-time despite tremendous fatigue, and the second week I worked full-time. At the end of the second week I had a second blood test, and it came back negative. The disease never progressed past the fatigue stage and went away in record time.

– Jessica F., Susanville, California

DIARRHEA AND DYSENTERY

Down Syndrome and Diarrhea

My son Zachary was born in 1993 with diagnosis of Down syndrome. He was pretty lucky except for his constant ear, nose and throat infections. He was always on antibiotics and had tubes put in his ears. He was very irritable and had escalating behavior problems because he was always ill.

Well, a little over a year ago I read an article about colostrum. We had tried virtually every natural product on the market, and his body often reacted with diarrhea (I think probably leaky gut syndrome). We had visited several specialists trying to stop the constant diarrhea. One doctor wanted us to try a potent antibiotic, and this time I put my foot down. So now I was ready to try colostrum. What if this was the answer?

Within a matter of weeks we began to see a difference, and now after a year and 3 months, it is just phenomenal. He is rarely sick, and when he is he gets better with a normal few days. The last time he had an infection was a year and 2 months ago. No more doctors, improved mood, all round better behavior. I will keep him on colostrum…

We also had his blood tested before starting colostrum. They measured the oxy-markers in his blood, an indication of free radicals. They called me up concerned about how awful his blood results were, concerned that he would get very sick and be in danger of contracting a serious disease (Down's children are more likely to get things like diabetes and leukemia, for example). After being on the colostrum 3 months we had him retested. The results were not a surprise because he was not getting sick any longer, but they showed a normal amount of free radicals compared to the normal population—not the Down syndrome population which have more free radicals than normal.

I would recommend this product to any child born with this. It is a godsend!

– Susan T., London, Ontario

INFLAMMATION

Bursitis

The bursitis in my left hip was so bad that my doctor was going to send me to a surgeon to have the bursa removed. I was crying every night from the pain. I could hardly walk.

I read some of the testimonials about taking colostrum, and one lady said her hip was improved in three weeks. Well, I had to try it. It took longer than three weeks for me. By the end of seven weeks, I felt like my hip was 95% better.

For two years my boss tried getting me to take colostrum. I'm just sorry I waited so long!

– Louise V., Omaha, Nebraska

Scalp Inflammation

I have an inflammatory scalp condition that no doctor has been able to properly diagnose. The condition causes inflammation on certain areas of my scalp that causes some of the hair to fall out. I read about bovine colostrum on a website and thought I'd give it a try. I was skeptical since nothing seems to help my condition. I've been taking it now for almost three weeks and am really amazed at how much the inflammation went down. I hope this is finally the answer I've been searching for. There are hardly any red areas on my scalp anymore!

– Kristen M., Drexel Hill, Pennsylvania

Brown Recluse Bite

A couple of years ago I was bitten by a brown recluse spider on the palm of my left hand. A sore formed with infection, and a hole was forming. My whole hand was swelling.

At the time I did not know of any treatment, so I mixed colostrum powder and aloe vera into a paste that I applied at least a dozen times a day. Believe it or not, within two days the swelling went down, and the near panic I felt was relieved. Healing had begun! Within two weeks, it was nearly healed.

Because amputation was the alternative, the healing was a wonder. Today there is no evidence of it at all. I love colostrum! It saved my hand.

– Patrick H., Sedona, Arizona

Poison Oak

A friend of mine told me that colostrum helped get rid of poison oak. My mom and daughter came down with it at the same time, so I told them to take the powder and mix it with a non-scented lotion to make a paste-like lotion and put it on the poison oak every 4 hours. It was gone in 24 hours. No one could believe it! I work at a school and this little boy came in one day covered in poison oak and his eyes were swelling shut. I ran home and got my colostrum and came back and put the lotion all over his poison oak. The school nurse saw him while I was putting the colostrum on him, and she thought it was so bad she took him to the doctor. By the time they got there, the swelling and redness was gone. When he came back to school, everyone in the office wanted to know what the doctor had given him. He told them, "Nothing." He had a prescription to go get filled and hadn't done it yet. Amazing!

– Nanette E., Willow Creek, California

AUTOIMMUNE DISORDERS

Chronic Fatigue

Before the colostrum, Jessica [my daughter] was seeing a doctor monthly or more frequently. She was on about ten or more different pills and supplements and on a very strict four-day cycle diet. Though we saw some improvement, it was very little. She is fifteen and is being home schooled. It was very difficult for her to finish a day of schoolwork. She would sleep at night and sleep five or more hours during the day. Even when she wasn't sleeping, it was difficult for her to do anything. Getting dressed was even a chore for her. Colostrum has given her her life back. Even though she is not yet well, she is able to complete a day of school work, go shopping and enjoy other things.

– Anne A., Carencro, Louisiana

Chronic Fatigue Syndrome/Fibromyalgia

In July of 1996 my wife, age 45 at the time, came down with a very mysterious illness that changed her entire life. Prior to July she was very active in the operation of our quarter horse business and only complained of the aches and pains that are expected with this kind of work. One particular day she began to get very weak and disoriented. She was rushed to the emergency room of a local hospital where they found no evidence of anything that should cause

She made very little recovery progress over the next ten days. Finally a new symptom surfaced, severe pain in the muscles and joints. Over the next six months she was seen by fourteen different doctors, and not ONE of them could put their finger on the problem. By this time orthodox medicine had her on several pain medications, and she stayed drugged to the point of all day sleeping all day.

I was introduced to colostrum and started her on it with her medications. After taking this product for three days I could see a noticeable difference in her pain and her energy. Being an individual that believes in natural body healing, I began to wean her from the conventional drugs until we got solely on the colostrum (this took me two weeks). She continued to take the colostrum and continued to improve. To eliminate any coincidence, I pulled her from the colostrum, and within two days she was going backwards again. After the second day, I returned her to the colostrum, and immediately she began to show progress again. She has been on the colostrum regularly ever since, taking four capsules in the morning and 4:00 in the evening. Today she is back working and doing things that were impossible prior to the colostrum.

She was finally diagnosed with chronic fatigue syndrome and fibromyalgia, and she does not take ANY drugs of any kind. Her last doctor was critical of the colostrum and suggested that we do away with it and take his recommended medications. We chose to terminate the doctor and his recommendations and continue on with the colostrum. This was in February of 1998, and she continues to do well.

– Dave S., Griffin, Georgia

Crohn's Disease

Kristen is a darling second grader with a huge challenge! At age six she was diagnosed with an autoimmune disease, Crohn's. As her mother, I was completely devastated when I heard the doctor give us the diagnosis. Where would I begin? How to begin helping my little girl live with this chronic illness? Kristen was having such a difficult time assimilating her food that her weight loss was alarming. The doctors had started her on large doses of steroids. My husband and I were frightened by the long-term effects of this medicine.

Late at night I would search the Internet for answers. Then I found colostrum. I called the company and asked a multitude of questions. They were so helpful and reassuring. Kristen has been on colostrum for three months now. She is steadily gaining weight, increasing the type of foods she can eat, and has not had a cold for eight weeks, which is absolutely exciting. At school she was always catching colds. We have been courageous enough to take her off the steroids.

– Tracey C., South Bend, Indiana

Multiple Sclerosis

Twelve years ago I was diagnosed with multiple sclerosis, and the neurologist who diagnosed this suggested I begin taking cortisone. Well, being the careful person I am, I began to do research about this drug. Upon finding information that indicated severe side effects and possible long-term damage to some major organs, I declined. So three years later I came upon alternative healing, i.e., herbs, vitamins, etc.

Even with this, I still had the major battle of locating a natural product to assist with my autoimmune disease. Thanks to all the information herb and vitamin stores gladly hand out, I came upon an article about colostrum. So again I did some intense research. After looking at all the materials and making phone calls, I decided to try colostrum. That was about three years ago, and thanks to the colostrum, my immune system is stronger than it ever was, even before my diagnosis of multiple sclerosis. I have also recommended colostrum to a couple of friends who also have multiple sclerosis, and their stories are just like mine—success!!!

It has also benefited my skin condition, eczema.

– Jude R., Green Bay, Wisconsin

Arthritis and Bone Disease

I am very pleased with the effects colostrum has had on my overall health. I began taking concentrated doses about two months ago and after one month reduced to the regular recommended dosage. I have noticed a few things. First, I soon felt in better health, with higher levels of energy than I had experienced before. Within a few weeks I reduced the amount of arthritis medications I took each day by half, with no increase in pain and no decrease in my activity level. I also experience less stiffness and pain in the morning upon awakening.

For whatever reason, about 1 ½ months ago I began to wonder if the colostrum was really helping me all that much and if I could do without it. Also, the daily drudgery of taking yet another pill began to wear on my patience. I stopped taking the supplements. Within a week I felt noticeably more tired, even badly for a few days. I began experiencing pain in my legs and had more general aches and pains than I'd been used to. I also realized that since beginning to take the colostrum I'd experienced no yeast infections, which had before been a monthly occurrence coinciding with the on-

set of my menstrual cycle. I of course immediately began taking colostrum again. With days I was feeling better and had the level of energy back that I'd so quickly become accustomed to. I have decided swallowing a few capsules a day is a very small inconvenience that has greatly enhanced my overall quality of life.

– CONNIE, FOGELSVILLE, PENNSYLVANIA

No More Scooters

My experience with colostrum has been very good for me in many ways. The first was the strengthening of my muscles to walk again. I have relied on a scooter for three and a half years and a walker to try to get some exercise around the house. I have arthritis in both hips, and one hip is worse than the other. Because of the fear of the hip giving out, it was easier to ride around. In the process of enduring this, the doctors prescribed Indocin, which I took for six years—I later read that it should be only prescribed for three months—which had the effect of my gaining weight. The good result of colostrum is the arthritis has left, I am losing weight, and I have a better disposition.

One day I was out on my scooter and hit something that caused my scooter to tip over, and I bruised my hip really bad. It was almost black and probably four inches by four inches around. I thought I would be really stiff the next day and my neck hurt the night before, but the next morning there was no stiffness at all and the bruise started to go away and was gone by the end of the week.

Because of these results several people are taking it because of what it has done for me. They were skeptics in the beginning.

– NANCY N., ROCKFORD, ILLINOIS

Osteoporosis

I am writing this letter to thank you for getting me to try colostrum. As you know, on June 15, 2000, I broke the L-1 vertebra bone in my back. I was out of work for twelve weeks. The bone and joint specialist sent me for a whole body scan, MRI, countless X-rays, and a bone density test.

The diagnosis was osteopenia [decreased bone density] throughout my body and spine. This is the last stage before full-blown osteoporosis. I was told by my bone and joint doctor that there was no cure for this bone disease. There were only two types of medicine available to treat this disease. The medicine I was placed on is called Fosamax. This drug is used to slow down the bone loss. The other is given if you have full-blown osteoporosis. I cannot tell you the pain got any better because it did not. It felt like my muscles were ripping away from my bones. I came to your office for my monthly visit. During our conversation, I told you of the problems with my back and the pain I was experiencing from the bone disease. You suggested I try colostrum.

But, being the skeptic that I am, I put you off for months. But you never gave up on trying to help me. Every time I came in, you said, "Please, just give them a try." First I bought some for my husband because they are good for his arthritis. He said he felt much better. The pain for me was getting much worse. On my next visit to your office I purchased a bottle and started to take them. About four to five weeks later I noticed a difference in the amount of pain I was experiencing. I have been taking colostrum for a year now. Today I got the best news. My doctor gave me another bone density test, and the test came back normal, no trace of osteoporosis. My spongy, thin bones are back to normal thanks to you and most of all thanks to colostrum.

– M. Hall, Lutz, Florida, from a letter to her chiropractor,
Dr. Donald Wolfe, DC, Bayonet Point, Florida

Of Cats and Sunburn

I have been taking colostrum now for two months. I have noticed improvement in a lot of areas, especially my joint pain. I also have been giving my cat colostrum who had a severe upper respiratory infection for two years that was finally killing him. I was told to put him down; there was nothing else to do for him. With a raw food diet and colostrum, my cat is healthier than I could have ever hoped for, and his coat is amazingly beautiful.

Two days ago I went to the beach to lay in the sun, and I was silly enough to stay too long. By the time I got home I was so burnt I was shocked to see myself in the mirror. I was in a lot of pain, and I knew this was serious. I was so frightened I started crying. Then I thought of mixing some colostrum with water and applying it to my burns. Almost right away I felt the pain lessen, and I reapplied some more. Within about fifteen minutes I was pain free. By the time my husband got home two hours later, I was exercising. He was not surprised after seeing what it has done for our cat. My burns healed. Without the colostrum I would have certainly ended up in the hospital.

– Johanne T., Richmond, British Columbia

Allergies

I have been using your brand of colostrum all through the pollen season, and I am still using it now to help with grass and mold pollen. This is the first time in many years I have found relief. I am very pleased and recommend it [colostrum] highly to everyone and anyone with allergies and sinus problems.

I used to have to take Claritin, a prescription drug, very expensive, with limited benefits and many side effects. I suffered from dry eyes, dry mouth, headaches and itching from taking Claritin. I have none of these side effects and great benefits from your colostrum, a great product!

– Anna M, Columbus, Georgia

Asthma and Allergies

I am a 72-year-old male. I have suffered with asthma, severe allergies and low blood sugar for the past ten years. I started using colostrum approximately two months ago. My allergies cleared up almost immediately. The only time I use my asthma medication is before exercise, i.e. treadmill, weight lifting, etc. This is a reduction of 90%. And my blood sugar is normal.

– Charles C., Henrietta, Texas

Hives

Prior to taking colostrum, I had hives throughout my body, both internal and external. My doctors were not able to determine the source and in frustration prescribed a strong medication to help alleviate the pain but could not and did not help with the symptoms. After taking colostrum, I immediately had an elimination of my allergic reactions. The hives are not entirely gone, but are 95% eliminated. For the first time in years I know can sleep, wear clothes comfortably, go to work, eat normal foods. The change in my life has been incredible. My wife thinks she's married to a new man. We cuddle, and it doesn't hurt! There are no words to express how incredible all this is and what it means to me. Because of colostrum I have my life back—plain and simple. Also, I sleep better, have more energy and am less moody than before.

– Warren D., Salt Lake City, Utah

Warts

My son had two warts on his foot for seven years that responded to treatment but always came right back. My sister had given me some colostrum to help speed up his recovery from strep throat. To my amazement, the warts just fell off! It has been two years, and the warts have not returned. I had a plantar wart that was not responding to treatment after four months, so I decided to try the colostrum. After two weeks the wart was gone and has not returned.

– Karen W., Hendersonville, Tennessee

Hemophilia

James [not his real name] was born with hemophilia. He is a fifteen-year-old Amish young man. Throughout his young life he has had several bleeding episodes from falls and injuries. He has always had to be very cautious, not playing hard like many of his friends did.

Approximately 18 months ago, James started taking colostrum powder. He mixed it in different foods and ate it very willingly. Soon James' brother was eating colostrum too. Colostrum has been the only supplement James has taken. No other vitamins, minerals, herbs or medications.

James has been working at a sawmill in Southern Indiana close to Bloomfield. One day his sleeve caught and pulled his forearm into the saw. The saw tore into his forearm making a deep and ragged wound. The ambulance was called. On the way to the hospital something began to happen: the bleeding slowed, slowed even more, and finally there was no bleeding. Actual clotting was taking place!

For James, his family and community, it was the "Miracle of Colostrum." James and his parents say the only thing different was the colostrum he was taking for the past many months because hemophilia is a frequent illness among the Amish people, they are now buying cases of colostrum. The Amish community is truly rejoicing for James and many others!

– S. Plew, Bloomfield, Indiana

COGNITIVE DISORDERS AND ALZHEIMER'S

Brain Damage

A lady we know has a boy, Casey, who at nine years of age was badly brain damaged in an accident with a pet donkey. He was in a coma on life support for some six months. He has slowly made a remarkable comeback. He can now walk but falls a lot. He has had bad memory problems and couldn't remember for even a few minutes what he was told to do. He also craved milk. His mother said he would "kill for milk." If allowed to, Casey would drink two gallons or more per day.

We gave this lady her first bottle of colostrum to see if it would help him, having read that colostrum would help brain damaged people. Within one week, she said Casey was so much better. It stopped his unreal milk cravings. He now drinks two or three glasses a day. He remembers so much better now, and is learning to take charge of his life. Also she says she has hardly had to help him up off the floor since taking colostrum.

The family was living in Modesto, California, and ran out of colostrum. After several days, Casey was falling again, craving milk, and the poor memory returned. She tried another brand from a health food store, but it didn't do the job. They then drove 700+ miles up here [to Idaho] to get some more colostrum. Needless to say, this customer is thoroughly sold on the product!

– Ken I., Melba, Idaho

Cancer

After becoming a cancer patient a couple of years ago, I began a journey to a healthier lifestyle, and much of that included the use of dietary supplements and vitamins. With all the immune boosting products out there and the hard sell many vitamin stores push to get you to buy things not necessarily in your best interest, I was still very excited to try colostrum. Furthermore, members of my online cancer group have been highly recommending many of your (colostrum) products as a good supplement to include in the anti-cancer arsenal.

– Cyd S., Littleton, Colorado

I believe it is worthwhile to tell you about the history and progress of Charles Kellum, a 57-year-old white male who was diagnosed with Non-Hodgkin's Lymphoma in September, 2005. Mr. Kellum, an RN, self diagnosed himself with splenomegaly at that time and a splenectomy was performed. Subsequent CAT scans revealed per-rectal lymph nodes and he was started on rituxin, velcaid, and sandostatin. He was plagued by diarrhea which the sandostatin relieved. He took chemotherapy from February 2006 through July 2006, and he had a weight loss of 50 pounds from 220 to170 pounds. He was extremely fatigued and suffered from diminished energy.

He was noted to have no change in lymph node masses via CAT scan. He was placed on more chemotherapy: rituxin, etoside, and cysblantin. This chemotherapy regimen began in April 2008 and finished four months later. His energy decreased significantly, his physical robustness diminished radically; he was only capable of staying in bed. His weight leveled off at 97 pounds. He was severely emaciated in appearance on May 11th, 2008 I wondered silently to myself when I saw him if would he survive for more than a month!

In April, 2008, I met you, and you told me about colostrum, the sublingual preparation. I said to myself—this polypeptide is worth a try. He was instructed to take the colostrum sublingually, beginning in the morning and evening for six months. When I saw him in May 2008, I called you and you said to have him take colostrum every 4 hours. In July 2008, he starting gaining weight, his weight currently is 137 pounds. He also became more physically active and was able to work at his hobby of repairing engines.

My clinical impression, which is not based on scientific fact but clinical observation of this patient, is that colostrum played a role in helping him battle with cancer. I know he is very grateful for the donated colostrum you have provided. I am also appreciative of the donation.

– Dr. John P. Miller, M.D.

Injury Recovery and Wound Healing

Before using colostrum repair cream, I would have a cut, scratch, wound, whatever take up to three months to totally heal and then would end up with a scar. Since I found this wonderful product—the repair cream—I apply it three times a day or more and have small wounds heal in about two to three weeks with no scarring. It is a terrific product and sure works well.

Also with reference to the colostrum capsules, they can be broken open and the powder patted onto cold sores with a healing, drying ability far surpassing any cold sore medication I've ever used, and with no symptoms of excessive drying and tightness as with other over-the-counter cold sore meds.

– Mimi P., Lewiston, New York

ATHLETICS

Muscle Building at 70

Golf is my game. When I retired, I thought playing on the golf course would keep me lean and toned. Did not happen. Then I started taking colostrum. Four weeks later I stepped out of my shower and looked in the mirror—a miracle had happened! I had muscles at 70! Nothing I had anticipated at all. But taking colostrum powder before my golf games had burned fat into muscles. Now I am exercising three times each week with weights and swimming at the gym. Colostrum energy is remarkable at my senior age. Thank you for the great surprise!

– Bill C, Ithaca, New York

PET HEALTH

Elderly Pets

Kindred Spirits Animal Sanctuary is dedicated to caring for elderly animals and, at the end of life, the Sanctuary offers compassionate hospice care. Prior to coming to the Sanctuary, most of our animals have suffered severe neglect, abuse and abandonment, and many are frail with a variety of ailments and disabilities.

The Sanctuary has always practiced high standards of nutritional care. However, about a year ago a holistic veterinarian suggested that the one real improvement we could make would be to add colostrum. I was concerned about the expense but decided to give it a try for our resident dogs. He was absolutely right. After only a few weeks, I noticed a marked improvement in their vitality. Minor eye and ear infections disappeared, wounds healed, and their coats gained a new luster. However, most of all they seemed to brighten in spirit. In fact, visitors often comment, "They all look so happy!" I feel that having added colostrum to their diets is a major improvement and has made a real difference in the lives of our senior dogs.

– Ulla Pedersen, Director

Kindred Spirits Animal Sanctuary and Eldercare Hospice, Santa Fe, New Mexico

Testimonial Snippets about PRP Spray

I have to say the biggest results I have seen are from my ninety-year-old father-in-law. He has five small tumors in his brain, and it has been affecting his balance and hearing. He also complains about headaches. He is taking medication for high blood pressure.

After the first day, his headaches and balance improved. He told me he now sleeps through the night, which he has never done. He has more energy than a forty-year-old. He has reduced his blood pressure medication. His blood pressure, which usually ran 158/115 with medication, now runs around 120/72. It's unbelievable. Also, his disposition is so much better. It's like a miracle drug for him.

My mother-in-law took it for a few days but went off it because it made her really tired. She blames the spray, but she wasn't feeling well before she took it. When she went to the doctor, her CBC came back showing infection, so I think it was that.

Paul, my Lou Gehrig's friend, has started to take it. He goes in for experimental treatments, which really took a toll on him, so we don't really see any major results. I would assume knowing his chronic condition it would take a really long, long time to show improvement.

My mom says her arthritis is better, and she has tons of energy. My granddaughter loves it. She is the only one from her pre-school who has not gotten sick. She has not had immunization shots, so this should keep her really healthy. I haven't heard from anyone else.

The spray has given me more energy then I had. I went to the doctor and found out I have something going on with my heart. I need further tests to figure out what. I have received your care package. Thank you, thank you.

I'm so thankful to have met you. You are a special person. My gratitude is so great just for the results my father-in-law is having. I have enjoyed the time that we have spent together. I am really thankful again to have met you. I know I already said it once, but I truly mean it.

I hope everything is going well for you...and you're out there saving the planet. I know you are.

– Colleen Kelly, Tucson AZ

A Collection of Letters from Richard Kolt of Tucson, AZ:

I met Richard Kolt in 2004. He is a retired successful businessman that is now dedicating his life to helping needy people become healthy. Colostrum has become his passion and he now spends much of his time in Africa providing colostrum products to the needy in Africa. Following are a collection of stories about his work.

Sunday, Dr. Catare and the group filmed the 30+ people at Reverend Bea's church. I had given colostrum to a woman and two children who are sickle cell victims. We took testimonies to be shown on TV, and the sickle cell child was well, just as had been reported. The interesting thing was that he only had one bottle of the PRP spray. They ran out in late January. It appears that a single bottle will reverse SCA? Now for the $64,000 question: how to expose this to the SCA community. Does anyone out there have an idea?

Sunday I had agreed to go to Rev. Bea's church. She is still in the Kwalangare slum, but she had to move into a building twice the size. Bea is quite a preacher. She reminds me of the movie about Amiee Semple McPherson who built the first entertainment-type church in LA in the '30s. Aimee passed the plate with clotheslines overhead where you clipped your bills. Change was not accepted, even then when a dollar was a dollar.

Bea's new church was on Church Row. Reminded me of the bars in Chicago, seven or eight on every block. The competition was from the music, the amplified speakers and a half-dozen talented preachers shouting and rolling. Since Bea started giving out colostrum, her flock has doubled. Location, location. Location or COLOSTRUM.

Bea's church starts at 9:30 AM with a half-dozen camp meeting hymns and rolls right into a couple of sermons by her helpers. Then for my benefit, I'm sure, she had testimonials from 12–15 people marveling about everything from HBP to arthritis and AIDS. I then spoke to the group again and received their thanks and gratitude. It's amazing what the product can do. Then I mentioned that we had been successful with a sickle cell anemia child and asked if anyone knew anyone with such a child. The first lady we had ever treated said there was one two minutes away. I asked her to go get the lady.

She was a pretty thirty-five-year-old woman with a two-year-old suckling and a ten-year-old boy, David. When she walked into the church, she had already heard the details from our friend, and she was sobbing. She has another thirteen-year-old son who is in a boarding school for sickle cell kids. She got the whole nine yards in Swahili translated by Bea. As she listened, she lit up. The whole thing was thrilling and unbelievable for her. We, of course, cautioned her that only one SCA child had been treated, but she said she had been praying and praying for years that something could help her babies.

We started the two kids on the spot. When I looked at her, she was awestruck and loving, focusing on the children while the whole congregation sang and prayed. She looked like she'd just won the lottery and spent two sputtering minutes thanking me. I again cautioned her that we had only worked on one, but she said, "It will work. God has answered my prayers." I'll never forget the eyes. Tough stuff! Made the rest of the three-and-a-half-hour service pretty tame. I asked each of the members to bring one other sick person with them next Sunday for some free samples, and they all promised.

I told Bea to start collecting more chairs.

■ ■ ■ ■

Just another Sunday in the Kwalangre (Nairobi) Slum.

I had forgotten to mention that Saturday I also saw Rev. Martin. I had met him around Christmas. He had fallen twice when his blood sugar was out of balance. He is a handsome sixty-year-old preacher of a small poor church outside Nairobi. He obviously has other income as he wears Seville Row suits, but he heard I was in town and came in to see me Saturday evening. He had completed the two bottles of PRP spray I had given him, had been taking two injections of insulin a day, and his eyesight was failing. According to him, "It's truly a miracle! Why doesn't everyone know about it?"

Monday morning at breakfast one of the waiters came up to me and told me quietly that his CD4 count was normal. He's been on PRP spray since January 10th!

At the office, Rhoda, the mayor's wife, brought Susan and Hassan. Hassan and her husband Iman had recently converted to Christianity. Their son, Hassan, had to have a shunt inserted in his brain because he had meningitis. After the operation he was paralyzed on his right side. He is five-years-old and has ADHD. Susan was concerned about the overactivity because they wouldn't let him stay in school. Also he was having convulsions three or four times per day.

I held the boy and told him we would have a party, four squirts for Hassan, four for GGP. Within two minutes Susan started to cry because Hassan's behavior was 90% normal. His teeth and gums were awful, so I gave us each four more squirts. She then told me that she needed spray for herself (ulcers, etc.), and her mom is a diabetic. They left the office higher than a kite.

I had eleven meetings/treatments/presentations ending with the final meeting at 6:30. Rhoda was still awestruck and told the four pastors what happened to Hassan. Two minutes after they left me walking down the hall, Hassan yelled, "Mom, look! I can move my hand!" A few steps later, "Mom, I can lift the water bottle to my mouth! Mom, look! I can walk without dragging the leg." Rhoda said, "All Susan could say was ***ni mujizza, ni mujizza, ni mujizza, ni mujizza...ni mujizza!*** *She cried all the way home!"*

Is it a miracle, is it the PRPs? I don't know, but it looks like what I've said before: colostrum fixes everything! Add meningitis to the list.

■ ■ ■ ■

Today an article in ***Parade*** talks about the work that Dr. Paul Law is doing on autism.

"I am currently using bovine colostrum on a group of 37 autistics in Nogales, Sonora, Mexico. I have been using colostrum for over two years on immune and autoimmune conditions in Africa.

"Almost by accident I gave colostrum to a grandmother here in Tucson who began treatment on her five-year-old grandson. His improvement was so stunning that the autistic program at the University of Arizona declared they had misdiagnosed the boy. The grandmother said, 'Isn't it amazing that he could never say my name?' And so forth.

"The boy at last report was acting normally. Keep in mind that the results were strictly anecdotal, but two months ago when I was in Africa one of my friends emailed

me to report that a woman with terminal cancer had had infant twin babies and was looking for someone to adopt them, and that my friend was starting colostrum therapy. She had terminal cancer, unable to work. My friend began colostrum on that lady and also a nine-year-old leukemia victim who had not eaten in days.

"The colostrum comes in a spray bottle. When the colostrum was taken to Mexico, an extra bottle was given to a neighbor child that was autistic. The results of all three were staggering. My friend made an appointment for me to meet the woman and sick child, who were back to work and back to school respectively, at an autistic house in Nogales. I am not at the computer to attach the results of my work there, but tomorrow from my office I will forward my letter.

"I have now used colostrum on the kids for three months, and copies of the parents' letters, which I just received Friday, will be translated from Spanish, and I will forward as well.

"I am a humanitarian and am spending my time and money helping people around the world to get well. I have never charged anyone, and pay for the products myself."

■ ■ ■ ■

Somewhere I have seen the phrase, "Expect a Miracle." Well, here's one.

In the past I have had many unbelievable experiences with colostrum. Yesterday was another Top Ten.

In Nogales, Sonora, Mexico, there is a day care home that cares for 37 autistics. I found the house through my friend, Myra, who is a friend of Alma, who is a friend of Fran, etc.—all colostrum missionaries. Myra had sent colostrum to Mexico to treat a woman who had terminal cancer. The woman had been looking for someone to adopt her twin baby daughters. I met her at the autistic house. The woman had been started on product four or five weeks ago. She is back to work!!

Also I met the nine-year-old that had leukemia; she was started on the product at the same time. Lupita was unable to eat and was bedridden for weeks. I held her and her mother while we all cried. Nobody can believe it but that's how it is. I will try to attach pictures of these people to this letter or send them later.

But that was just an extra on this trip. Sandra and her husband Jesse Tapia picked me up in Nogales, Arizona, and took me across the border to the house. The house is run by the parents and has no other funding. They have 37 people, mostly 4–12 years old, but with three or four adults. They have a medical doctor who has computerized the information. They have a supplement that is marketed by Kirkman who specializes in diet and supplements for autisics.

When I entered the house, it was organized bedlam, even though the most disruptive were in a separate population upstairs. After introductions and translations (my seventh grade Spanish, their seventh grade English), they assembled about 25 of the more sedate kids, and I outlined colostrum and expected results. When I asked one of the three women who were in charge, Maria, which was her child, she told me he was upstairs with the most disruptive kids. I insisted that all of them should assemble in the little entry area. I then sat on the floor with all the kids. It was bedlam. We then gave bottles of colostrum to each parent and had them apply the first dose. Some day I hope to be organized enough to capture these experiences on tape, but the worst case boy, Maria's son, is about fourteen. He couldn't control his arms and legs and had to be restrained from eating his arm. He had large, open scars on his arms from his teeth. He also is blind in his right eye where he had tried to gouge it out.

Within a minute, the bedlam was not from the kids but from the parents. Each of the kids was visibly less active. Marie's son actually sat still some of the time, and there was probably a 70–80% reduction in the activity of each of the kids. The parents were amazed! They were chattering like magpies about what they had witnessed. I had seen this before with an autistic kid in my office, but never with 37 people. It was simply indescribable.

We then met with the MD and the head women and reviewed the computerized records. The doctor had started, like many people, withdrawn and skeptical. After witnessing the first application, he was enthralled.

The hair sample tests show that all of them had very, very heavy contamination of heavy metals, aluminum, mercury, and eight or ten others. He showed me the reduction that had been achieved with the Kirkman supplement, which was impressive, but not enough to noticeably reduce their overactivity.

We outlined a test, and they agreed to place a group of six or eight of the same age kids on colostrum and the supplement and another group on just colostrum. We talked about doing a test without colostrum, but we all agreed that the results we had just seen indicated that it would be wrong to exclude any kid that could be helped. So my test may not fit Big Pharma parameters, but it can help them decide on what's best for the kids.

Please tell everyone you know about the miracle of colostrum. Sandra has journal-

ized all the results so far, and each parent has promised to record individual results. Somehow I suspect that we will have the best efforts of 37 poor, less distressed people. When I have the results, we will print and distribute them.

With everyone's agreement I renamed the house ***La Casa de Tranquilla****—The Quiet House. I promised to return November 20th as soon as I return from my two weeks in Africa. They are planning to have newspaper and TV reporters there to record the happenings. Hopefully it will be a non-event because I expect all the kids to be much more sedate.*

■ ■ ■ ■

Today I meet with fifteen autistic kids and their parents from Tucson in my office. So expect another miracle soon.

On November 27th, exactly one month from the beginning of treatment of the 37 autistics in Nogales, Sonora, Mexico, we returned for our second visit.

Myra's sister, Sue, had arranged for Mexican newspaper and TV stations to be there to report on the first month's results. Of the 37 clients, only two failed to show much progress. Those two were older children that had habituated their different behaviors, and although they may have improved medically, they will require mental therapy.

Every one of the others had significant improvement. Marie's son, the most unmanageable of the group, was almost placid. Marie reported that the best part was he was much happier and easier to manage. I have pictures of him hugging and playing with Marie, which was previously impossible. (I'll try to forward the pics later.)

A number of the mothers were interviewed with me by the paper and the TV reporters. Each related their particular story, and the most poignant perhaps was Maria #2. In Spanish, of course, she said that her six-year-old daughter was epileptic as well as autistic. She said that the daughter had experienced half as many epileptic incidents in the last month, and that every one was two-thirds less severe. She said that the best part was that she was able to sleep, because in the last six years she seldom had a good night's sleep due to the daughter's attacks. Since colostrum she had only one major attack and that was a day when she had forgotten to give the child the colostrum. She then hugged me and said, "You aren't ever going to let my child run out of colostrum, are you?" And as you can imagine, that will never happen.

Clinically, the parents agreed that the improvement has been progressive, so it will be interesting to follow.

The only flaw, remember, is that there is an MD on staff who was originally skeptical then supportive. He had agreed to test a group of kids with and without colostrum. Unfortunately, the Medical-Industrial Complex reared its ugly head once again. He said he was concerned about being involved because of possible professional conflicts and elected not to do it. We will just have to wait a few months, let him see the continued improvement, and twist his tail again. He is still supportive and very positive but just pharmaceuticalized. It's truly amazing how deep the fear of Big Pharma goes.

– Richard Kolt, Tucson AZ

To contact Richard Kolt about his experiences please call (520) 981-3575

Professional Testimonials

We are so excited about the results we are having from the colostrum. Here are four wonderful healing results we have to share with you. There are a lot more that will be using this colostrum. This truly is a wonderful product for those who are fighting to regain health and wholeness. Please share these healing testimonies with others who need healing.

One young twelve-year-old boy in California was suffering from a severe case of mucosa colitis and losing weight. He was literally dying. His doctor was planning surgery to remove his colon. His father called me and asked what could be done naturally. I recommended that he start taking double doses of colostrum. After 5 days, the bleeding from the rectum ceased, and within 7 days he began to have normal bowel movements. From that point on he has gained 32 pounds of weight. His parents were most delighted to see the change.

Here in our town of Cottage Grove, Minnesota, a local minister had uncontrollable diabetes and was taking three insulin injections daily. I shared with him the benefits of colostrum, and several months later he came back to me and was convinced that something besides injections had to be done. He purchased the colostrum, and within one week the miracle of healing kicked in and he was no longer giving himself insulin injections. Now he will not go without colostrum to regulate his insulin secretion. He is totally convinced of the benefits of taking colostrum.

Then his wife came to see me. She had a staphylococcal infection and numerous ulcer-type sores on her body. We placed her on double doses of colostrum and natural zinc ointment. Within two days the sores began to heal, and in one week they were gone. She had visited no less than two medical doctors who could not help her. Now her countenance has changed with joy and health restored.

A lady in our church had bouts of heavy asthma-like breathing. We put her on colostrum, and she noticed how easy her breathing became. She found that she has more energy and continues her daily schedule with ease and comfort.

– Michael McCann, ND

McCann Wellness Center, Cottage Grove, Minnesota

Miss C.B., age eleven, has suffered from severe juvenile rheumatoid arthritis since age one. She has also been under the care of a pediatric rheumatologist since age one. This rheumatologist has tried every nonsteroidal anti-inflammatory agent available with no great improvement. When she presented to my office three weeks ago, she was taking Celebrex 200 mg daily, which is widely known to be the best treatment available. The rheumatologist was planning to place C.B. on methotrexate and steroids if no improvement was seen.

When I saw C.B., she was wearing braces on her lower legs, had swollen joints, to include her knees, elbows, neck, and back. I placed her on colostrum 4000 mg daily (4 capsules every 12 hours), and three weeks later she no longer needed her braces. She had no more pain or swelling in her joints. Her recovery was nothing short of miraculous. She is continuing to take her colostrum as directed, and she has had no relapse of symptoms. Her rheumatologist is shocked and amazed. I continue to see wonderful results in my patients. Keep up the good work. If every person were taking (colostrum), most of the medical community as we currently know it would dry up and blow away. Very few people would get sick.

– Gary Mezo, ND, PhD

Westchase Alternative Medicine, Inc., Tampa, Florida

M.T., a seventy-year-old female, complained of "bowel trouble all my life." Constipation requiring continuous use of laxatives, stool softeners and enemas might last several weeks, followed by diarrhea for a few weeks. Then the cycle would repeat.

She had seen many doctors, had many tests, including barium enema X-rays, colonoscopy, etc. Her most frequent diagnosis was irritable bowel syndrome and slight iron deficiency. No treatment, diet or drug therapy was effective.

M.T. is an active person of normal weight and is a competitive barrel racer on the rodeo circuit. There were times when she had to drop out of competition due to explosive bouts of diarrhea. She complained of ongoing pain in her abdomen and chronic fatigue.

I started her on broad spectrum colostrum, and within two weeks she noted a good improvement. By the end of the third week she had completely normal gastrointestinal function. No more diarrhea. No more fatigue. No more constipation. The slight iron deficiency has normalized, and she has, in her own words, "energy to burn."

I feel your colostrum is the only truly effective product on the market today. We have in past years used several other brands of colostrum with little or poor results.

– E.W. McDonagh, DO
McDonagh Medical Center, Kansas City, Missouri

My use of bovine colostrum is based on good science, experience, and common sense as I was introduced to veterinary medicine while working on a dairy farm during high school and later as a milk test supervisor for the University of Georgia Dairy Department. I have been a veterinarian for 52 years—the last 44 years in small animal practice—and have been involved in numerous clinical trials. I have seen old, favorite treatment modalities replaced with new and better protocols. The use of bovine colostrum in my practice has favorably impacted a greater diversity of diseases than any other product except the "silver bullet," cortisone.

Jake, a 125-pound Rottweiler, was presented with a sarcoma half the size of a tennis ball just lateral to the fetlock. Excision necessitated transpositioning the skin to cover the defect. Ten days post surgery the graft had failed, and the exposed tissue appeared to be a recurring tumor. Treatment consisted of debriding dead tissue, two capsules of colostrum twice a day, and powdered colostrum liberally applied under bandage to the wound every other day. Healing was complete after six weeks. Six months later there has been no evidence of recurrence of tumor, and no further surgery was needed.

Nancy is one of those unfortunate women who are addicted to picking up strays. In spite of reasonably good care, antibiotics and appropriate vaccines, she was continually plagued with upper respiratory infections in both kittens and puppies, nonresponsive to anything except tincture of time. Addition of colostrum to her regimen had kept Nancy happy for the last ten months.

For about six months now, we have been seeing an unusual number of cats with recurring cystitis in spite of various antibiotics or diets. Approximately two months ago, we started giving these cats one capsule of colostrum twice a day, maintaining them on the cystitis diet and discontinuing antibiotics. To date all have responded (at least 2–3 per week).

The most gratifying results have been in "curing" inflammatory bowel disease and controlling the many forms of allergic dermatitis/otitis/pododermatitis and the accompanying yeast and/or bacterial infections. Clients continue to amaze me with their reports of the improved quality of life in their senior citizen arthritic dogs and cats.

– B.S. Austin, DVM, Longwood, Florida

I have a number of patients who are arthritic, and bovine colostrum dispensed for the treatment of rheumatoid and osteoarthritis has provided them with amazingly good results. One small-boned elderly gentleman who was terribly overweight did suffer in total agony from rheumatoid arthritis. He could hardly walk. I put him on colostrum, about a bottle of 120 capsules per week, and he soon reached the point where he could walk without pain even though he did not lose the weight.

I used bovine colostrum for the arthritic treatment of my fifty-six-year-old mother. Her left knee exhibited a lot of inflammation as the result of having been damaged in a prior automobile accident. I had tried a number of different therapies such as shark cartilage and MSM without success, but when I added the bovine colostrum she was pain free in three days. She now takes it religiously.

In Mexico, my staff and I do a lot of work with cancer, and two-thirds of my cancer patients are taking colostrum. About half of my patients are poverty-stricken, and I stretch my resources to help them by dispensing colostrum to them at little or no cost. For those who can afford it, I typically have them take five or more 480-milligram capsules a day—that's over 2000 mg. Colostrum really does seem to make a beneficial difference for my cancer patients. They have more energy, and it keeps down some of their infections as a complication of the illness.

I am giving colostrum to hepatitis C patients. One of these people living in Northern California who found it impossible to come to Mexico consulted me by telephone. His situation was really serious because he had a hepatitis C viral load of 8 million. I put together a protocol for him of bovine colostrum, calcium orotate, reduced glutathione and protease enzymes. Within two months, this patient returned for laboratory testing and discovered that his hepatitis viral load had plummeted to 100. Since the patient did not take treatment with anything else, this is convincing proof to me that bovine colostrum works synergistically in a combined nutritional protocol. I've gone on to successfully treat many more cases of hepatitis C.

– Stephen Hynes, ND

Dr. Hynes runs a clinic in Ciudad Acuna, Mexico,
just across the border from Del Rio, Texas.

Scientists have long known about the increased resistance of breast-fed babies to certain infections, particularly to intestinal disorders. However, because of changing cultural values, many post-war mothers didn't breast-feed their babies, and now many of these grown-up babies are dealing with prevalent and difficult-to-treat immune-compromised conditions. Part of this problem is due to the breakdown of the environment and the nutrient-deficient food we eat. Furthermore, many older people have fragile immune systems due to a multiplicity of factors, including stress, illness, viruses, diseases, toxin-laden food and polluted air. Colostrum may well be one of the most important immune system nutrients to come along in the last fifty years, since more and more illnesses and disease conditions are linked to a suppressed or compromised immune system.

– James Wilson, DC, ND, PhD

We have had this man on heavy colostrum from three or four months. He is riddled with cancer but continues to improve. I have been treating Charles, using the standard protocol with colostrum but on higher doses.

Two weeks ago Charles had a septic knee that was treated with antibiotics successfully. His weight was 100 pounds, but he now weighs 120 pounds and is regaining his vigor! I find it astounding that he didn't die.

– John Miller MD

PART II

PROLINE-RICH POLYPEPTIDES

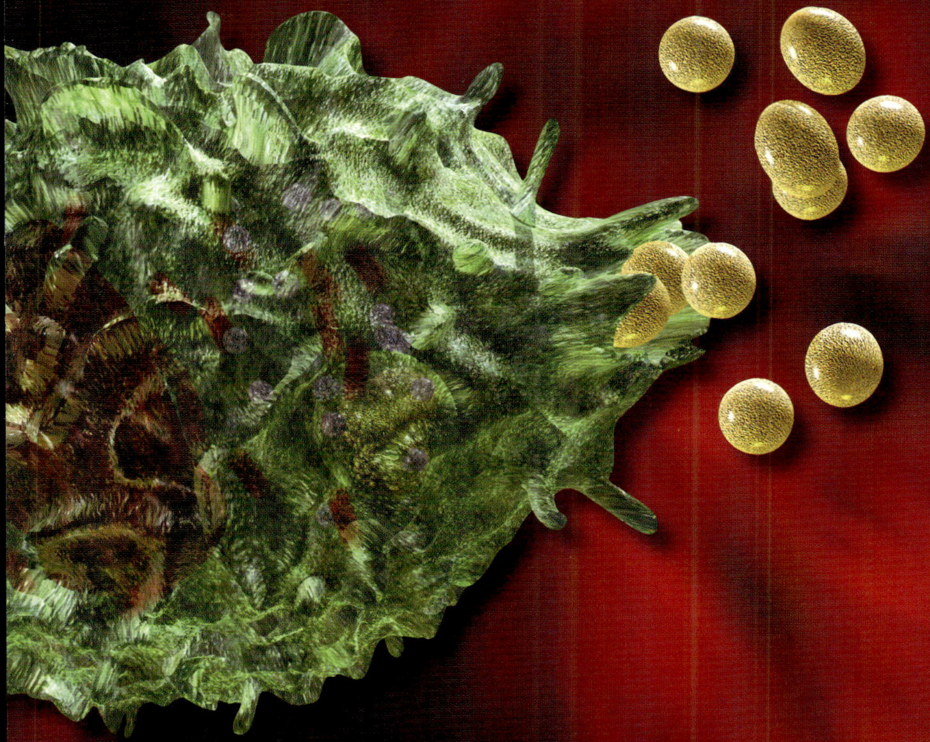

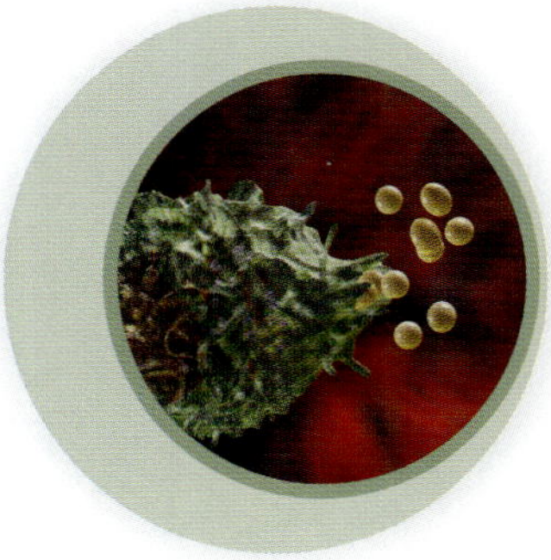

CHAPTER 8

BOVINE LIQUID COLOSTRUM WITH PRPS: A PHYSICIAN'S CLINICAL EXPERIENCE WITH AUTOIMMUNE DISEASES AND OTHER CONDITIONS

By Kenneth J. Frank, M.D.

In my 19 years of nutritional research, I have never come across anything with an effect as powerful, rapid, and far-reaching as liquid bovine colostrum with PRPs (Proline-rich Polypeptides). This supplement has far-reaching effects on overall health. While there is an abundance of scientific literature supporting the use of colostrum with PRPs to treat many disease states, in this chapter I would like to explain why, as a clinician, I have been so impressed by my personal experience with PRPs.

PRPs are specialized peptides or very small polypeptides (chains of amino acids found in the colostrum of all mammals). The most common source of these PRPs is cow's colostrum.

PRPs are powerful and very fast-acting immune signalers. In this capacity, they signal the immune system to upgrade its actions to fight infections, including those of viral (including AIDS and hepatitis), bacterial (including highly antibiotic resistant bacterial strains), parasitic (including malaria), and fungal origins. These PRPs also upgrade immune activities that are known to help prevent and fight cancer. On the other hand, they can downgrade certain actions of the immune system that may become overactive, thus rapidly reversing symptoms of autoimmune diseases. In many disease states, they aid in stopping chronic pain.

And that is not all. In my clinical experience, I've also seen that in most people who use them, PRPs have a powerful effect on restoring energy levels. They also stand out as a number one choice in treatment plans for people who seek relief from chronic fatigue, or for people who simply want to feel more energy. For many, this is the most important affect of colostrum. Additionally, PRPs have far-reaching protective effects on the gastrointestinal tract. They are useful for the treatment of colitis in its many forms (including ulcerative colitis and Crohn's disease) and to prevent the damage done to the gastrointestinal tract from chronic use of NSAIDs (non-steroidal anti-inflammatory drugs) such as aspirin, ibuprofen, and naproxen – the most commonly used treatments for joint pain.

As if this were not enough, in my clinical experience, I have observed people who have remarkably improved from symptoms of numerous autoimmune diseases such as rheumatoid arthritis, lupus erythematosus, Sjögren's syndrome, and multiple sclerosis. I have also witnessed its positive effects on ankylosing spondylitis and spinal stenosis.

Let me share with you how I came to learn about the PRPs in liquid bovine colostrum and the clinical experiences I've personally had that confirm the benefits of this nutritional supplement.

I am a physician (NYU Medical School, 1972) who has always been interested in alternative approaches to health and healing. During my practicing years, I personally saw or oversaw as a medical director over 300,000 patient visits. Having spent long enough in the practice of modern allopathic medicine to fully grasp both its incredible benefits and its tremendous liabilities, I made the choice to engage full-time in the research, development and distribution of nutritional products. Over the years, I had seen that many drug treatments caused harm due to side effects. News stories in the past 20 years have borne this out: that drugs, which are made to have highly specific action in the body can cause harm or even death—even when used correctly.

This happens much more often than the public is aware. As the scale of the use of medications expands farther and farther—it is estimated, as of this writing, that almost half of the U.S. population has taken at least one prescription drug in the past month—adverse events and side effects become increasingly prominent issues in medicine. Drugs most commonly linked with deaths or serious side effects are in the classes of pain medications (non-steroidal anti-inflammatory drugs, also known as NSAIDs) and those that alter the function of the immune system (e.g. drugs administered to treat symptoms of autoimmune diseases).

In a meta-analysis of studies published in 1998 in the ***Journal of the American Medical Association*** (JAMA), researchers found that around 100,000 deaths occur each year in hospitals due to drug side effects.[383] Five percent of hospital admissions are due to drug side effects.[384] In fact, when a patient visits his or her doctor for a new problem, a good physician always considers the significant possibility that this problem may be from a drug side effect.

Nowhere is this problem worse than in the arena of pain treatment with the most commonly prescribed NSAIDs. Most gastrointestinal bleeds and ulcers are side effects of NSAIDs[385,386]. Even more surprisingly, studies show that 50 percent of those who take an NSAID according to recommended daily doses within days of initiating therapy exhibit damage to their upper GI tract[387,388,] and that after two weeks (depending on the NSAID and the study), from 15 to 30 percent show signs of ulcer development[389].

Unfortunately, almost all NSAID-induced ulcers are asymptomatic. As a result, the first indication of their presence may be a GI bleed. Symptomatic ulcers of the upper GI tract occur in 2.5 to 5 percent of NSAID users each year, and significant complications such as upper GI bleeding, obstruction, and perforation occur in one to 1.5 percent of users each year. Considering current concern about the extraordinary cost of health care in this country, it is even more amazing to consider that this GI bleeding results in about 100,000 hospitalizations per year (according to data from the 1990s) with about 10 percent mortality. Some experts have calculated that for every dollar spent on NSAIDs, between sixty-five cents and $1.25 is spent on treating GI adverse effects associated with these medicines.

My immediate family has fallen prey to several severe drug side effects. In 2002, during her third trimester of pregnancy, my daughter, a stable, highly productive mother and successful business woman developed severe depression feeling overwhelmed with her life and emotionally removed progressively worsening over two months. Multiple doctors including psychiatrists could not figure this out and put her on anti-depressants. Finally, after she could no longer even get out of bed because of severe lethargy, I looked closely at her medications. Among her medications was one that was commonly prescribed for acid reflux from pregnancy, and, once this was stopped, she returned to normal in one day. I was admitted to the hospital in 2004 because of an upper GI bleed due to overuse of NSAIDs. These aren't the only drug side effects my family has experienced—just the most serious.

I saw, back in the late 1980s, that natural products were safer than drugs and that they had the potential to be equally or more effective in some cases. I knew that the funding for drug research far outweighed any potential funding for research into natural products—this, due to the fact that a synthetic drug can be patented and sold at far higher prices than natural products, which cannot be patented. For the same reason, it is also more difficult to gather adequate funding to conduct the same kinds of research studies on natural products than on synthetic drugs, which has made it difficult for such products to gain the respect they truly deserve in the practice of medicine. Still, the research I had seen on natural therapies and their relative lack of side effects and drug interactions drew me to make a big shift in 1993 from full-time practicing MD to full-time researcher, developer, and distributor of nutritional products. Interestingly, some of the therapies upon which I have focused much of my energy have yielded supplement products designed to relieve many of the same symptoms relieved by the most dangerous classes of drugs. Some of these supplements can relieve symptoms that modern, mainstream medical care cannot do well, such as chronic fatigue. Even more importantly, these supplements do not come close to causing the negative side effects that often occur with pharmaceutical medicines.

Sometimes, through a long process of research and investigation, I find supplements that work to help my customers. At other times, I find out about an exciting supplement by accident. My discovery of bovine colostrum was just such a fortunate accident.

How I Discovered Bovine Colostrum

One fateful day, I connected with a fascinating 80-year-old humanitarian named Dick Kolt. On the phone, Dick told me about his philanthropic work, much of which centered around a particular health product: a liquid form of bovine colostrum, the first food made by a cow for its newborn calf. It wasn't long before Dick learned from me that I had developed several natural products for pain relief—an arena in which he also had an interest.

Dick continued to speak at length about this colostrum product, and while he told me about its ability to stop pain in people who had autoimmune diseases —a special area of interest for me—he centered his discussion on treating AIDS orphans in Africa. He told me that he had seen this supplement rapidly (within hours) stop severe diarrhea and then, in the following weeks, quickly reverse the wasting aspect of AIDS so that these children gained weight and their energy was restored. He said a lot of things about colostrum to me that, at the time, seemed preposterous, but his passion and transparent honesty kept me on the phone.

I knew from experience that something with such amazing healing properties ***could*** exist without the public at large knowing about it. Stringent FDA rules about health claims for natural products have made it extremely difficult to inform the public about these products, even when they seem to be a slam-dunk in terms of risk-to-benefit ratio. Gradually, as Dick and I conversed, I began to see how my particular decade-old interest in natural therapies for inflammation and pain relief might bring me to investigate colostrum—particularly, the liquid version of colostrum that Dick was telling me about—more fully.

Dick recommended that I connect with a scientist named Andrew Keech, PhD—the author of most of this book. Dr. Keech had been supplying Dick with colostrum to take to Kenya and other parts of Africa, where he was using it to help people with life-threatening diseases like AIDS and the resulting diarrheal wasting disease these people developed. When I connected with Dr. Keech, I found that he had an incredible volume of knowledge and enthusiasm about the health benefits of bovine colostrum in both powdered form and in a liquid form rich in a particular immune-signaling substance called ***Proline-rich Polypeptides,*** or PRP (also referred to here as PRPs).

From Dr. Keech, I received thick packets full of information about colostrum and PRPs, including hundreds of scientific studies regarding the health-promoting, healing, and therapeutic properties of this first food made by any mammal for its newborn. I was most struck by the research into PRPs, which are covered in depth in this book. As it turned out, Dr. Keech had discovered a way to process fresh liquid colostrum that would ensure a very high content of PRPs. I always approach these kinds of seeming natural health breakthroughs with skepticism, but the scientific literature describing the benefits of PRPs was very impressive—an eye-opener to me.

I examined the information on colostrum that Dr. Keech had given me, along with doing some of my own independent investigation, and said to myself, "Wow!" I saw that it could really help our customers who were seeking pain relief but did not respond as well as hoped to my natural products for pain. I also realized it could be an incredible aid to our many customers who have autoimmune diseases and chronic fatigue.

In the past decade, I have decided that no matter how good the scientific literature appears to be regarding the positive health benefits of a supplement, it is best to observe the supplement's effects first-hand before releasing it to the public. The next step I took was to obtain Dr. Keech's PRP colostrum and to use it myself. Immediately, I was pleased by how easy it was to use—simply spray beneath the tongue, hold there, and swallow.

I had already developed four other products with a similar delivery system, so I was well aware of its benefits of delivering ingredients rapidly and effectively through the mucous membranes of the mouth, tongue, and throat into the bloodstream. Beneath the tongue, many blood vessels lie immediately under the mucous membranes; spraying the product under the tongue maximizes absorption in this location. Much is also absorbed through the mucous membranes in the rest of the mouth.

I was aware that powdered colostrum had been used for many years as a health food and that it certainly had some health benefits. Liquid colostrum has been used less frequently. While there are cases of Third World countries having used liquid colostrum directly from cows, almost all colostrum used by the public has been in powdered form.

While powdered colostrum is of huge value and has many health-promoting effects, my interest was most piqued by PRPs. I came to realize that PRPs are very powerful immune signalers and that small amounts can have far-reaching effects. I also recognized early on that PRPs are most available in a liquid colostrum form. Here's why: when powdered colostrum is swallowed, the gastrointestinal tract in the process of digestion destroys many of the active ingredients, including PRPs. On the other hand, when the liquid colostrum is sprayed into the mouth, held there, and swallowed, the PRPs are, for the most part, absorbed intact into the bloodstream early in the digestive process through the mucous membranes of the mouth and esophagus. They are protected against digestive enzymes and acids that would otherwise break them down.

As I used the PRP liquid colostrum myself, I also handed it to as many others as possible: friends, family, employees, and other volunteers who were willing to give it a try. Over time, I began to make it available to the tens of thousands of customers who buy nutritional products from my company every month.

I told my staff to inquire, whenever someone called to make a purchase, as to what health conditions might be affecting the customer on the line. If these individuals had a health condition that was on the long list of issues given to me by Dr. Keech (which you'll find on pages 57-60 of this book), I instructed them to give me the phone. I particularly looked for those who had autoimmune diseases, since these are notoriously difficult for physicians to treat. I also looked for other diseases that PRPs were touted to work for and that are also notoriously hard for physicians to treat, such as spinal stenosis and fibromyalgia. I would tell the customer about this remarkable colostrum and would give him or her the option to try it. Thereafter, I did my best to follow up with any customer who tried the product to track the benefits or problems they might encounter.

In these follow-ups, the promise of the scientific literature I had seen—particularly, the research Dr. Keech had sent to demonstrate how PRPs might impact specific diseases—was confirmed. Since that time, I have personally been witness to reversal of symptoms for many (over 40) cases of autoimmune diseases including multiple sclerosis, rheumatoid arthritis, Sjögren's disease, lupus erythematosus, ankylosing spondylitis and fibromyalgia (which is believed by some to be an auto-immune disease) with liquid bovine colostrum. This also reduced pain for many with garden-variety osteoarthritis. I've seen huge changes in people who were sick constantly before starting on the PRP supplement and who have more than halved or completely stopped their yearly episodes of bacterial and viral infectious illnesses while using the supplement and shortened the course of them if they did occur. I received reports of cold sores healing much more quickly; of stubborn warts disappearing; and of persistent, antibiotic-resistant ***Staphylococcus aureus*** infections dissipating with regular use of PRPs.

Commonly, users reported pronounced boosts in energy levels and relief from mood swings (some even reported that their PMS symptoms disappeared, including pain and moodiness). Trying to understand this better, I delved deeper into the biochemistry of the immune system and the PRPs, and learned that in most situations there was a reasonable explanation for how the PRPs worked to alleviate the myriad symptoms for which they seemed to be so effective.

Some of the most astounding results I have witnessed have been for those with autoimmune diseases. While the literature on PRPs supports the use of colostrum for these diseases, I decided I had to prove its value for these diseases for myself. I have personally witnessed cases of people with autoimmune diseases (lupus, multiple sclerosis, Sjögren's disease, rheumatoid arthritis, and more) who, in many cases, showed significant levels of improvement on multiple levels. Some enjoyed complete reversal of symptoms of fatigue and pain. About 25 percent of customers with autoimmune disease whom I tracked did not experience any detectable change that they could attribute to the colostrum. For those who did respond, the loss of fatigue usually occurred as the first sign of the PRPs doing their work. This was usually quick, with a pronounced decrease in as little as one day for many and within a week for most. The reversal of pain was more variable, but usually, when it occurred, it became evident in three days to two weeks. Some who had skin manifestations of their disease noticed changes within a week, and some showed complete disappearance in one month.

The History of Colostrum and Transfer Factor

For 50 years, scientists have known that colostrum contains a substance that was believed to transfer immunity from one animal to another—thus its name, ***transfer factor***. Curiously, the actual identity of transfer factor was, for many years, a mystery. Scientists knew that something in colostrum could have profound effects on the immune system, but they didn't know exactly what that something was. At the time of this initial research, they also knew that what they were calling transfer factor could be obtained from white blood cells.

Sherwood Lawrence, MD, was a professor of mine at NYU Medical School 36 years ago. He was one of the first scientists to study transfer factor. I still remember him saying that there was something in the plasma of an animal that could transfer immune activity to another animal when the plasma was injected into the bloodstream of that other animal, but that his research team had not yet identified the exact substance.

In 1974, a group of Polish scientists isolated peptides and small polypeptides from cow's milk that further research showed acted very much like what scientists had been calling transfer factor. It turns out that these peptides and polypeptides, called ***colostrinin*** by the Polish scientists after their origin in colostrum, were, in fact, this mysterious transfer factor. Transfer factor later came to be called Proline-rich Polypeptides (PRP or PRPs). Polypeptides and peptides are the building blocks of proteins, built from various configurations of amino acids; these particular polypeptides, as the name suggests, are rich in the amino acid proline

PRP is actually not a single peptide, but rather a group of similar peptides that function as cellular signaling molecules. Approximately 85 have been identified in bovine colostrum. Many of these PRPs are identical to those found in human colostrum. In the case of colostral PRPs, these peptides modulate the immune system by suppressing it if overactive or stimulating it when underactive when it has been weakened or compromised—or when the immune system needs to be more active to overcome infection or cancer.

While it was originally thought that transfer factor transferred immunity to an individual, it is now believed that what actually happens is somewhat different, that transfer factor does not actually transfer immunity. Rather, it stimulates a weakened or underactive immune system, which then creates stronger immune system activity than would have occurred without the use of the PRPs. It kicks the immune system into gear.

PRPs, on the other hand, have the ability to suppress an overactive immune response, such as in an autoimmune condition. This suppression was not initially noted by scientists as they tried to figure out what this transfer factor was; they only recognized the immune stimulation effect. As it turns out, PRPs can play a dual role: both immune enhancer and immune downregulator, and they can play both roles at the same time.

Literally thousands of papers have been written about colostrum by scientists at major universities and research centers in over 25 countries. A subset of these papers that deal with PRPs/transfer factor has found that administration of transfer factor may confer benefit in over forty disease conditions. It appears that the best way to deliver high concentrations of PRPs is with a liquid supplement.

All in all, over 4,000 of my customers have used PRP liquid colostrum. Several thousand reorder it regularly. My staff and I have followed up with as many of these customers as possible. Here are a few of the many stories I've heard from happy users of PRP liquid colostrum.

Anne: In Need of an Immune Boost

Anne, one of my employees, used to get sick quite often. "At least once a month for five or six days," she reports, "and I'd get strep throat three or four times a year." She had very low energy, and her doctors had started her on antidepressants to try to boost her mood and give her more 'get-up-and-go.' Even though some aspects of her immunity seemed to be less than effective, she also had severe eczema—a symptom of an overactive immune system. In other words, Anne's immune system just wasn't functioning well. It wasn't kicking in enough when it was really needed, and it was overshooting at other times. This made her a perfect candidate for PRP colostrum, which is able to move these two extremes of immune dysfunction back towards a balance point that improves health.

A week after Anne began working in my office, she caught a bug and stayed home. I sent over some PRP liquid colostrum. She took it as directed and was pleased to find that her illness only lasted for three days rather than the customary week. Anne kept using the spray and found that over the next year or so, she only got sick once or twice—a reduction in bouts of illness of over 50 percent. The strep throat infections also stopped coming, and when I interviewed her for this story, it had been a year and a half since her last bout of strep.

Anne's eczema had been a major problem. It had covered her forearms and itched terribly. This recurrent eczema has disappeared since she began to use the PRP spray. She was amazed to find that a wart she'd had for ten years disappeared within two months of starting this spray. (My own grandson, Mason, had this same experience. He had a stubborn wart on his hand that a physician had tried to remove and that had returned. Once he began the PRP spray, the wart went away and never reappeared.)

"One thing that really surprised me with the PRP spray was the energy I felt," she told me. "Before, I was chronically fatigued. I was always tired during the day and sleepless at night. This was so frustrating for me—I was motivated to get things done, but I always felt like I was up against this solid wall of fatigue." She experienced a boost in energy after starting PRP. "I had more energy, and I was sleeping better. I started to wake faster in the mornings and napped less. The energy I feel is ***even***—no more drastic ups and downs like I used to have. And my emotions, too, don't swing up and down so dramatically." Her regular doctor decided that she could taper off the antidepressants. When we had our interview, she had been off of them for a year.

Anne decided to give the PRP spray to her daughter and even to her pets. Her daughter, who got sick often as well, had a dramatic decrease in her bouts of infectious illness—from four to five times per year to one to two times per year.

What is it about PRP colostrum that could have all of these diverse effects in one person? That's what this book explains in great detail in other chapters, but the short version goes something like this: PRP and other ingredients of colostrum have balancing, modulating effects on the immune system. These effects can boost aspects of immunity that are flagging—such as Anne's ability to fight off infectious "bugs" and to mount an immune reaction against a wart, eliminating it—and they can reduce over-activity in other aspects of immunity, such as those that cause eczema.

Why the increased energy? So far, we aren't completely sure about the full picture here. From my experience, I know that increased energy is one of the most common effects people report with the use of the PRP-rich colostrum. Users report fewer ups and downs in energy and mood; less stress, better sleep, less need for daytime naps, and enhanced daytime alertness.

We know that constantly fighting a losing battle against infections can be very depleting; perhaps the immune boost from the PRPs allowed Anne's body to conserve energy for other things. PRPs are messenger peptides that signal cells to produce another group of messenger molecules—small proteins called cytokines. It is these cytokines that, in the end, mediate and regulate the specific activities of the immune system. Different types of cytokines can upregulate or downregulate the immune system's function. It is believed that a certain mix of cytokines promoted by the PRPs enhances energy.

Colostrum is also very good for the digestive tract, helping to promote better digestion and assimilation of foods; this could help the body obtain nutrients needed for high-energy lifestyles that have previously been lacking. PRPs improve nutrient absorption quite significantly, resulting in much healthier hair, skin and nails. Most noticeable in my experience for myself and others is much stronger nails after three months of PRP use.

Colostrum contains dozens of compounds (including PRP, growth factors, antibodies, cytokines, interferon, lactoferrin, and retinoic acid) that may affect energy levels and sleep quality. Some of these are only contained in the powdered form of colostrum.

The PRP liquid form created by Andrew Keech has larger molecules removed so that its main active ingredient is the PRPs. You will learn far more about these compounds and the overall health effects of colostrum as you move through this book—which is a veritable 'bible' on the subject!

Monique: Colonized by Dangerous Staph Infection (MRSA)

Another employee, Monique, had recurrent ***Staphylococcus aureus*** infections. These infections could not even be eradicated with methicillin, the antibiotic recognized as the best treatment for this type of infection; in other words, she was fighting a MRSA (Methicillin-Resistant Staphyloccus Aureus) infection. Her doctor had told her that she would continue to develop abscesses because her skin had become colonized, and no medication was able to stop this.

Staph is no picnic to begin with, and when one becomes infected with a strain that is resistant to the antibiotics normally given to tame them, a difficult battle can ensue. The infection can linger on and on and even endanger the life of the person. Understandably, Monique was frightened. She was leaving to return to school around the time I first discovered PRP liquid colostrum.

When she left my employ, she stocked up on the PRP liquid colostrum. I instructed her to use it every four hours to assist the immune system in knocking out the staph infection (the general dose for restoration of energy and pain relief is lower—just twice daily). She stayed on the regimen I suggested for several months and then, when satisfied that the infection was gone, continued at twice per day. My strong feeling that it would help her was confirmed. Her staph infection disappeared and stayed away. One year later, she continues to use the PRP spray and has not developed further abscesses.

Cold Sore Help

I've seen PRP liquid colostrum do wonders for people with recurring herpes infections that show up as cold sores or shingles. Its stimulating effect on antibody production seems to help squash an outbreak in far less time. Kayvon, an employee at my offices, showed up one day with a big cold sore on his lip. I ventured to ask him about it and offered the PRP spray. He had almost immediate relief from the tingling and itching characteristic of cold sores, and the sore resolved completely in about four days with no scab formation. (Cold sores usually form scabs and take at least a week to heal.)

When the five-year-old son of a colleague who was using the PRP spray got his first cold sore, she began to give him the spray. Customarily, a first outbreak of herpes virus is intense—a large sore forms with a lot of discomfort and a lingering scab. Sometimes there are other, flu-like symptoms such as fever. "I started the spray as soon as the sore was recognizable as a cold sore," she told me. "The next day, it was ***gone,*** leaving just a red blotch that went away soon after that." She had similarly good effects with a cold sore while taking PRP. It went away in half the usual time and never scabbed over.

In fact, I've heard about and witnessed many cold-sore reversals with the PRP spray. The product has also worked well for people with genital herpes infections. Several people with chronic frequently reoccurring genital herpes infections report that with daily use of the PRP liquid colostrum, their recurrences have ceased. In some cases, these customers have had no outbreaks for 18 months and counting.

Amy: An Immune System Out of Balance

Amy is an extremely friendly and engaging owner of a company with which my company does regular business. She likes to stay on top of things and generally has lots of energy and enthusiasm. Over a year ago, I began to hear about her health problems, which began in the early 2000s. Those problems went on for at least four years. I was concerned, but believed that I might have a way to help her with the PRP liquid colostrum.

The first thing she noticed was digestive problems, including constipation and bloating. Soon after that, she began to gain weight and complained of just "not feeling right." Her father passed away in 2003, and that was when she first noticed these issues—which she chalked up to stress, as people often do when their doctors can find no cause for their problem.

But as her life began to fall back into place after her loss, she still wasn't feeling well: "I was tired. I had always been a high-energy person." Visits to doctors got her diagnoses of irritable bowel syndrome (IBS) and 'general stress.' She had symptoms consistent with low thyroid activity (hypothyroidism), including hair loss, but her thyroid tests appeared normal. No one seemed to think her problems merited drug therapy. Amy tried probiotics and other supplements, but nothing was helping her to move into feeling like her old self.

In 2007, after Amy had been feeling poorly for about four years, she had a colonoscopy to see whether her digestive issues might have a hidden source; the test was negative. She had gained about 18 pounds on her small frame—extra weight with which she felt very uncomfortable. And then, to add to her woes, she found a lump in her breast that doctors called "suspicious."

Amy underwent a breast biopsy that, thankfully, revealed no cancer. What it did reveal was something less dangerous but far more confusing: An uncommon lesion that doctors call ***lymphocytic lobulitis.*** This is a finding that the doctors believe is indicative of some kind of autoimmune disease, such as lupus or rheumatoid arthritis, but Amy's medical team couldn't put their finger on which autoimmune condition might be affecting her. (It isn't uncommon for doctors to inform patients that they suspect an autoimmune disease, but that they cannot identify a specific one.)

At that point, I had just begun to get excited about PRP liquid colostrum. I sent her a bottle as soon as I heard about her travails. Meanwhile, blood work could not lead to the identification of any specific autoimmune disease, leaving Amy without a clue as to exactly what was causing the symptoms that were interfering with her quality of life.

Doctors told her that they didn't want to do any more testing, but Amy knew that something was wrong. With nothing to lose, Amy started on the PRP spray. "Not even one day since then have I looked back," she told me with characteristic enthusiasm. "I started the PRP spray on a Friday morning and by Monday I was bouncing out of bed! I was back to my normal self within three weeks of taking the PRP, three sprays twice a day. My energy's back. My digestion is great. I lost six pounds and have no more constipation. I can go to bed at 10:30 instead of 8:30 and have plenty of energy the next day. And even when my trainer was out of town, I kept up with my workouts!"

Amy's turnaround was pretty amazing, but in light of what I had come to understand about colostrum and PRPs by that time, I wasn't all that surprised. I knew that colostrum had healing effects on the gut that could counteract so-called "leaky gut syndrome," where food sensitivities or NSAIDs (non-steroidal anti-inflammatory drugs) erode the protective lining of the small intestine, allowing food particles that have not been completely broken down to pass into the circulation and inhibiting absorption of nutrients. The immune system then reacts against those particles, creating a state of inflammation in the body and causing irritable bowel symptoms further down the line.

Seventy percent of the immune system cells are located in the walls of the gastro-intestinal tract. This is primarily due to the Peyer's patches, which are collections of lymphocytes that make antibodies. Peyer's patches reside in the walls of the intestines. This may explain why colostrum is so effective in helping people with gastrointestinal diseases such as the various types of colitis. Colostrum has been shown to protect the GI tract from damage by NSAIDs, the dangers of which I discussed earlier in this chapter. Throughout the remainder of this book, you will learn a great deal more about the positive effects of colostrum on GI health.

My experience with PRPs has included customers finding relief from symptoms of some rare immune related conditions such as ankylosing spondylitis. This chronic and usually progressive condition primarily involves pain and inflammation of the joints and usually strikes in early life with the potential to cause severe limitations of movement and pain. I have also received anecdotal reports from people with more common auto-immune diseases such as rheumatoid arthritis, lupus erythematosus, multiple sclerosis and Sjögren's disease.

Autoimmune diseases are so difficult to treat because they are caused by the body's immune system targeting its own cells and organs for destruction. Medical treatment usually involves drugs that turn the immune system way down or off with immunomodulating drugs, chemotherapy drugs, and powerful steroid medications, all of which have a long list of potentially devastating side effects—as any patient using these medications will tell you. I feel confident that PRP can have a significant role in the healing process for anyone with autoimmune problems.

Marlene: Help with Lupus-Related Exhaustion

Marlene is a 72-year-old customer who had just completed a move from Phoenix to Southern California—"it's just too hot in Phoenix!" she told me—and soon after getting settled, she developed the characteristic rash seen in lupus patients. The rash, which came up on her legs and hands, was severe enough to leave scars. After many tests in her rheumatologist's office, she was told that she had lupus.

She knew one thing for sure: she was exhausted. "Whenever I wanted to walk anywhere, I had to stop and take a breath," she told me. "It took forever to get out of the car." She had trouble getting out of bed. Her right foot became numb and the pinky finger and third finger on her left hand also became numb. Then, she saw one of my advertisements on television and called; she began to take my pain relief spray and found herself regaining some feeling in those areas.

One day, I had occasion to speak with Marlene on the phone and suggested the PRP spray. She tried it, and found her symptoms of fatigue much improved. Then, a bout of heart failure brought her a one-and-a-half-month hospital stay. "I couldn't take the immune spray while I was there, and I felt the difference. I couldn't wait to get back on it when I got home." Within a couple of weeks, she reported, the PRP spray had restored her energy. (Of note is that I have followed others with lupus who have had skin and joint problems that have responded well to the use of PRPs.)

Corina: Fibromyalgia, Osteoarthritis and Chronic Fatigue

Another employee, Corina, had spinal osteoarthritis in her neck and low back. On top of this, she developed fibromyalgia, a painful condition with unknown causes that results in daily, total-body, severe muscle pain. As often happens with fibromyalgia, Corina also developed debilitating chronic fatigue that was diagnosed as chronic fatigue syndrome (CFS). "For a year," she told me, "getting out of bed or walking were so, so hard." Not surprisingly, she fell into very low spirits feeling depressed as her health declined.

I started her on some natural products, and she found that her fibromyalgia and osteoarthritis pain improved by about 50 percent. Still, she suffered from chronic fatigue and low mood. I added the PRP spray to her supplement plan. "Then, I was 80 to 90 percent pain-free," she told me. "My energy returned and my depression lifted."

The first couple of weeks on the PRP spray, she had some sleep disturbance—a circumstance that occurs in a limited number of PRP liquid colostrum users, and one I'll discuss a little later in this chapter. All in all, however, she slept better with PRP as her pain no longer woke her up. Once she got through the initial couple of weeks of disturbed sleep while taking the supplement, she found she could sleep more soundly than ever for as much as eight to 10 hours a night—something that had been impossible before.

Convinced of the value of PRP-rich colostrum, Corina began to give it to her daughter, Amanda. "Amanda had been constantly sick with chronic middle ear infections. She was about to get tubes in her ears. But after a month and a half on PRP spray, she had no more earaches." At the time we had our interview for this chapter, it had been a year since Amanda's last ear infection. She still suffered some from allergies but had been able to reduce her use of allergy medication while taking PRP colostrum.

Tammy: Multiple Sclerosis Help

I was happy to hear from Tammy, a 38-year-old mom from Halifax, Nova Scotia, about her PRP experience. She was diagnosed with multiple sclerosis (MS) in her 20s, and although she is not confined to a wheelchair, she had been suffering pain, stiffness, shaking, and fatigue due to her disease. Just prior to using the PRPs her symptoms had gotten so severe that she basically had become homebound and had given up on her workout program. Her doctors were frustrated because none of the medications they were trying seemed adequate to stop Tammy's pain.

Tammy describes herself as someone who doesn't like to take pills. She had resigned herself to using one medication to relieve the muscle spasms characteristic of people with MS. Within a few days of starting to take PRP spray, she noticed reduced fatigue and improved energy. Her pain and stiffness disappeared altogether.

She wrote to me in an e-mail, "I want to thank you for this wonderful product. It is giving me the opportunity to work out again to keep me from a wheelchair, and a chance to live my life again. I have an 11-year-old, a husband, a three-story home, and a large black lab, and using your products gives me enough energy and relief of MS symptoms to take care of my family. THANK YOU!"

Tammy is one of eight customers with multiple sclerosis who I have followed. Most of them showed quick improvement and continued to improve more and more over time. What they appreciated the most was how rapidly their energy levels turned around.

Support for Those With HIV/AIDS

When I got that fateful call from Dick Kolt, he told me about his use of colostrum to help African communities stricken by infectious diseases, including the AIDS virus. AIDS reduces levels of T cells, which are essential immune factors; PRP supplementation has been found, in a few studies performed in Kenya, to raise T cell count and decrease viral load and slow weight loss in people with AIDS.

In these same studies, symptoms like nausea, malaise, diarrhea, and vomiting were significantly reduced with the use of PRP. Other common sequelae of the AIDS virus, such as tuberculosis, fever, cough, and nerve damage (paresthesias), were also reduced. (These studies are covered in detail later in this section of the book.)

Alex: Raging PMS

Alex worked for me for some time, and she complained of having the full gamut of PMS symptoms around that time of the month. "Restless legs, mood swings, cramps—every symptom imaginable," she sighed. I gave her the PRP spray and told her, "Let's see if it helps."

It did help her. Her cramps and mood swings were much reduced. She found herself sleeping better as well. She began to use it just around her periods. During an episode of bronchitis that turned to walking pneumonia, she found it helpful as well; she offered some to her mother-in-law during a bout of shingles. "Usually, shingles lasts a long time," she told me, "but with the PRP it was gone in a few days."

Alex wasn't the only person in her family who benefited from PRP. Her husband, a building contractor, was in constant pain from spinal stenosis. In this condition, the spinal canal narrows, impinging on the nerves that emerge from the cord to the rest of the body. The result is nerve pain that can be severe. He found that PRP helped his pain, stiffness, and lack of sleep, and it proved helpful in only a matter of days after he started to use it. Even Alex's beloved pet Pomeranian, Neil, ended up using PRP: he had patellar luxation, where his kneecap would slip out of place, causing inflammation and a limp. Alex observed that regular use of this spray stopped his limp.

When asked why PRP spray might help with PMS symptoms, I have to admit that I don't really know. It may be that more conditions are related to the immune system than we are currently aware of. It may have to do with decreased inflammation, more energy, reduction in the body's production of stress hormones, or better sleep. At this juncture, we simply don't know. But as long as the product is safe—and colostrum is safe, as has been shown by research where very high doses are given to try to gauge how much is too much—it makes sense to use it when it seems to help.

Side Effects and Warnings

Some people who go on the PRP liquid colostrum find that as their daytime energy improves, their sleep is also disturbed. This is the most common side effect I have encountered with this product. In some instances, this shows up as insomnia; in others, people go to sleep as they normally would, but then awaken three or four hours later and have trouble getting back to sleep.

This almost always resolves within three weeks, but that can feel like a very long time if sleep is frequently disrupted. What I recommend is to reduce the dose. My initial instructions are to use it in the morning and the evening with three sprays under the tongue at each time, and if this causes sleep disturbance, I instruct them to start with only one spray in the morning. If they don't have sleep disturbance at this dose, I advise them to increase the dose by one spray every two to three days. Then, I advise that as they gradually increase the morning dose, they introduce the afternoon or evening dose, starting with one spray and increasing gradually to the target dose as long as there is no sleep disturbance. If increasing the dose brings back the sleep disruption, I recommend reducing again until the body can adjust. This has worked for all except three people who, even at one dose per day, had sleep disturbance and could not continue.

Nursing mothers need to be careful about using PRP colostrum as it may cause sleep disturbance in a newborn. I don't recommend it for pregnant mothers since it could theoretically lead to rejection of the fetus. People who have had organ transplants should avoid it, as it could promote organ rejection.

In other parts of this book, and in the ensuing chapters, particularly, there is detailed explanation about PRPs and the complex mechanisms by which they work to balance (enhance or suppress, as needed) the immune system. Clearly, the value of understanding and using these remarkable substances is tremendous. While PRP liquid colostrum is an extraordinary tool for the practicing physician to use in the treatment of so many difficult-to-treat medical problems, these PRPs are available for anyone to try. Few who do so fail to find some benefit.

As a physician and formulator of natural products, I'm convinced that PRP liquid colostrum is safe, effective, and of great value. I have seen how many diseases that are very common and difficult to treat—and becoming more common every day—can be successfully addressed with PRP colostrum. I encourage you to read on to understand these remarkable substances in greater detail.

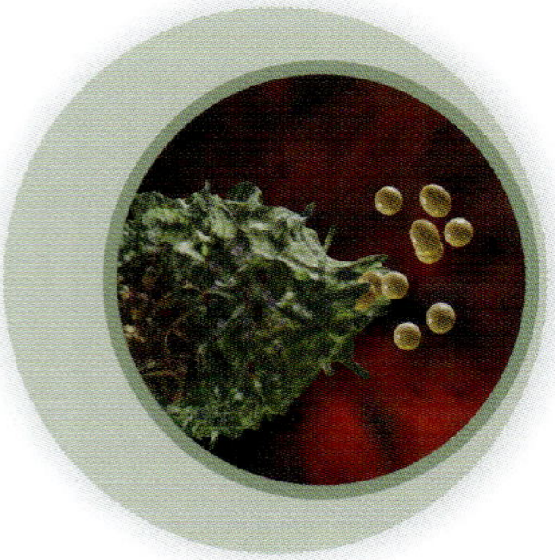

CHAPTER 9

WHAT ARE PROLINE-RICH POLYPEPTIDES?

Proline-rich Polypeptides (PRPs) are one of the components of colostrum, as discussed in Part I. They function as signaling peptides that control the production of specific proteins, such as immunoglobulins, in cells of the immune system. Such signaling peptides are found throughout the body and are the main regulators of protein synthesis in cells for those proteins which are involved in extracellular functions, such as immunoglobulins.

Signaling peptides function as messengers in the body. They are how a cell keeps up with the latest news and events occurring in other parts of the body. If an infection of cold viruses is discovered in the lungs, for example, the cells of the immune system need to be informed of this so that they can join in the defense. So in this case the signaling peptides are like the alarm box in the firehouse. They warn the cells of the immune system that there is a problem and that they are needed to help fix it.

PRPs have the unique ability to modulate the immune system, increasing its activity level in the case of a challenge, such as an infection or a wound, and decreasing its activity level when the challenge is controlled. When an infection is detected by scout immune cells, chemical signals go out to mobilize other cells to come to the defense and fight off the infection. PRPs are one of the primary signals to go out at this time. And later, when the infection has been contained, PRPs are again one of the primary signals to call down the inflammatory response to the infection.

Thymocytes—lymphocytes which develop in the thymus gland in the neck—have PRP receptors on their surface membranes.[390] These thymocytes are stimulated by PRPs to either differentiate into helper T cells,[391] which are part of the inflammatory response to infection, or suppressor T cells[392] which inhibit the inflammatory response. PRPs regulate the differentiation and maturation of monocytes and macrophages, cells normally found in the bloodstream and connective tissue which are involved inflammation.[393] PRPs also induce resting B lymphocytes—lymphocytes that develop in the bone marrow—to differentiate and form mature B cells.[394] B cells are the only cells which produce immunoglobulins (antibodies).[395]

PRPs regulate the production of various cytokines, which are signaling molecules that regulate the immune response. These include IL-6 (interleukin-6), IL-10, INF-γ (gamma interferon) and TNF-α (tumor necrosis factor-alpha).[396] This is one of the ways in which PRPs regulate the inflammatory response to infection. Both IL-6 and IL-10 are anti-inflammatory cytokines, but TNF-α is the main cytokine controlling the entire inflammatory cascade of cytokines. INF-γ is an inflammatory cytokine as well. It is particularly effective against viruses as it interferes with the genetic ability of viruses to replicate.

The inflammatory response consists of a complex series of events in which the body mobilizes its defenses to the site of the infection. PRPs are involved in that mobilization effort as well as controlling the production of immune proteins by immune cells. PRPs stimulate the production of leukocytes (white blood cells) which are a principal component of the inflammatory response.[397] PRPs increase the permeability of the blood vessels in the skin allowing immune cells and antibodies to enter the tissue space to fight off the infection.[398] PRPs stimulate natural killer (NK) cells, which are a specialized type of hunter-killer lymphocytes. They are the first responders in case of an infection and will attack and destroy anything they encounter that is not identified as "self."

PRP has been shown to be a potent stimulator of NK cell activity. Dr. Daryl See, MD, Director of the Bioassay Laboratory at the Institute of Longevity Medicine, conducted a comparative study of 196 dietary supplements that claimed immune system enhancement, broad-spectrum antimicrobial activity and antioxidant action. Bovine colostrum was shown to promote significant NK cytotoxicity.[399] Later studies by Dr. See showed that transfer factor (PRPs) increased NK cell cytotoxicity by up to 400%. Among other natural products that increase NK cell cytotoxicity, none exceeded a 50% increase.[400] Another study by Dr. See showed that a combination of nutraceutical products, including transfer factor (PRPs), increased the cytotoxic activity of NK cells in patients with late-stage cancer.[401]

PRPs are immunoregulatory, however, so their function is not limited to calling out the troops in case of infection. They also come into play when it is time for the troops to stand down. If the inflammatory response to infection were allowed to continue once the infection has been controlled or isolated, then normal tissues would come under attack by the activated immune cells. Antibodies would be produced against proteins of the body rather than foreign proteins. This is exactly what happens in autoimmune conditions when the body begins attacking its own proteins, causing serious consequences. Thus the immunoregulatory effect of PRPs is just as important as their ability to mobilize the immune system to fight an infection. Due to this ability to both stimulate and dampen the immune response, PRPs have shown a great deal of promise in treating autoimmune conditions such as lupus, rheumatoid arthritis and Type I diabetes.

However, before we examine the benefits of PRPs in greater detail, let's take a look at the structure of PRPs and how signaling peptides actually work in the cell in order to give us a better idea of the process.

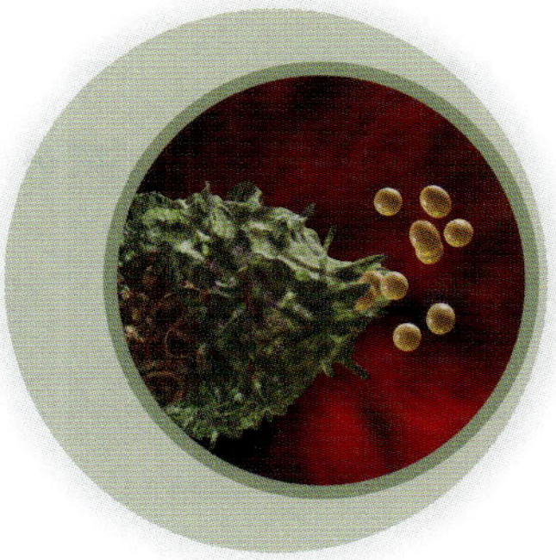

CHAPTER 10

STRUCTURE OF PRPS

A size exclusion ion-exchange column in a High Performance Chromatography Unit effectively separates the aqueous proteins in a liquid colostrum sample. The following pages in this chapter illustrate this peptide separation. Figure 1 shows an HPLC IX printout of a raw bovine liquid colostrum sample. Figure 2 shows the same colostrum sample, a liquid PRPs isolate, that has had the major colostrum components removed, leaving only the PRPs. By removing the other components of the beginning colostrum liquid, as shown in Figure 2, the peptides are now able to move more freely in the aqueous water solution, increasing the PRPs mass transfer coefficient, and thus transfer faster to our immune cells in our body, reducing molecular steric hindrance.

From Figure 2, the PRPs can be grouped by size into PRPs1 (larger, 2,500–5,000 molecular weight), PRP2 (1,000–2,500 molecular weight), and PRPs3 (500–1,000 molecular weight). PRPs1 are the non-protein nitrogen component of colostrum, also seen in mammalian milk, and is biologically inactive. Figure 3 is a close-up of Figure 2 PRPs.

Using Proteomics (Gas Chromatography/Mass Spectrometry combined with an extensive peptide database) there have been many PRPs identified in colostrum. Figure 3 shows the molecular appearance of PRPs2 and PRPs3 peptides.

HPLC Individual Sample Report

Reported by User: System   Project Name: IgGDetermination

SAMPLE INFORMATION

Sample Name:	Raw Colostrum 112905	Acquired By:	System
Sample Type:	Unknown	Date Acquired:	11/30/05 2:58:15 AM
Vial:	1	Acq. Method Set:	IgG_Method_Set2
Injection #:	1	Date Processed:	11/30/05 3:28:26 AM
Injection Volume:	30.00 ul	Processing Method:	IgG_Process2
Run Time:	30.0 Minutes	Channel Name:	280nm
Sample Set Name:	051129_PRP	Proc. Chnl. Descr.:	PDA 280.0 nm

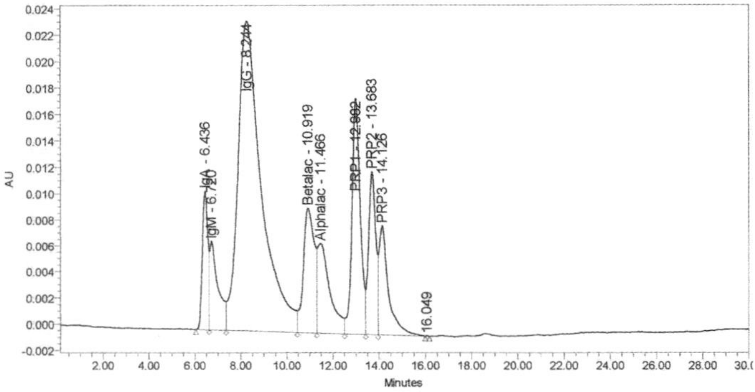

	Peak Name	RT	Area	% Area	Height	Amount	Units	Percent_IgG
1	IgA	6.436	175689	4.93	10629			
2	IgM	6.720	175551	4.92	6782			
3	IgG	8.244	1679042	47.08	23569	113.955	mg	67.5
4	Betalac	10.919	315423	8.84	9542			
5	Alphalac	11.466	262375	7.36	6870			
6	PRP1	12.982	449356	12.60	17973			
7	PRP2	13.683	269095	7.54	12457			
8	PRP3	14.126	239875	6.73	8372			
9		16.049	240	0.01	38			

FIGURE 1. HPLC OF RAW COLOSTRUM

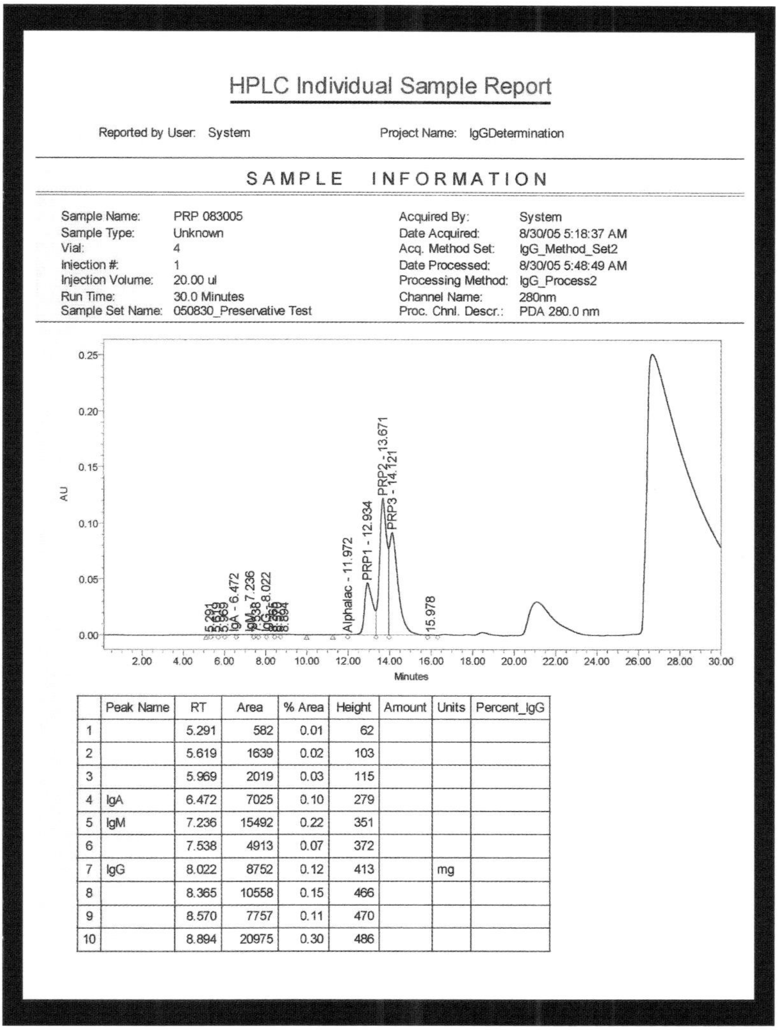

HPLC Individual Sample Report

Reported by User: System Project Name: IgGDetermination

SAMPLE INFORMATION

Sample Name:	PRP 083005	Acquired By:	System
Sample Type:	Unknown	Date Acquired:	8/30/05 5:18:37 AM
Vial:	4	Acq. Method Set:	IgG_Method_Set2
Injection #:	1	Date Processed:	8/30/05 5:48:49 AM
Injection Volume:	20.00 ul	Processing Method:	IgG_Process2
Run Time:	30.0 Minutes	Channel Name:	280nm
Sample Set Name:	050830_Preservative Test	Proc. Chnl. Descr.:	PDA 280.0 nm

	Peak Name	RT	Area	% Area	Height	Amount	Units	Percent_IgG
1		5.291	582	0.01	62			
2		5.619	1639	0.02	103			
3		5.969	2019	0.03	115			
4	IgA	6.472	7025	0.10	279			
5	IgM	7.236	15492	0.22	351			
6		7.538	4913	0.07	372			
7	IgG	8.022	8752	0.12	413		mg	
8		8.365	10558	0.15	466			
9		8.570	7757	0.11	470			
10		8.894	20975	0.30	486			

Figure 2. HPLC of PRPs liquid isolate

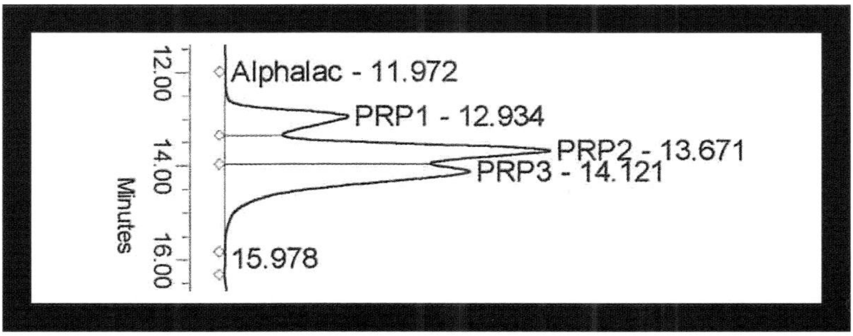

Figure 3. Close-up of PRPs1, PRPs2 and PRPs3 peaks.

	MW	Class	Approx. Volume	Amino Acid
				A= Ala= Alanine
Asp - Lys - Glu	390	PRP3	472	T = Thr Threonine
Leu - Asn - Phe	392	PRP3	474	V = Val = Valine
Ser - Glu - Gln - Pro	459	PRP3	555	C = Cys = Cysteine
Val - Val - Met - Glu - Val	576	PRP3	697	L = Leu = Leucine
Phe - Pro - Pro - Pro - Lys	585	PRP3	708	Y = Tyr = Tyrosine
Ser - Glu - Glu - Met - Pro	592	PRP3	716	I = Ile = Isoleucine
Pro - Gln - Ser - Val - Leu - Ser	630	PRP3	762	N = Asn = Asparagine
Asp - Ser - Gln - Pro - Pro - Val	642	PRP3	777	P = Pro = Proline
Val - Leu - Pro - Pro - Asn - Val - Gly	695	PRP3	841	Q = Gln = Glutamine
Asp - Pro - Pro - Pro - Pro - Gln - Ser	737	PRP3	892	F = Phe = Phenylalanine
Met - Gln - Pro - Pro - Pro - Leu - Pro	779	PRP3	943	D = Asp = Aspartic Acid
Ser - Trp - Met - His - Gln - Pro - Pro	882	PRP3	1067	W = Trp = Tryptophan
Ala - Phe - Leu - Leu - Tyr - Gln - Glu	883	PRP3	1068	E = Glu = Glutamic Acid
Arg - Gly - Pro - Phe - Pro - Ile - Leu - Val	898	PRP3	1087	M = Met = Methionine
Lys - Tyr - Lys - Leu - Gln - Pro - Glu	905	PRP3	1095	K = Lys = Lysine
Ser - Leu - Pro - Gln - Asn - Ile - Leu - Pro - Leu	994	PRP3	1203	G = Gly = Glycine
Val - Glu - Ser - Tyr - Val - Pro - Leu - Phe - Pro	1050	PRP3	1271	R = Arg = Arginine
Thr - Gln - Thr - Pro - Val - Val - Val - Pro - Pro - Phe	1084	PRP3	1312	S = Ser = Serine
Val - Tyr - Pro - Phe - Thr - Gly - Pro - Ile - Pro - Asn	1104	PRP2	1336	H = His = Histidine
Gln - Pro - Leu - Pro - Pro - Thr - Val - Met - Phe - Pro	1126	PRP2	1362	
Met - Pro - Gln - Asn - Phe - Tyr - Lys - Leu - Pro - Gln - Met	1397	PRP2	1690	
Leu - Phe - Phe - Phe - Leu - Pro - Val - Val - Asn - Val - Leu - Pro	1405	PRP2	1700	
Phe - Leu - Leu - Tyr - Gln - Glu - Pro - Val - Leu - Gly - Pro - Val - Arg	1531	PRP2	1853	
Val - Leu - Glu - Met - Lys - Phe - Pro - Pro - Pro - Pro - Gln - Glu - Thr - Val - Thr	1713	PRP2	2073	
Met - His - Gln - Pro - Pro - Gln - Pro - Leu - Pro - Pro - Thr - Val - Met - Phe - Pro	1717	PRP2	2078	
Asp - Leu - Glu - Met - Pro - Val - Leu - Pro - Val - Glu - Pro - Phe - Pro - Phe - Val	1729	PRP2	2092	
Leu - Lys - Pro - Phe - Pro - Lys - Leu - Lys - Val - Glu - Val - Phe - Pro - Phe - Pro	1786	PRP2	2161	
Leu - Gln - Thr - Pro - Gln - Pro - Leu - Leu - Gln - Val - Met - Met - Glu - Pro - Gln - Gly - Asp	1925	PRP2	2329	
Ser - Leu - Thr - Leu - Thr - Asp - Val - Glu - Lys - Leu - His - Leu - Pro - Leu - Pro - Leu - Val - Gln	2016	PRP2	2439	
Leu - Gln - Pro - Glu - Ile - Met - Gly - Val - Pro - Lys - Val - Lys - Glu - Thr - Met - Val - Pro - Lys	2024	PRP2	2449	
Asp - Gln - Pro - Pro - Asp - Val - Glu - Lys - Pro - Asp - Leu - Gln - Pro - Phe - Gln - Val - Gln - Ser	2067	PRP2	2501	
Ala - Thr - Phe - Asn - Arg - Tyr - Gln - Asp - Asp - His - Gly - Glu - Glu - Ile - Leu - Lys - Ser - Leu	2136	PRP2	2585	
His - Lys - Glu - Met - Pro - Phe - Pro - Lys - Tyr - Pro - Val - Glu - Pro - Phe - Thr - Glu - Ser - Gln	2191	PRP2	2651	
Leu - Ser - Gln - Pro - Lys - Val - Leu - Pro - Val - Pro - Gln - Lys - Ala - Val - Pro - Gln - Arg - Asp - Met - Pro - Ile - Gln	2470	PRP2	2989	

TABLE 1. AMINO ACID SEQUENCE OF PRPs2 AND PRPs3s.

Using Proteomics (Gas Chromatography/Mass Spectrometry combined with an extensive peptide database) there have been many PRPs identified in colostrum.

Figure 3 shows the molecular appearance of PRPs2 and PRPs3 peptides.

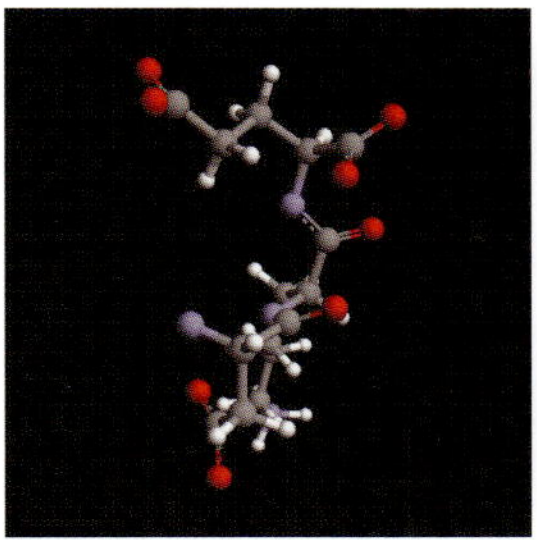
DKE

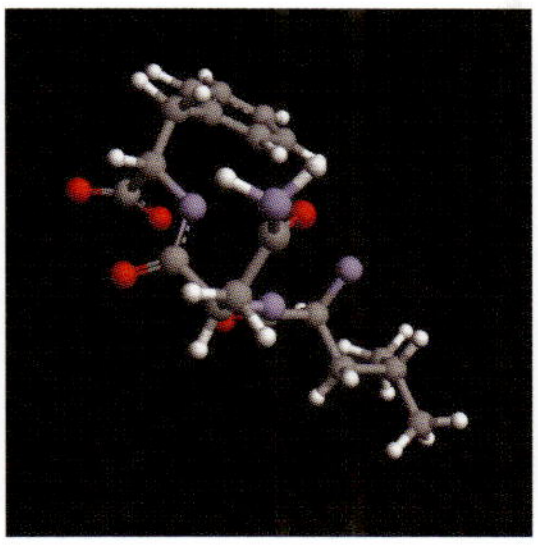
LNF

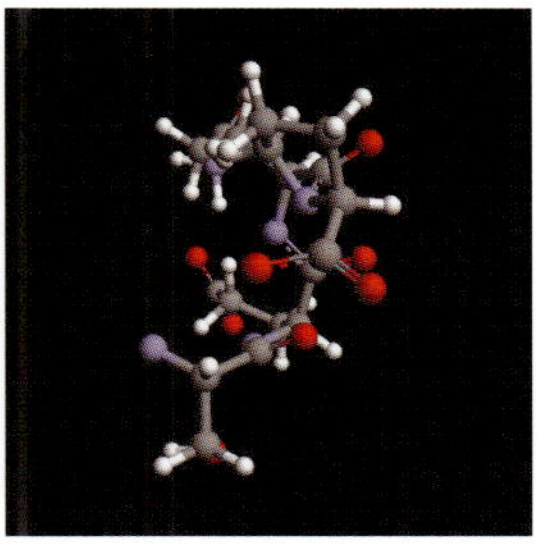
SEQP

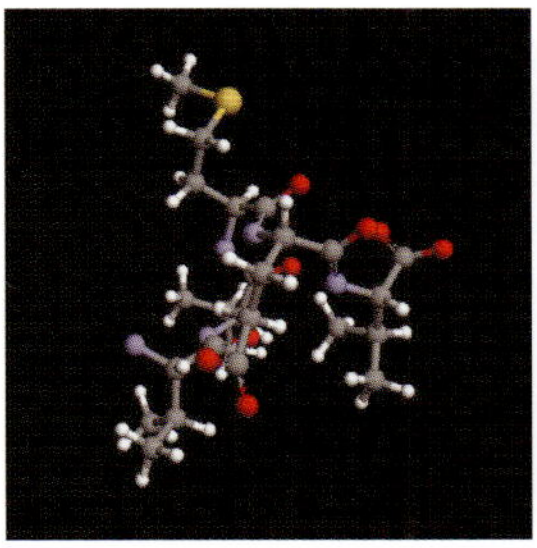
VVMEV

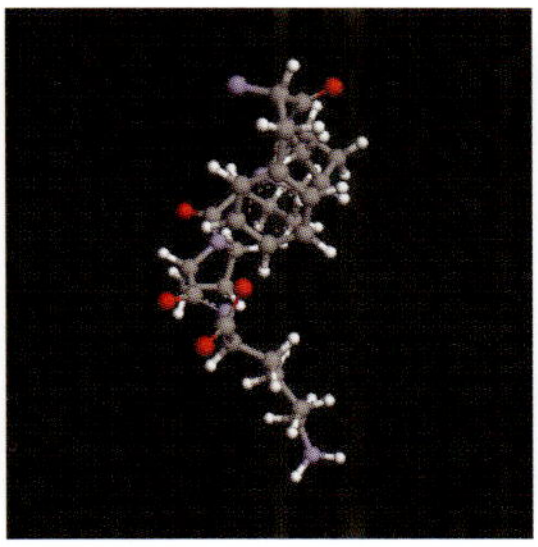
FPPPK

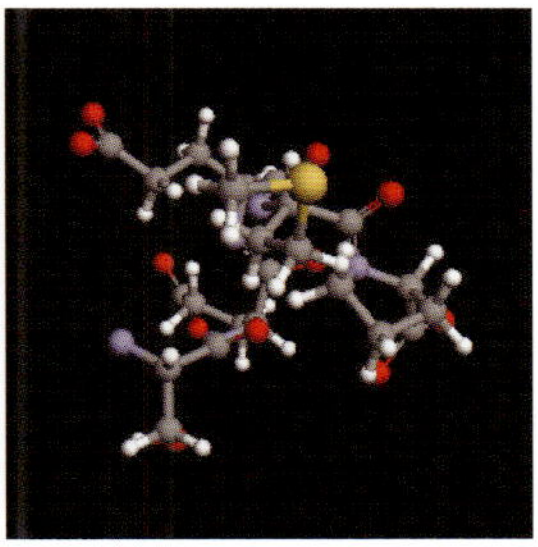
SEEMP

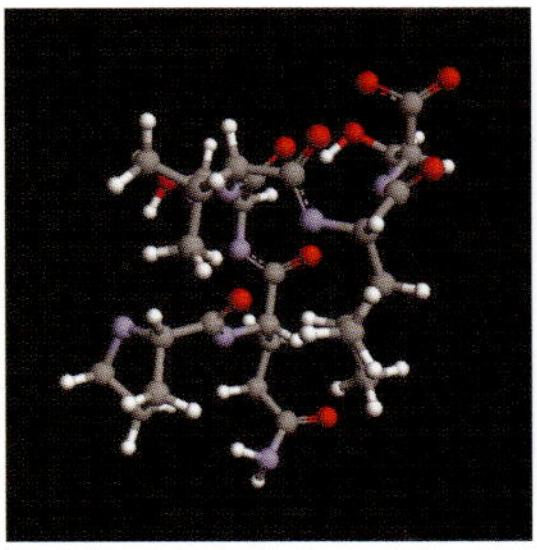
PQSVLS

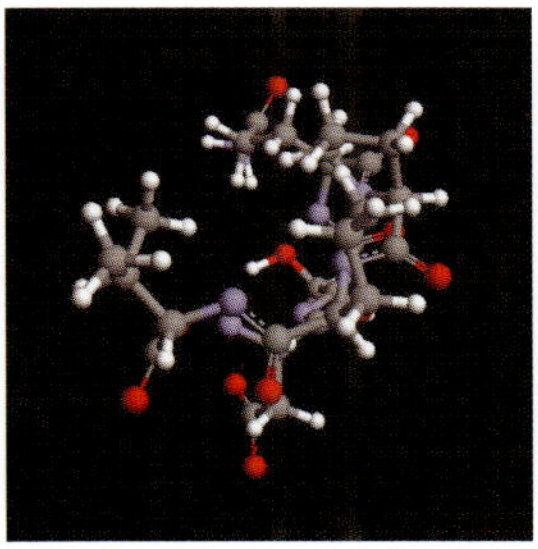
DSQPPV

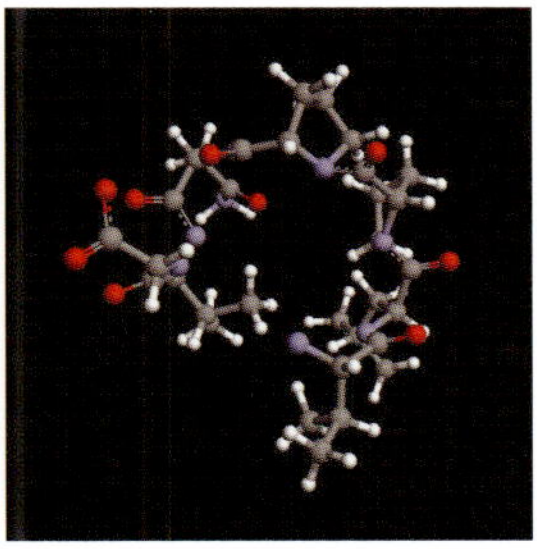
VLPPNVG

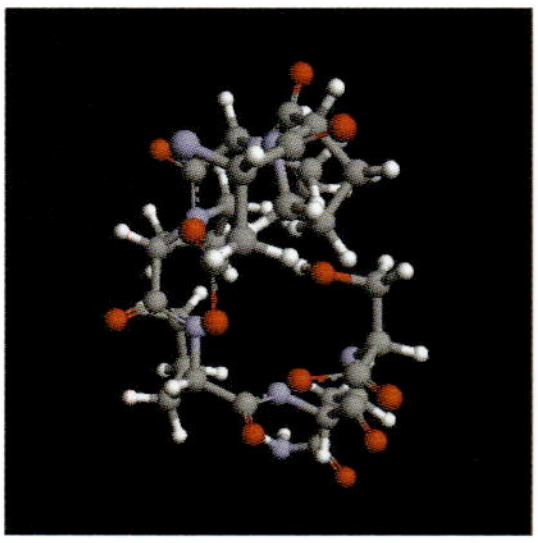

DPPPPQS

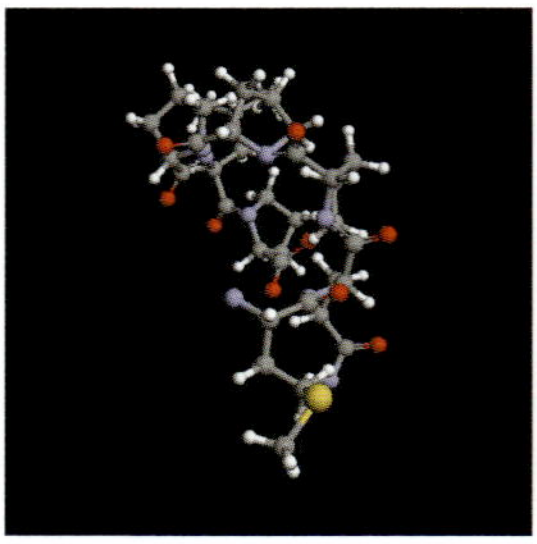

MQPPPLP

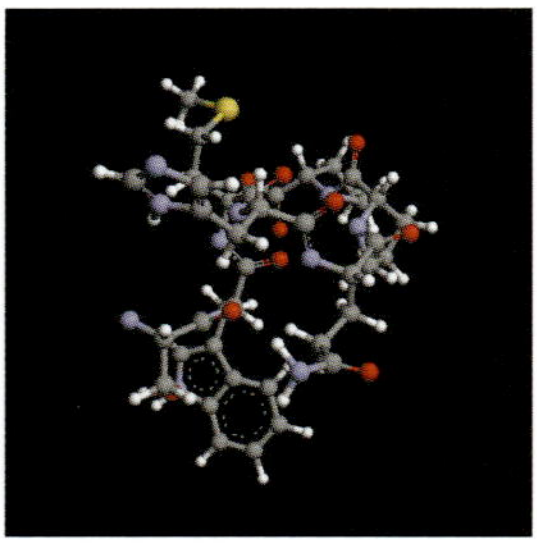

SWMHQPP

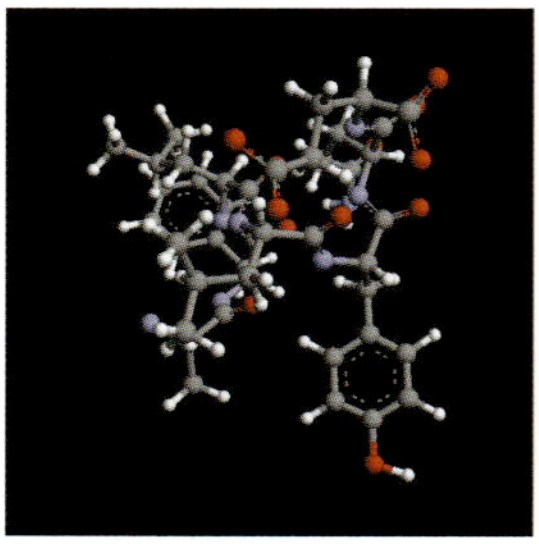

AFLLYQE

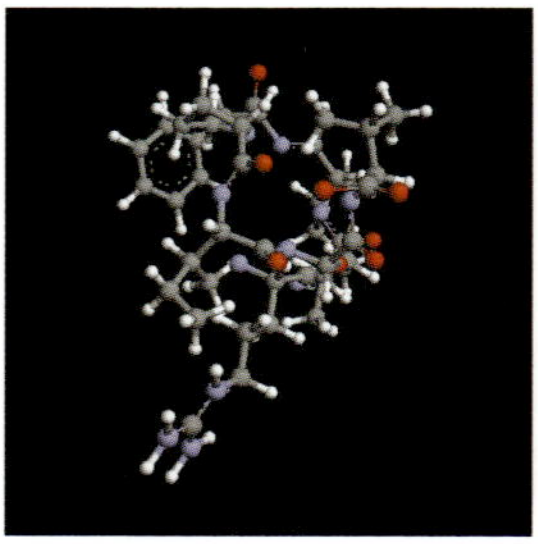

RGPFPILV

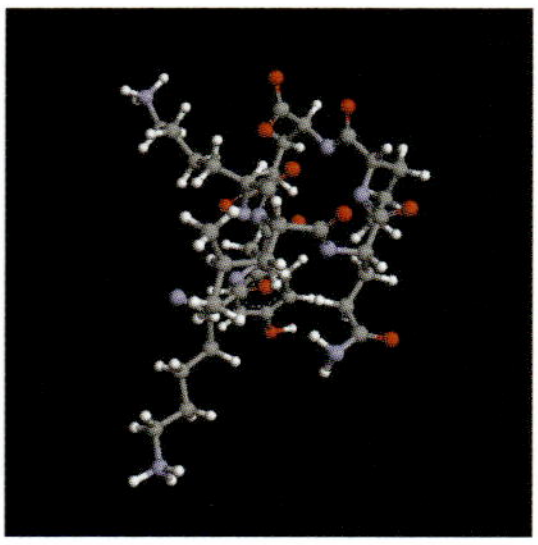

KYKLQPE

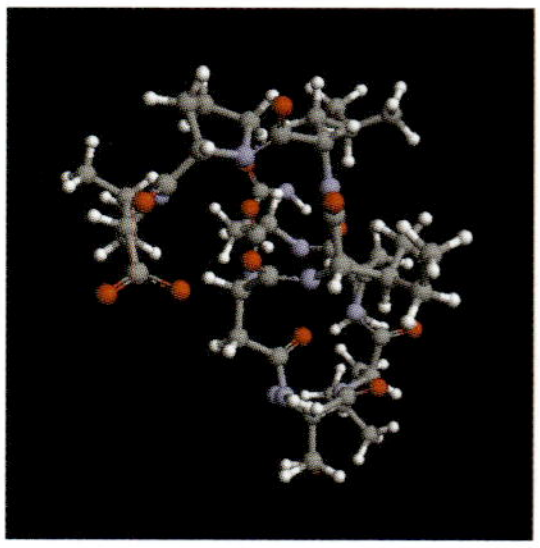

SLPQNILPL

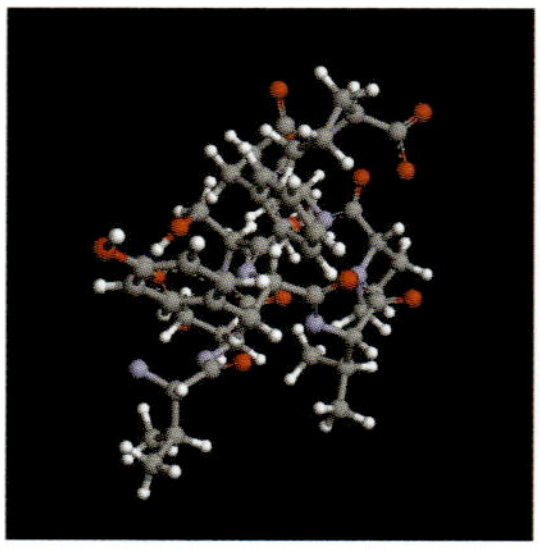

VESYVPLFP

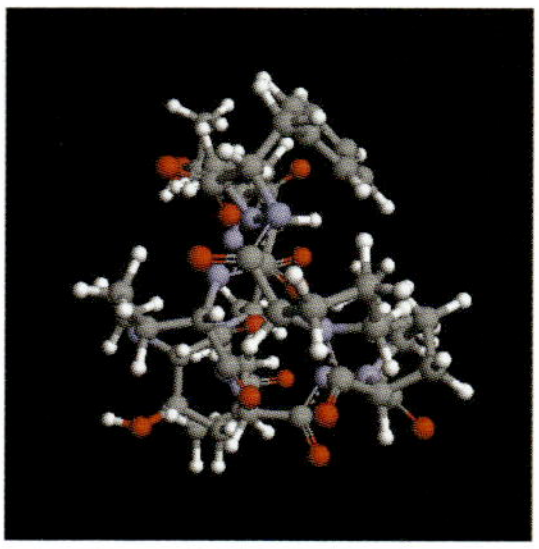

TQTPVVVPPF

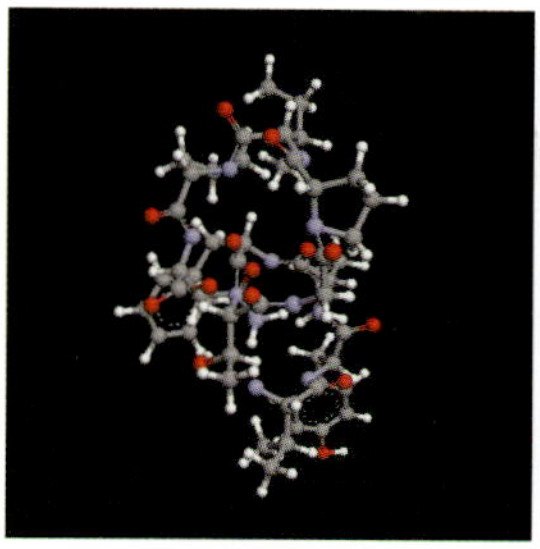

VYPFTGPIPN

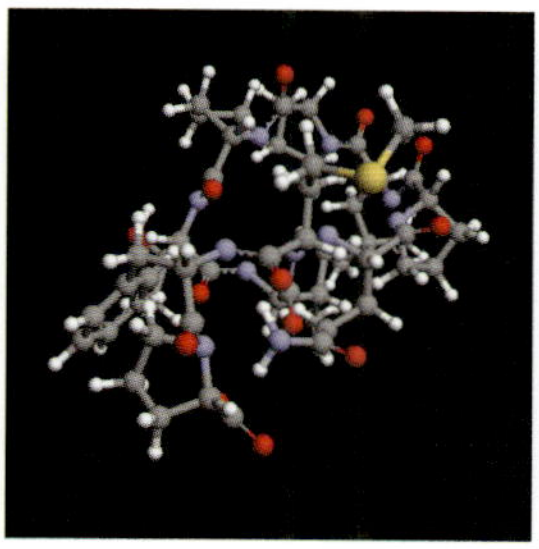

QPLPPTVMFP

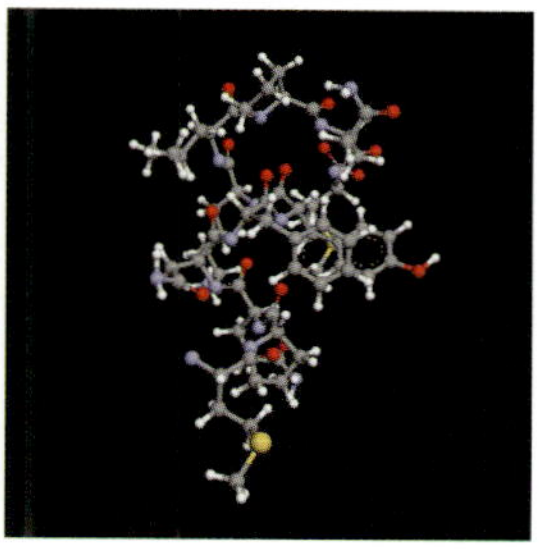

MPQNFYKLPQM

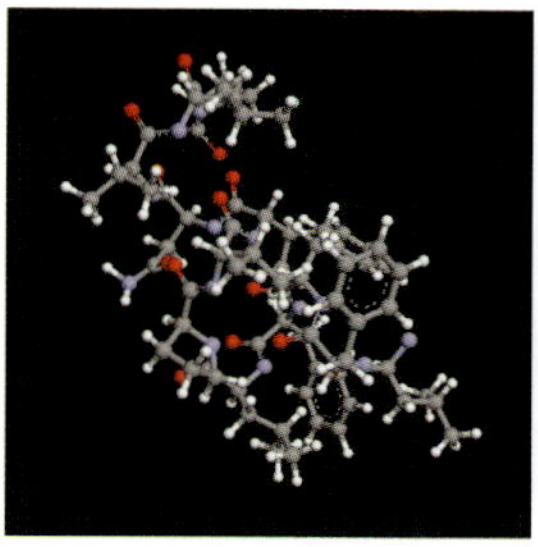

LFFFLPVVNVLP

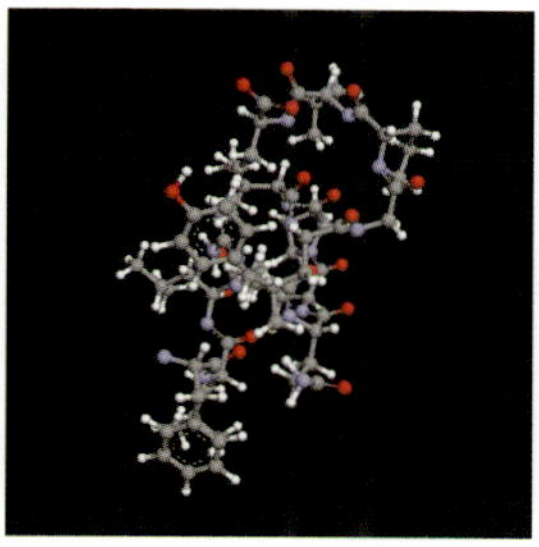

FLLYQEPVLGPVR

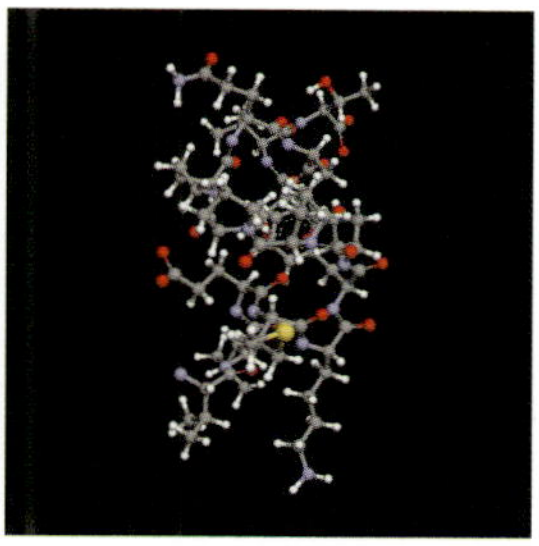

VLEMKFPPPPQETVT

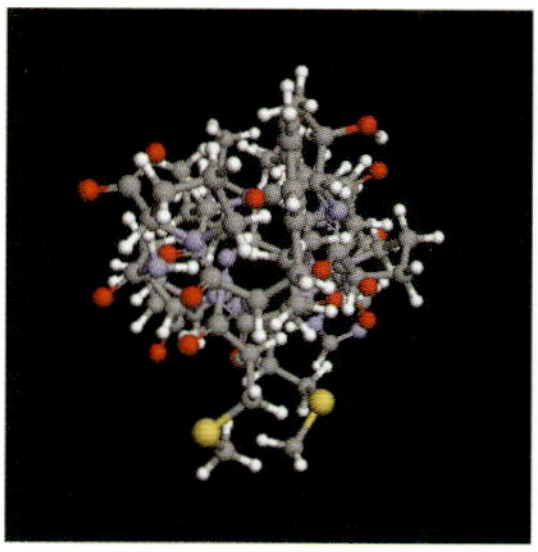

MHQPPQPLPPTVMFP

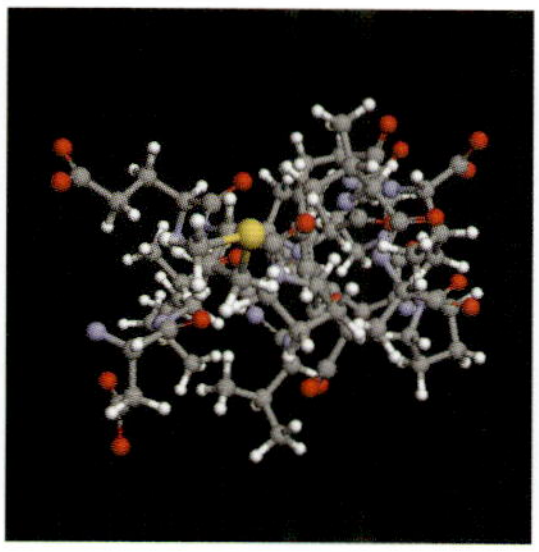

DLEMPVLPVEPFPFV

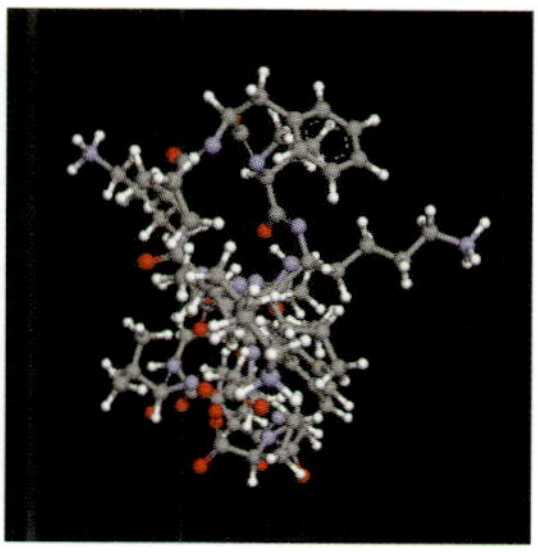

LKPFPKLKVEVFPFP

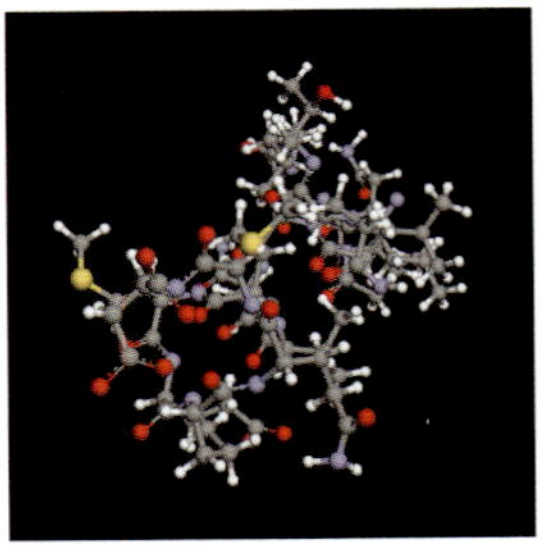

LQTPQPLLQVMMEPQGD

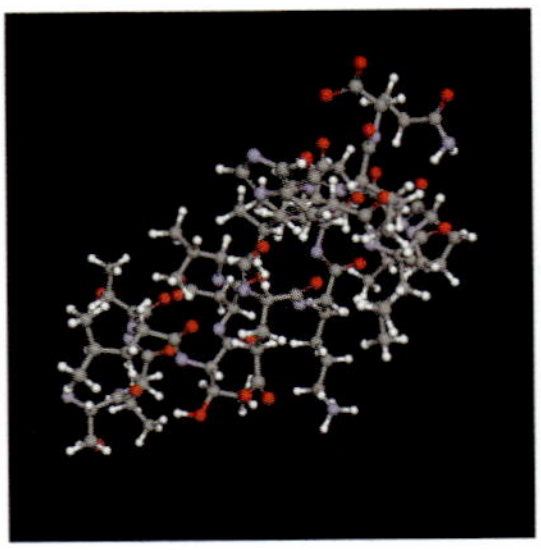

SLTLTDVEKLHLPLVQ

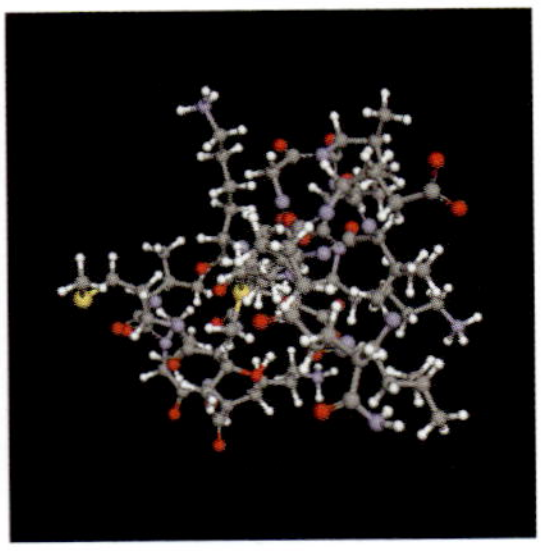

LQPEIMGVPKVKETMVPK

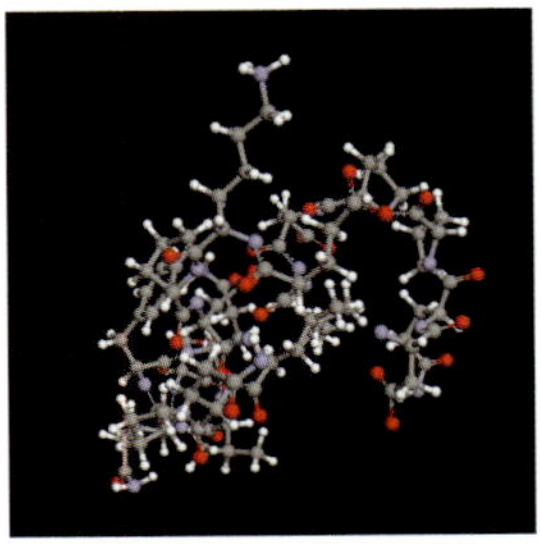

DQPPDVEKPDLQPFQVQS

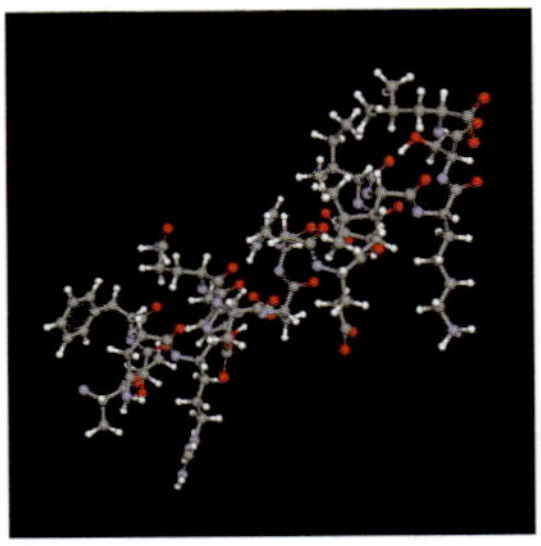

ATFNRYQDDHGEEILKSL

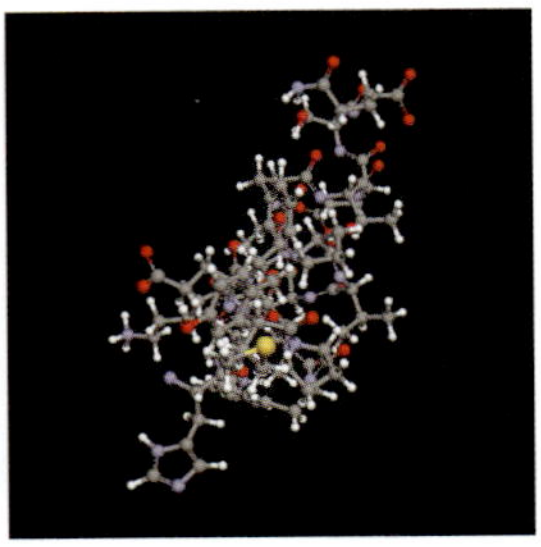

HKEMPFPKYPVEPFTESQ

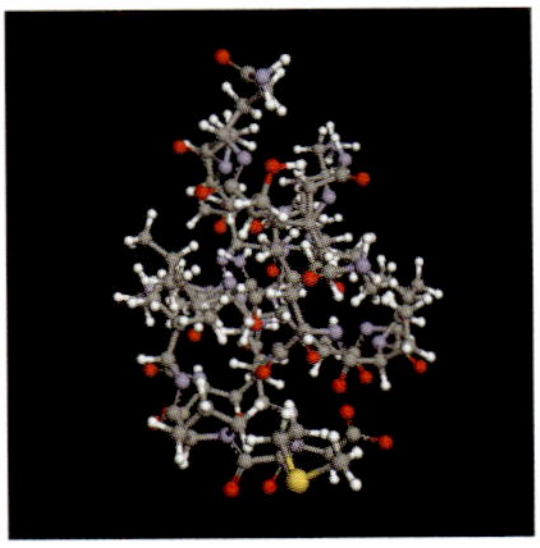

LSQPKVPVQKAVPQRDMPIQ

FIGURE 3. MOLECULAR APPEARANCES OF PRPS2 AND PRPS3 PEPTIDES.

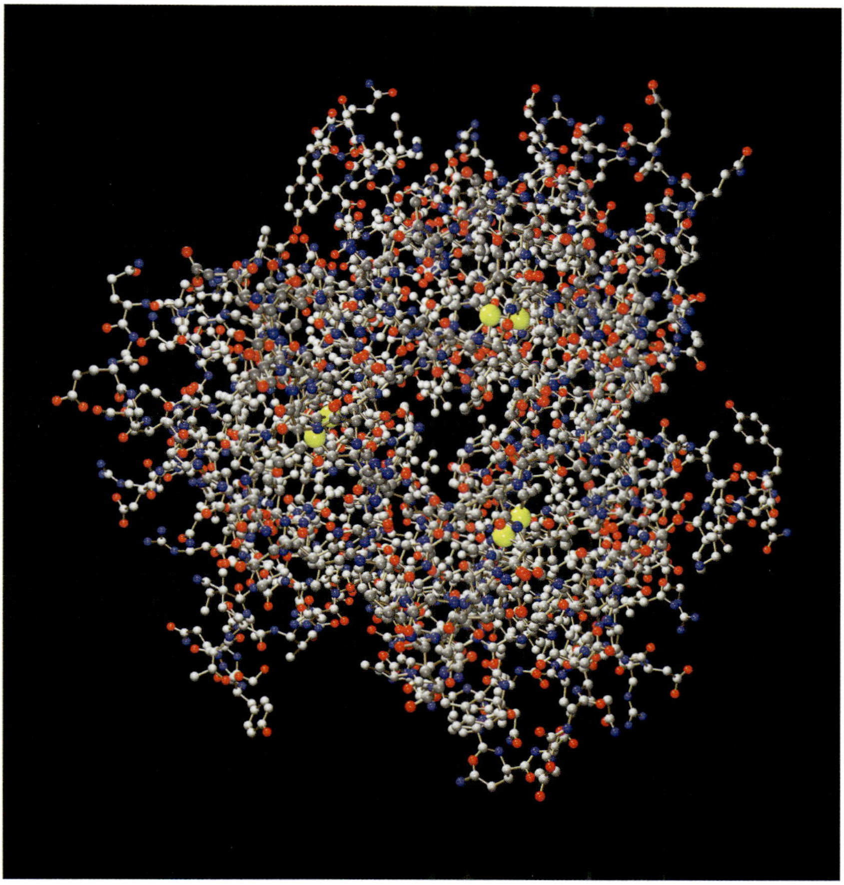

DR. MARK J. WINTER / PHOTO RESEARCHERS, INC

FIGURE 4. TUMOR NECROSIS FACTOR-ALPHA (TNF-ALPHA), COMPUTER MODEL. ATOMS ARE REPRESENTED AS SPHERES AND ARE COLOR-CODED: CARBON (GREY), HYDROGEN (WHITE), OXYGEN (RED) AND NITROGEN (BLUE). DISULPHIDE BRIDGES ARE YELLOW. THIS PROTEIN GENERALLY EXISTS AS A TRIMER (A MOLECULE CONSISTING OF 3 IDENTICAL SMALLER MOLECULES, SEEN HERE). IT IS RELEASED BY WHITE BLOOD CELLS, MAINLY MACROPHAGES, DURING INFLAMMATORY IMMUNE RESPONSES, AND ACTS AS A SIGNALING MOLECULE. ITS RELEASE IS TRIGGERED BY INJURY OR BACTERIAL ENDOTOXINS. ONE OF ITS ACTIONS IS TO KILL TUMOR CELLS, HENCE ITS NAME. TNF-ALPHA IS ALSO INVOLVED IN A NUMBER OF INFLAMMATORY ILLNESSES, INCLUDING RHEUMATOID ARTHRITIS, PSORIASIS AND CROHN'S DISEASE.

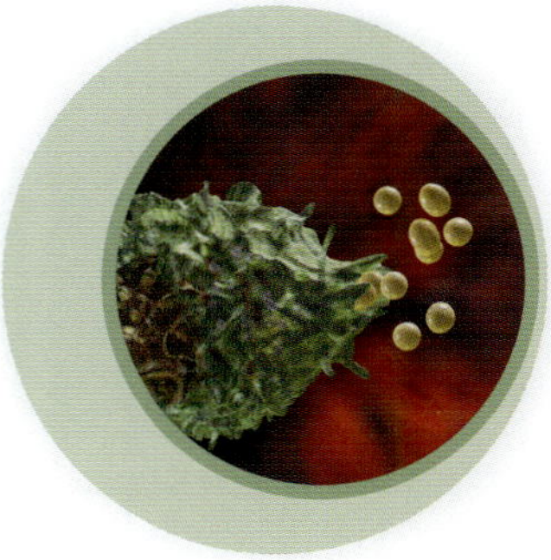

CHAPTER 11

SIGNAL TRANSDUCTION

When a peptide messenger attaches to a receptor on the surface of a cell, a series of biochemical reactions take place that result in some action occurring in the cell, such as a specific protein being produced by the cell. This process is called signal transduction. It may be worthwhile to take a look at how this process takes place to understand how PRPs and other signaling peptides function in the body.

The membranes that surround all cells in the body are composed of phospholipids—long fatty acid chains with hydrophilic (water-loving) and hydrophobic (water-fearing) areas that when assembled into a bilayered membrane form a selectively permeable barrier. The membrane is also composed of proteins that are embedded in the phospholipid and that function as receptors, channels and structural components of the cell. The receptors for PRPs and other signaling peptides are found in this pospholipid bilayer.

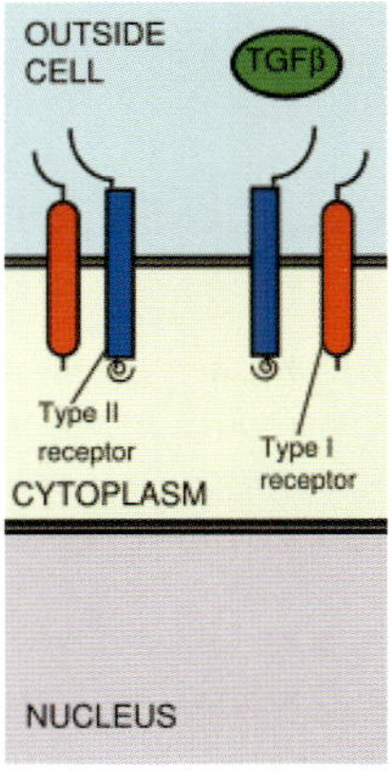

FIGURE 1 TGF-β AND ITS RECEPTORS IN THE CELL MEMBRANE. (DRAWINGS BY JEROME WALKER)

For an example of how signal transduction works, let us look at the signal transduction pathway that transforming growth factor-beta (TGF-β) activates.[402] First, the TGF-β molecule, known as a ligand (or binder), binds to the TGF-β receptor in the cell membrane of the target cell (re-

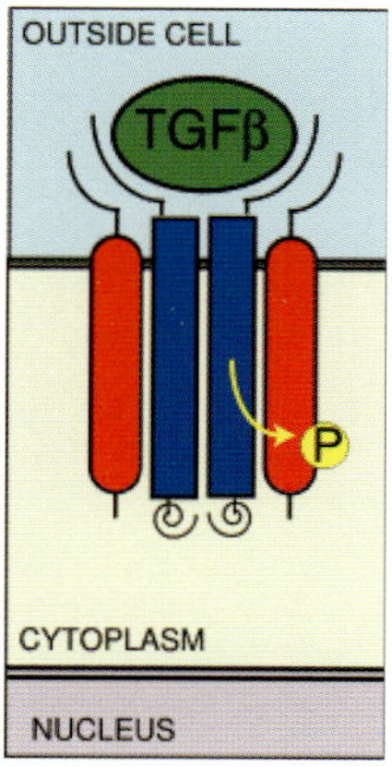

Figure 2
The ligand-receptor complex.

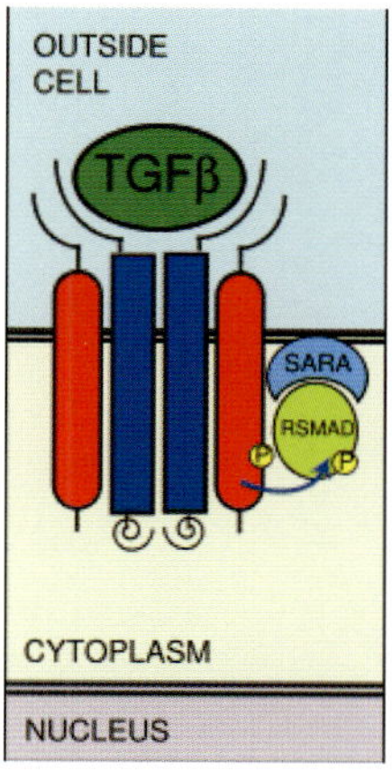

Figure 3
Phosphorylation of RSMAD

ceptors for TGF-β are found on virtually every cell in the body), as shown in Figure 1. The Type 2 receptor shown is the TGF-β-specific receptor. The TGF-β molecule binds to two Type 2 receptors, and this action recruits two Type I receptors, which are not specific to TGF-β. These all bind together with the TGF-β molecule to form a complex (Figure 2).

The binding of these molecules together causes the Type 2 receptors to rotate to expose the enzymatically active portion of the receptor. When this happens, the Type 2 receptor phosphorylates (donates a phosphorus atom) the Type I receptor. This activates the Type I receptor protein. Meanwhile a protein in the cytoplasm of the cell, called SARA (SMAD anchor for receptor activation), brings another protein called RSMAD to the Type I receptor and facilitates its binding to the receptor (Figure 3). The phosphorus atom the Type I receptor received from the Type II receptor is then passed to the RSMAD. The result of this

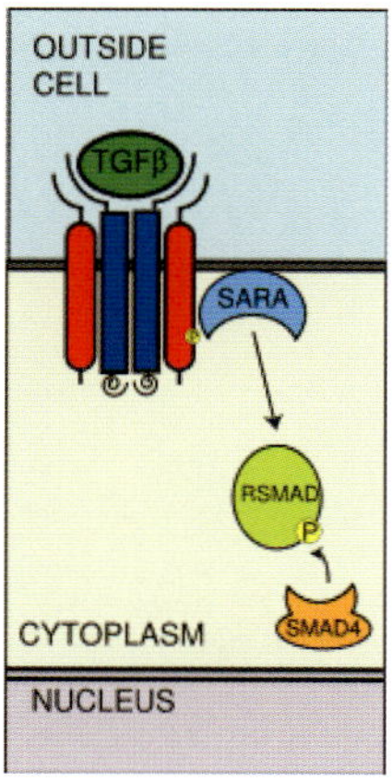

Figure 4
RSMAD release from receptor complex

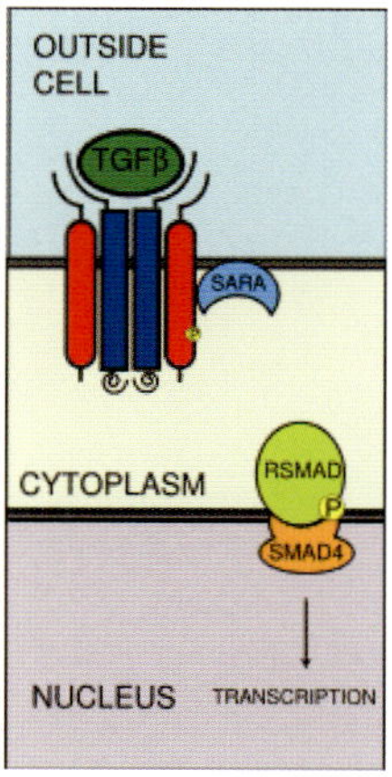

Figure 5
RSMAD-SMAD4 complex enters cell nucleus to initiate mRNA transcription

phosphorylation of the RSMAD is that it changes conformation and is released from the TGF-β-receptor complex (Figure 4). The RSMAD moves through the cytoplasm of the cell and binds to a coSMAD, in this case SMAD4. The combination of the RSMAD and coSMAD enter the nucleus of the cell (Figure 5) where it binds with transcription promoters and cofactors to cause the transcription of mRNA (messenger RNA), which then is used to synthesize the protein in the ribosomes of the cell. In the case of TGF-β, the protein would be one of several that TGF-β initiates, including proteins involved in apoptosis (programmed cell death), extracellular matrix formation, and immunosuppression.

This brief (and simplified) description of how signal transduction works inside the cell illustrates what a complex process is involved. With so many different steps and proteins involved, there are many places where regulation of the process can—and does—take place. This is how PRPs are able to modulate the immune response, by the action of regulatory proteins at different stages of the signal transduction cascade of events.

Now that we have some idea of how PRPs work, let us explore further the benefits of PRPs.

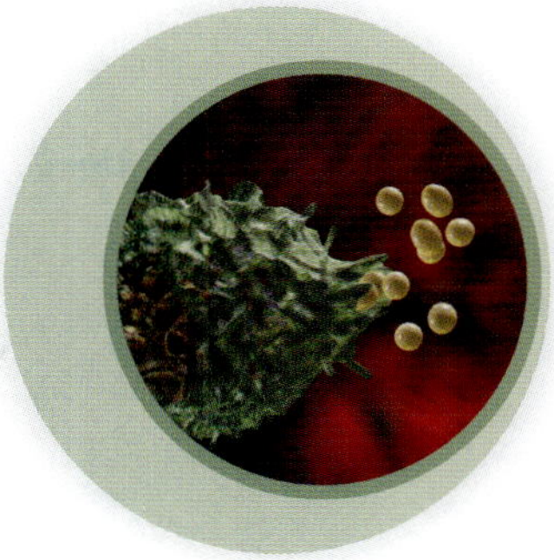

CHAPTER 12

THE ROLE OF PRPS IN TH1/TH2 CYTOKINE BALANCE

Role of Th1, Th2

Before one can understand the usefulness of PRPs, it is helpful to have an understanding of the Th1 helper/Th2 helper paradigm.[403] T helper lymphocytes develop along two lines of cell populations. Th1 cells, which modulate cell-mediated immunity, produce the cytokines IL-2, IFN-gamma, and TNF-alpha. Th2 cells, which modulate humoral immunity, or antibody production, produce IL-4, IL-5, IL-6, IL-10, and IL-13. Once you're familiar with the particular Th1/Th2 predominant phenotypes in a patient, you can more easily identify certain constellations of diseases or conditions and tailor your therapies.

Cell-mediated, or Th1 helper responses, are important in the body's ability to defend itself against viruses, fungi, parasites, cancer, and intracellular organisms. Cell-mediated immunity can be tested by:

1. Skin tests–delayed hypersensitivity skin testing;
2. Response to non-specific mitogens, such as phytohemagglutinin (PHA), concavalina, or pokeweed mitogens;
3. Response to specific mitogens, such as diphtheria, tetanus, or candida;
4. Response to alloantigens—mixed lymphocyte reaction;
5. T cell subsets;
6. IL-2R;

7. NK cell level;
8. NK cell activity;
9. IL-1 assay; and
10. IL-2 and interferon gamma, and other cytokines.

If one has a Th2-dominated condition with decreased cellular immunity and heightened humoral immunity, the conditions that tend to prevail are:

1. Allergies
2. Chronic sinusitis
3. Atopic eczema
4. Asthma
5. Systemic autoimmune conditions such as lupus erythematosus and mercury-induced autoimmunity
6. Vaccination-induced state
7. Certain cases of autism
8. Hyperinsulinism
9. Pertussis vaccination
10. Malaria
11. Helminth infection
12. Hepatitis C
13. Chronic giardiasis
14. Hypercortisolism
15. Chronic candidiasis
16. Cancer
17. Viral infections
18. Ulcerative colitis

A Th1-dominated picture would include the following medical states:

1. Diabetes Type 1
2. Multiple sclerosis
3. Rheumatoid arthritis
4. Uveitis

5. Crohn's disease
6. Hashimoto's disease
7. Sjögren's syndrome
8. Psoriasis
9. Sarcoidosis
10. Chronic Lyme disease
11. Helicobacter pylori infections
12. Entamoeba histolytica

Pregnancy is a Th2-dominant state. This is an advantage during pregnancy, since a Th1-dominant state, or cell-mediated immune response, would induce rejection of the fetus and placenta. Because it stimulates a Th1 response in most cases, PRPs should not be used in pregnancy. Certain autoimmune conditions, such as multiple sclerosis and rheumatoid arthritis, which are Th1-dominant states, are ameliorated during pregnancy.

Th1-dominant states are generally helped by PRPs. Many of them, such as rheumatoid arthritis, multiple sclerosis, and Crohn's disease, are thought to be possibly caused by an infection or reaction to a pathogen. If the Th1 response is an inadequate attempt of the immune system to fight off a microbe, then PRPs would augment that process and be effective in certain cases. Clinically, this is seen in certain cases, e.g., Crohn's disease, multiple sclerosis, and chronic Lyme disease, where PRPs help a Th1-dominant condition.

PRPs augment cell-mediated immunity or push a Th2 to a Th1 state. This is useful in Th2-dominated conditions. Normally, on exposure to gut-related microbes and childhood infections, a child's Th2-dominated immune system is subject to Th1 stimulation and Th1/Th2 balance ensues.[406] If TH2 dominance remains, this can lead to atopic (allergic) states. We see this in the increased incidence of allergic symptoms, postnasal drip, asthma, etc, in clinical practice.

The other side of this Th2 state is a decreased Th1 or cell-mediated immunity. With this, we see an increased incidence of viral infection, fungal infection, and cancer. Vaccinations tend to push the immune system toward a Th2-dominant state.

To help overcome this tendency, we can use PRPs pre- and post-immunization.

Cancer, Cell-mediated Immunity, and PRPs

Since cancer can be associated with a Th1-deficient state, use of PRPs should be considered as part of immune augmentation therapy. Factors that decrease cell-mediated immunity and increase Th2 dominance are age, cytotoxic cancer treatments, post-surgery stress, metastatic disease, etc.[407] Cell-mediated immunity (CMI) can be a predictor of morbidity and mortality over the age of sixty. In patients with liver metastases or colon rectal carcinoma, CMI is predictive of survival.[408] Decrease in cell-mediated immunity, along with an increase in circulating immune complexes, indicates unfavorable prognosis in cancer patients.[409] Studies show that patients who have multiple skin cancers had impaired CMI.[410] In a study of gynecological cancer patients compared to control groups, those on chemotherapy had a decrease in immune parameters (i.e., refractory decreased cell-mediated immunity), whereas the group getting immunotherapy (in this case, thymopeptin) maintained their immune parameters at normal levels.[411,412]

Immunologically deficient cancer patients are susceptible to infection by viral pathogens, such as herpes zoster and cytomegalovirus (CMV). Infection occurs as a result of cytotoxic therapy and deficiency of cell-mediated immunity.[413] Th1-dominant states, characterized by increased amounts of IL-2 and IFN-γ, are immuno-stimulatory and limit tumor growth. In contrast, Th2-predominant patterns, characterized by IL-4 and IL-10 cytokines, are immuno-inhibiting and stimulate tumor growth. HIV progression to HHV-8 infection with Kaposi's sarcoma, ulcerative colitis, progression to colon cancer, and obesity with increased incidence of carcinoma are all associated with the increased Th2 state (and decreased cell-mediated immunity). Studies suggest that this shift to Th2 dominance precedes the cancerous transformation. As the cancer grows, it becomes increasingly hypoxic. This leads to further suppression of cell-mediated immunity, allowing decreased immune surveillance. Studies show that a Th2 immune response is associated with a proangiogenesis state, which facilitates cancer growth.[414]

PRPs have been shown to improve cellular immunity in patients with immune defects.[415] Since they augment Th1 or cell-mediated immunity, PRPs are helpful in these situations. For example, by conveying cell-mediated immunity against bladder and prostate tissue-specific antigen, PRPs were efficacious in the treatment of stage D3 hormone-unresponsive metastatic prostate cancer. Follow-up showed increased survival rates in fifty patients, with complete remission in two, possible remission in six, and no progression of metastatic disease in fifty-eight.[416] PRPs were shown to improve survival as an adjunct to resection in non-small cell lung carcinoma.[417]

Before PRPs were derived from colostrum, it was obtained from dialyzed leukocyte extract (DLE). The literature has many citations of DLE of an antigen-specific nature being used for various viral conditions, autoimmune conditions, and certain cancers. It has been found that DLE facilitated immunity to tumor-associated antigen. Fudenburg showed that PRPs could, from selected donors, increase the cell-mediated responses to tumor-associated antigens in human osteogenic sarcoma patients.

One of the compromises on our cell-mediated immunity is environmental stress (e.g., chemical or heavy metal pollution). It has been shown that long-term exposure to polychlorinated hydrocarbons suppresses phagocytosis, decreases NK cell activity, and reduces lymphocyte response to mitogens in mice.[418] Alterations in immune dysregulation, with a predominantly Th2 response, occurs with lead and mercury exposure. This leads to impaired cell-mediated immunity, increased incidence of infectious disease or cancer, and can end with an autoimmune disease.[419]

Viral Infections

Currently in medicine, we are seeing increased problems with viral infections, such as otitis media, measles, chronic fatigue, Epstein-Barr virus (EBV), cytomegalovirus (CMV), acquired immunodeficiency syndrome (AIDS) due to human immunodeficiency virus (HIV), hepatitis, and West Nile virus. Treatment regimens range from interferon to azidothymidine (AZT), ribavirin, and relenza. However, even with all the high-tech immune weapons available, we are still losing the battle.

In the treatment of viral infections, PRPs provide a modality that works at a fundamental level. They have been shown to induce interferon in patients with viral infections.[420]

Viral infections tend to have increased Th2 and decreased Th1. This is also seen with fungal infections, parasitic diseases, and cancer. Bacterial infections are associated with decreased Th2-dominant states.

By stimulating Th1, PRPs may be advantageous in the treatment of hepatitis. In hepatitis C, the activation of the Th2 dominance plays a role in the development of chronic hepatitis changes. Th1 stimulation may result in clearance of viral particles and improvement in the hepatitis.[421,4122] Studies show that severe complicated measles has been treated successfully with non-specific PRPs. Symptoms were ameliorated within 24 hours, without side effects.[423]

One theory claims that one of the mechanisms involved in autistic spectrum disorders is an immune imbalance toward a dominant Th2 pattern, resulting from measles, mumps, and rubella (MMR) vaccination. Currently, a study is ongoing to test the efficacy of PRPs to act as an immune modulator in this disorder.

It is well-known that viruses play an important role in the etiology of acute otitis media (AOM) in children. In a study of AOM, 75% of the children were positive for viruses such as respiratory syncytial virus (RSV), parainfluenza, and influenza, and 48% had the causal viruses in the middle ear effusion.[424] These viruses probably act as antecedents to the bacterial infections typical of AOM.[425] This could account for the excellent results seen in early treatment and prevention of otitis media using PRPs.

A certain percentage of asthmatics have their symptoms precipitated by respiratory infection, most of these secondary to viral infections. A study conducted with PRPs and asthmatic patients showed that approximately 50% discontinued their steroid medication and the other half decreased their steroid use. Overall, there was a decrease in hospital admissions. Administration of PRPs improved cellular immunity. No adverse effects or allergic reactions were observed.[426]

An increased incidence of infection, such as parainfluenza virus, syncytial virus, adenovirus, etc, may be precipitating factors in children who have asthma. It was also found that children with asthma have a propensity toward frequent infection.[427] Twelve of fifteen children exhibited defects in T cell immunity, many of which were not drastic[428]. This should emphasize that functional, suboptimal defects in cell-mediated immune function can be a factor in viral illnesses, as measured with sensitive immunological testing. Once again, we see that PRPs can help in conditions with increased susceptibility to viruses, a dominant Th2 (decreased cell-mediated) profile.

It was found that women with extended human papilloma virus (HPV) infections have defective protective mechanisms of cell-mediated immunity.[429]A pronounced shift from Th1 to Th2 cytokine pattern is associated with more extensive HPV infection. Increased gynecological problems are found secondary to HPV. The potential of PRPs in HPV infections needs to be further explored.
Chronic Infection

The addition of PRPs can help an impaired immune system that is subject to chronic infections. How many practitioners see this scenario? A child comes down with recurrent bronchitis or tonsillitis, starting shortly after birth, necessitating frequent courses of antibiotics. This can then lead to symptoms of chronic candidiasis. A history of chronic eczema or allergic diathesis can also be found. Immunological or skin testing shows a mild defect in cell-mediated immunity, but no abnormalities. Grohn reported on several similar cases and obtained successful treatment with administration of PRPs.[430] Here we see that PRPs are helpful for elevated Th2 states, allergy, chronic candidiasis, and eczema.

PRPs have ameliorated cases of recurrent, non-bacterial cystitis (NBRC) when treatment with antibiotics and nonsteroidal drugs was unsuccessful, and cell-mediated immunity to herpes simplex and candida was decreased.[431]Various studies show positive results with PRPs in chronic mucocutaneous candidiasis.[432]
In Lyme disease, cytotoxic production of a Th2 phenotype is correlated to resistance, while that of a Th1 phenotype is correlated to susceptibility.[433] This suggests that certain people have an immune glitch that makes their immune system

prone to either the Th1 or Th2 pattern, and therefore more susceptible to different diseases. This may be precisely where PRPs, having immunomodulating activity, can be helpful. For instance, in Lyme patients we usually see a Th1 dominated pattern, but PRPs work very well for certain subsets of Lyme patients.

Chronic Fatigue

PRPs have been used in chronic fatigue immune dysfunction syndrome, especially if a viral etiology can be found. It has had varied success, although one may need to use increased dosages. If polyvalent PRPs are not successful, the use of antigen- or disease-specific PRPs may need to be explored.[434]

In elderly patients with cellular immunodeficiency and chronic fatigue syndrome, age-related decrease in recovery occurred after treatment with PRPs[435]. Success with PRPs in chronic fatigue syndrome secondary to human herpes virus-6 (HHV-6), genital or labial herpes, and recurrent ocular herpes has been well-documented.[436,437,438] A study on the effect of PRPs on the course of multiple sclerosis showed that it retarded the progression of the disease in mild to moderate cases.[439]

The Treatment

Treatment with PRPs is dose-dependent. In viral infections, one usually starts with three sprays three times a day. The dose is then tapered down to one spray three times a day. That dose is maintained in cases of chronic viruses, chronic herpes infection, chronic fatigue secondary to CMV or EBV, chronic colds and impaired resistance. If there is any flare-up in viral infections, the dose can be increased to three sprays three times a day. Usually patients report decreased susceptibility to colds and decreased nasal symptoms (for instance, postnasal drip and chronic sinus symptoms). In allergic conditions, an adult starts with two sprays three times a day, increasing to three sprays three times a day if symptoms worsen. Again, the dose is tapered to a maintenance level with amelioration of allergic symptoms.
In cases of chronic fatigue syndrome, patients start on three sprays three times a day. One may need to increase the dose depending on the response. Doses of

four to five sprays three times daily can be used as an adjunct cancer treatment for patients undergoing chemotherapy and/or radiation therapy, with a resulting decrease in cellular immune function.

Various immune function tests, especially those measuring CMI, can be done to gauge maintenance dosage. One can also perform a cytokine panel, measuring IL-2, IL-4, IFN-γ, IL-10, etc. An elevated IL-2 and IFN-γ would indicate a TH1-predominant state, while an elevated IL-4 and IL-10 would point to a TH2-dominated state. NK cell activity, which is usually decreased in cases of cancer, is increased secondarily to PRP administration and can be periodically measured. Occasionally when a patient starts PRPs, he or she may experience flu-like symptoms, nausea or gastrointestinal symptoms. Since PRPs are small peptides and do not contain milk protein, allergic reactions are rare. These symptoms are usually classified as Jarisch-Herxheimer reactions, and they probably signify a direct reaction of PRPs on gut or systemic pathogens. If patients are informed of these possible mild adverse reactions, they are more likely to continue treatment.

PRPs and Other Alternative Therapies

In complicated immune cases or in adjunct cancer treatment, it is advantageous to add complementary classes of herbs and nutrients to augment the immune-stimulatory effects. These auxiliary factors boost natural killer cell activity, increase phagocytosis, increase maturation of T cells, enhance general immunity, and trigger the complement cascade, helping cytotoxicity. Compounds that act synergistically with PRPs include thymic protein factors, Chinese herbs (such as astragalus, cordyceps, shiitake, maitake, and reishi mushrooms), inositol hexaphosphate, melatonin, 1-3 beta glucan, glutathione, and associated antioxidants. Vitamins A D, and B_6 promote the Th2 pattern, while vitamins E, C and folate support the production of a Th1 response.[440] Vitamin B_{12} suppresses the Th1 response.[441] In addition, acupuncture has been found to increase the immune perimeters of CMI. Levels of CD3+, CD4+, CD4+/CD8+ and beta-endorphins were found to be increased in patients with malignant tumors after a course of acupuncture treatment.[442]

Thymic factors cause maturation of naïve T cells and increase cell-mediated immunity. It is known that PRPs are more effective in post-thymic cells. Therefore both thymic factors and PRPs are recommended for mild thymic primary immunodeficiency.[443,444] A recent study by Dr. Daryl See showed that PRPs enhanced natural killer cell cytotoxic activity. The effect of PRPs was greater than that observed with other well-known NK cell activity enhancers, such as echinacea, acemannan, 1-3 beta glucan, IP-6, and certain Chinese mushrooms. Colostrum had one-quarter the potency. Other immune parameters, such as T cell function and test of cellular immunity, were not done in this particular study.[445]

Conclusion

Immune system functioning is at the heart of the increasing infectious and immunologic disorders seen in clinical practices. Through its unique properties and activities, PRPs are an extremely useful, relatively risk-free alternative and adjunctive therapy for treatment of cell-mediated or Th1-deficient conditions. Think of its potential use in illnesses such as cancer, chronic fatigue, viral infections, allergies, fungal infections, chronic infections, and autoimmune conditions.

[The Role of PRPs in TH1/TH2 Cytokine Balance, courtesy of Dr Steven J. Bock. Dr. Bock has been practicing alternative and integrative medicine for over 20 years. He has extensive experience in the integrative treatment of Lyme disease. Dr. Bock is a certified acupuncturist. He is medical director of The Rhinebeck Health Center, The Center for Progressive Medicine, and PatientsAmerica.com. He is the author of Natural Relief for Your Child's Asthma *and* Staying Young the Melatonin Way *(New York: Plume Books, 1996).]*

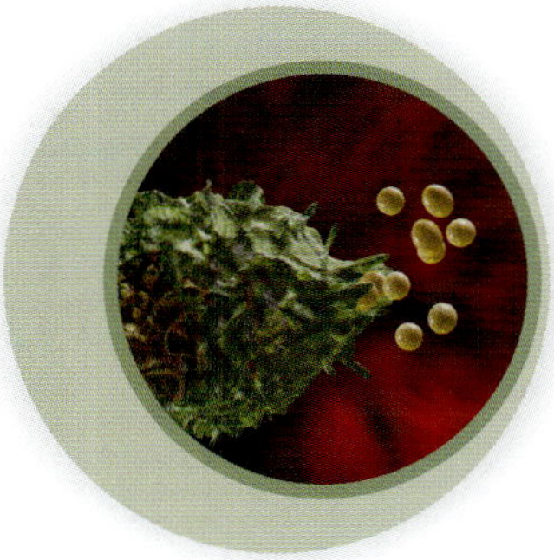

CHAPTER 13

BENEFITS OF PRPS

So far we have talked about how PRPs work in the body and how they affect the immune system. Now let us look more closely at the benefits PRPs provide.

PRPs contain a set of messaging molecules that convey immune information within an individual's immune system. Nature also uses PRPs to carry immune information from one individual's immune system to another individual. PRPs are signaling peptides or **Proline-rich Polypeptides (PRPs)** that have the ability to transfer immunity from one person to another. This immune information is vital to our health.

PRPs are small immune messenger molecules that are produced by higher organisms. Their role is to transfer immune recognition signals between immune cells and thereby assist in educating naïve immune cells about a present or potential danger. PRPs are natural, microscopic molecules that are found in all animals. They are messenger molecules, passing information about the presence of an immune threat—whether external or internal—and how to properly respond, from immune cell to immune cell.

In the harsh and hostile environment in which a baby suddenly finds itself, invading microorganisms could rapidly overcome and destroy the new life. Nature has provided a procedure to rapidly educate the infant's naïve immune system. Prior to delivering a baby, the expectant mother prepares a natural immunizing cocktail that she includes in the first milk (colostrum) she provides to her new baby. PRPs provide a key part of this process.

Dr. CH Kirkpatrick determined that blood contains small peptides of about eight amino acid residues.[507] Eighteen different amino acids have been represented which may combine to create billions of different PRPs. These very small PRP molecules contain the essence of the immunological message.

PRPs do not elicit an allergic response and are not species-specific. What this means is that PRPs peptides produced by a cow are just as effective in humans as they would be in another cow. This exciting ability could spark a revolution in medicine and has prompted the following statement: "PRPs [have] an important role to play in modern medicine which, from AIDS to Ebola, faces the emergence of new viruses or the resurfacing of old pathologies such as tuberculosis"[508] PRPs have been successfully used to treat the following conditions: viral, fungal, neurological and parasitic infections, malignancies challenges, and autoimmune conditions.

PRPs are potent antivirals. Viruses are immune to antibiotics as antibiotics attack bacteria but not viruses. Going to the doctor to get antibiotics for a viral infection, such as a bad cold or the flu, is actually worse than counterproductive. Taking antibiotics unnecessarily kills off the flora in the intestines, which can lead to overgrowth by harmful bacteria or fungus, such as ***Candida***. This leads to leaky gut syndrome, poor nutrition and more disease. Furthermore overuse of antibiotics results in resistant strains of dangerous bacteria which no longer are susceptible to antibiotics. This can have fatal results. And you still have the viruses to contend with.

PRPs are known to provide immunity to a number of dangerous viruses.[446] These include all types of herpes viruses,[447,448,449,450,451,452,453] which are notoriously difficult to treat with standard pharmaceutical means. They are also effective against HIV,[454] measles,[455] and other viruses. Epstein-Barr virus (EBV) is a form of herpes virus that has been associated with infectious mononucleosis, Burkitt's lymphoma, nasopharyngeal cancer and autoimmune conditions, including chronic fatigue syndrome and multiple sclerosis. Anti-Human Herpes Virus-6 (HHV-6) PRPs have shown some promise in the treatment of multiple sclerosis, while both anti-HHV-6 and anti-EBV demonstrated some efficacy in the treatment of chronic fatigue syndrome.[456] PRPs have been used in the treatment of hepatitis B,[457] which is caused by the hepatitis B virus. PRPs are effective in the treatment of epidermodysplasia verruciformis (EV), a chronic viral infection of the skin caused by a variety of human papilloma viruses that is very resistant to standard treatments.[458]

There are also clinical reports of PRPs being used successfully against difficult bacterial and fungal infections. These include lung infections with ***Mycobacterium fortuitum***[459] and ***Mycobacterium tuberculosis***[460] (the causative agent of tuberculosis), cryptosporidiosis diarrhea in AIDS patients,[461,462] typhoid fever,[463] and melioidosis, a tropical infection found in immunocompromised individuals caused by ***Pseudomonas pseudomallei.***[464] PRPs are particularly effective against ***Candida*** fungal infections.[465,466,467]

PRPs have shown promise in the treatment of some cancers, though these studies are still in the early stages. These include mycosis fungoides[468] (lymphoma of the skin), nasopharyngeal carcinoma, renal cancer,[469] prostate cancer,[470] non-small cell lung cancer,[471,472] Hodgkin's disease,[473] melanoma metastatic to lung,[474] and osteogenic sarcoma.[475]

As part of their function to balance the immune system, PRPs have also been shown to prevent allergic responses to common indoor and outdoor allergens, including ragweed pollen and dust mites. PRPs decreased IgE and IgG1 production, significantly decreased airway eosinophilia (the accumulation of eosinophils, a type of white blood cell associated with inflammation, in the airway), and decreased mucous production and hypersensitivity to allergens.[476]

Oral supplementation of PRPs quickly modulate or balance the body's cytokine panel, particularly IL-4, IL-10 and IL-14. By down regulating these pro-inflammatory cytokines, food, airborne, and environmental allergens are then not recognized as allergies by the body's immune system. Thus the cytokine cascade immune response to these allergens does not result in the production of IgE antibodies.[477]

Atopic dermatitis, an allergic skin condition, responds favorably to treatment with PRPs, resulting in statistical improvement in all four clinical parameters (erythema, eczema, pruritus, and papulae).[478] PRPs have also proven effective in the treatment of asthma,[479,480] again by the down regulation of particular cytokines, e.g., IL-5 and IL-9.

It is this property of modulating the immune system that can be used to advantage in the treatment of autoimmune disorders with PRPs.[481] Autoimmunity occurs when the body makes antibodies against its own proteins. There are many autoimmune conditions, such as rheumatoid arthritis, diabetes type 1, lupus erythematosus, multiple sclerosis, Sjögren's syndrome, pernicious anemia, Addison's disease, and so forth. PRPs have shown promise in treating these conditions by turning down the immune response to normal levels.[482,483] Laboratory trials in an experimental system using mice with induced hemolytic anemia showed that supplementation with PRPs resulted in longer lives and less evidence of the disease. Those mice started on treatment earlier in the progression of the disease had better results, suggesting that PRPs may induce suppressor T lymphocytes that control the development of the disease.[484] In another experimental trial, PRPs restored normal immune functioning.[485] Moderate success was found in treating multiple sclerosis.[486] PRPs were used successfully in a clinical trial with rheumatoid arthritis.[487] PRPs produced a "dramatic clinical and immunologic response" in lupus.[488] They have shown benefit in the treatment of Behçet's syndrome[489,490] as well as chronic fatigue syndrome.[491] An autoimmune-like disease called sarcoidosis, characterized by the formation of granular inflammatory nodules in various organs and thought to be caused by an alteration in immune function, also responds to treatment with PRPs.[492]

PRPs have shown great promise in slowing and even reversing the effects of Alzheimer's disease and other neurodegenerative disorders. There is some indication that some such disorders have a basis that resembles autoimmunity as there are remarkable similarities between the central nervous system and the immune system. A chemical that stimulates B cell replication and function in the immune system was tried in patients with Alzheimer's who had atrophy of the frontal lobe and immune dysfunction with dramatic response both immunologically and clinically.[493] Later studies have confirmed that PRPs significantly improved the condition or stabilized the progression of the disease.[494,495,496] PRPs have been successfully used in the treatment of epilepsy[497,498] as well, indicating that they may potentially be of benefit in a variety of neurological conditions.

PRPs are an immune modulator, that is, a substance that produces differential responses in different classes of immune cells. This is different from strict immune stimulants and suppressors. Strict immune stimulation can lead to immune system exhaustion and can lead to immune compromise and ineffectiveness. PRPs are a true immune modulator since they also contain inducer and suppressor fractions and demonstrate different effects on various immune cell populations. This is in keeping with the differential functions of PRPs.

It is important to point out that PRPs appear to produce immunity by stimulating cell-mediated immunity rather than by transferring immunity, say, from a cow to a man as was originally believed. This was discussed in detail in Chapter 8. The fact that PRPs provide immunity to certain viruses, such as herpes and HIV, does not mean that they will not stimulate immunity to other types of viruses as they are doing so by stimulating the immune system to develop immunity, not "transferring" immunity from one organism to another.[499] It is also important to note that in all of these studies no side effects, adverse reactions or drug interactions were noted. PRPs are safe to use.

The immunomodulatory effect of PRPs may prove lifesaving if the threat of avian influenza ("bird flu," the H5N1 strain of influenza virus) becomes a reality. Health authorities are concerned that this deadly strain of flu could make the jump from birds to humans with deadly results—a global pandemic similar to the one in 1918 that killed millions. The bird flu virus kills by short-circuiting the immune system, disabling the feedback system that turns the immune response off before it can damage the body. The inflammatory response remains turned on, pumping out pro-inflammatory cytokines. The lungs become filled with fluid from the inflammatory process. The result is that the patient dies, not from the flu, but by literally drowning in his or her own fluids.[500] By modulating the immune system to normal levels, PRPs may be able to prevent this result, allowing the flu virus to be handled normally by the immune system.[501]

PRPs are also cytokine modulators. Cytokines are a diverse group of soluble proteins and peptides that act as humoral regulators at nanomolar to picomolar concentrations and which, either under normal or pathological conditions, modulate the functional activities of individual cells and tissues. These proteins also mediate interactions between cells directly and regulate processes taking place in the extracellular environment. Cytokines IL-1 and -6, interferon-γ and lymphokines have been shown to stimulate the lymph glands and are thought to be highly effective antiviral immune substances. Interleukins regulate the duration and intensity of the immune response and are responsible for cell-to-cell communication as well as boosting T cell activity and the production of immunoglobulins.

In summary, PRPs present an alternative to standard, pharmaceutical drug-based medicine and offer hope against otherwise difficult to treat or untreatable conditions. They are safe and come from a trusted source—cow's colostrum. Now we shall explore a real-life trial of PRPs in the fight against AIDS.

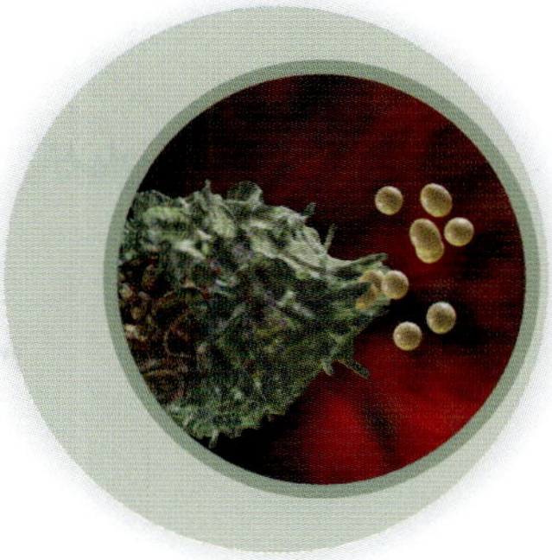

CHAPTER 14

PRPS AND AIDS

Since AIDS first appeared in the early 1980s, over 25 million people have died from the disease and an estimated 33.2 million people are infected with the HIV virus, according to WHO. In 2007 alone, approximately 2.1 million people died from the disease, including around 330,000 children under fifteen. Hardest hit of all is sub-Saharan Africa. Over three-quarters of all deaths from AIDS in 2007 occurred in this region.[502] Whole areas of some countries have been emptied of inhabitants, and the number of orphaned children continues to skyrocket. It is estimated that one in three people in Botswana are infected and life expectancy has declined from 65 pre-AIDS to only 40 today.[503]

While more effective remedies for treating AIDS have become available, the high cost of such remedies effectively prevents the people of so-called Third World countries from receiving these remedies. If an effective alternative could be found to the high-priced pharmaceutical drugs currently being used in the West, many lives could be saved which might otherwise be lost.

AIDS is an unusual viral infection in that the virus, a retrovirus known as Human Immunodeficiency Virus (HIV), attacks the very cells that normally would protect the body against a viral attack, the CD4+ lymphocytes (T cells), macrophages, and dendritic cells of the immune system. Infection by the virus kills cells in three ways: direct viral killing of the cells when the virus replicates; increased rates of apoptosis (programmed cell death) of infected cells; and targeting by CD8 cytotoxic lymphocytes that recognize infected cells and kill them. Eventually the T cell levels degrade to such low levels that cell-mediated immune function is lost. This leaves the body open to opportunistic infections, such as ***Pneumocystis pneumonia*** or Kaposi's sarcoma. These secondary infections are what eventually kill the victim. As PRPs are known to be immunomodulatory, up-regulating the immune system when it is underperforming and down-regulating it when it is hyperactive, it was hypothesized that giving AIDS patients a PRP supplement might counteract the effect of the HIV and restore T cell levels.

Synthetic peptides can also be used to help with HIV infection. Researchers developed Peptide T. Peptide T is a synthetically produced protein derived from gp120—the protein on the surface of HIV particles that binds to the CD4 molecule on the surface of some human cells. Peptide T was discovered in 1986 when scientists were screening for gp120 derived peptides which might block HIV infection. However, using synthetic peptides does not work as effectively as natural peptides because the synthetic peptides often do not fit into natural human cell receptors.

Based on the premise of using a PRP supplement to combat AIDS, a Phase I trial was carried out with several AIDS patients at the Infectious Disease Clinic in Dayton, Ohio, in 1996. A spray PRP preparation called PRPs™ was given to AIDS patients in a dosage of three sprays every four hours. Patients were initially assessed as to severity of the disease and clinical symptoms, such as diarrhea, nausea, vomiting, fever, cough, and so forth. Based on the success of these initial trials, two Phase II trials were carried out at the University of Nairobi, Nairobi, Kenya, in 2000.[504]

Results of these trials were very encouraging. All participants in the study experienced a rise in T cell levels. None had levels below 300 at the end of the study, while at the beginning of the study levels were well below normal (median 275). Over half of the patients had CD4+ levels in normal ranges (500–1500) by the end of the study (Tables 1–4).

	Before		After	
	No.	%	No.	%
150-200	17	29%	0	0%
201-250	10	17%	0	0%
251-300	21	36%	0	0%
301-400	4	7%	8	14%
401-500	4	7%	19	33%
501-600	2	3%	12	21%
601-1000	0	0%	19	33%
Totals	58		58	

TABLE 1 . CD4+ COUNTS IN 58 EXPERIMENTAL SUBJECTS BEFORE AND AFTER APPLICATION OF ORAL PRPs SPRAY.

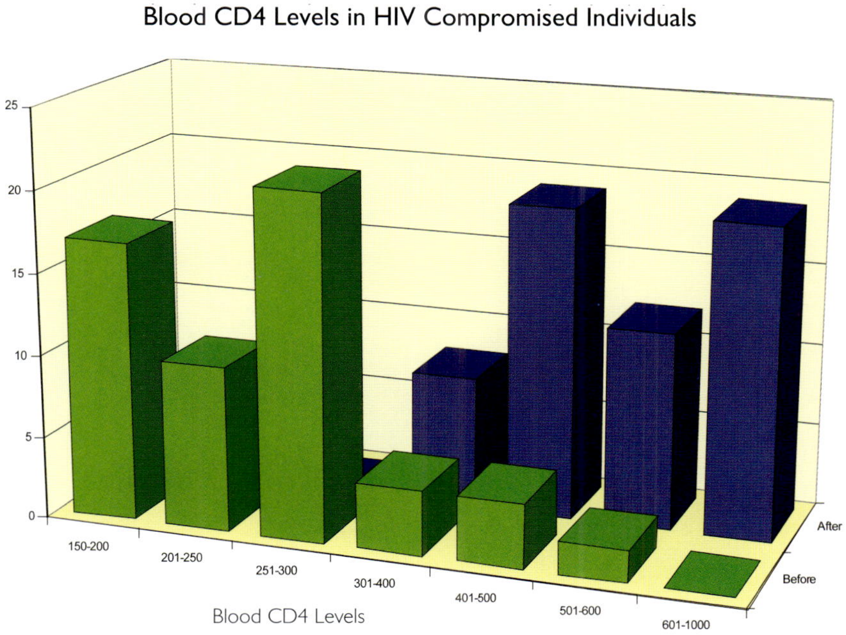

TABLE 2. CD4+ LYMPHOCYTE LEVELS IN HIV COMPROMISED INDIVIDUALS BEFORE AND AFTER TREATMENT WITH PRPs ORAL SPRAY. THIS BAR GRAPH CLEARLY ILLUSTRATES THE MARKED INCREASE IN CD4+ LYMPHOCYTE COUNTS IN PATIENTS WITH LONG-TERM HIV/AIDS AND SEVERELY DEPLETED CD4+ COUNTS AFTER ADMINISTRATION OF ORAL PRPs SPRAY. RESULTS FROM TRIAL 1 HELD IN NIGERIA.

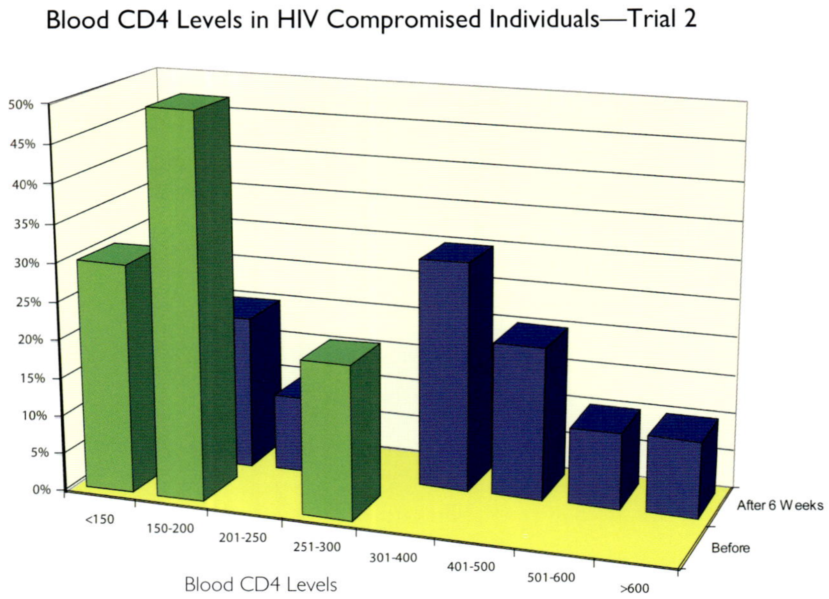

TABLE 3. CD4+ LYMPHOCYTE LEVELS IN HIV COMPROMISED INDIVIDUALS BEFORE AND AFTER TREATMENT WITH PRPS ORAL SPRAY. THESE RESULTS ARE FROM TRIAL 2 HELD IN KENYA.

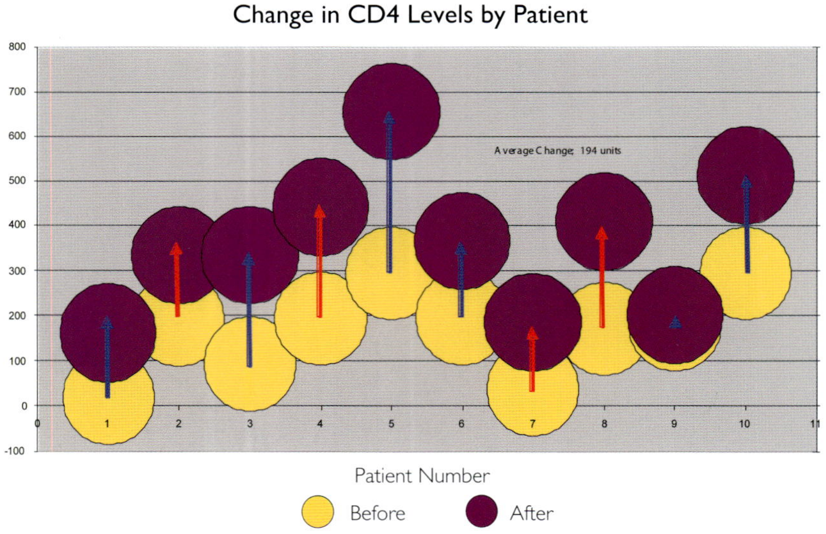

TABLE 4. A GRAPHICAL REPRESENTATION OF CHANGES IN CD4+ LYMPHOCYTE LEVELS IN PATIENTS PARTICIPATING IN TRIAL 2. WHILE LEVELS FOR SOME INCREASED OVER 100% IN SOME CASES, WHAT IS PARTICULARLY SIGNIFICANT IS THAT LEVELS INCREASED FOR ALL PARTICIPANTS IN THE STUDY.

Clinical symptoms also showed dramatic improvement over the course of the studies. All clinical parameters improved dramatically or were eliminated in the participants. These results are summarized in Tables 5 and 6.

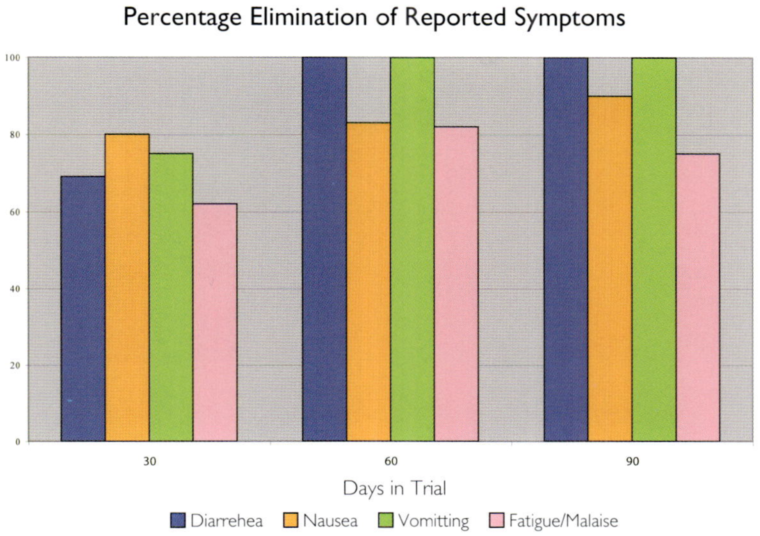

TABLE 5. RELIEF OF DIARRHEA, NAUSEA, VOMITING, AND FATIGUE/MALAISE IN TRIAL PARTICIPANTS OVER THE 90 DAYS OF THE STUDY

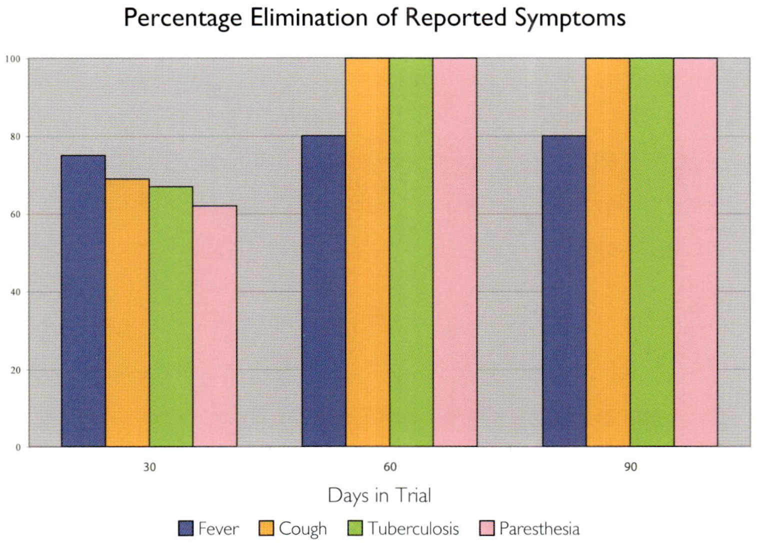

TABLE 6. RELIEF OF FEVER, COUGH, TUBERCULOSIS AND PARESTHESIA IN TRIAL PARTICIPANTS OVER THE 90 DAYS OF THE STUDY.

Viral load also decreased dramatically in study participants, most likely as a result of the increase in T cells. These data are presented in Table 7.

	Initial Total	30 Day Total	60 Day Total
	92,448	9,755	445
	28,049	625	n/a
	33,093	239	n/a
	439	n/a	175
	59,821	n/a	320
	40,381	180	n/a
Expected Phase III % Reduction		<1,000	<500 (<250 at 90 days)

Table 7. Viral Load. Viral load counts in six patients from the Phase II trial.

Patients in the studies also experienced significant weight gain, another marker of improved health (Table 8). Patients receiving PRPs showed an average weight gain of 3.4 kg over the course of the study, while those receiving anti-retrovirus therapy (ART) averaged only a 0.3 kg weight gain.

These results show that supplementation with PRPs can significantly affect the course of viral disease, in particular one caused by a deadly virus like HIV. They also indicate that PRPs can be a valuable adjunct therapy for AIDS patients, greatly increasing quality of life, reversing the progress of the disease, and presumably increasing life expectancy. Phase III trials of this product are currently underway.

A recent study indicated an increase in lytic readings in 10 women and 10 men by an average of 248%[505] when given dialyzable leukocyte extract, a form of PRP. Lytic readings are an indication of the function of the body's natural killer cell activity. This may explain why PRPs are so successful against viral infections. However, much work remains to determine the actual mechanisms of action. A discussion of natural killer cell function follows.

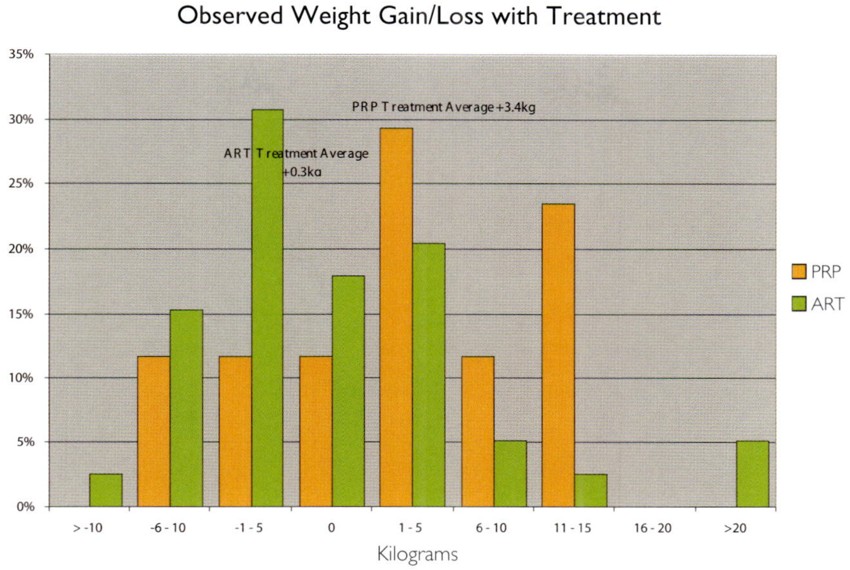

TABLE 8. WEIGHT LOSS/GAIN FOR PATIENTS ON ORAL PRPs OR ANTI-RETROVIRUS THERAPY (ART).

What Are Natural Killer Cells?

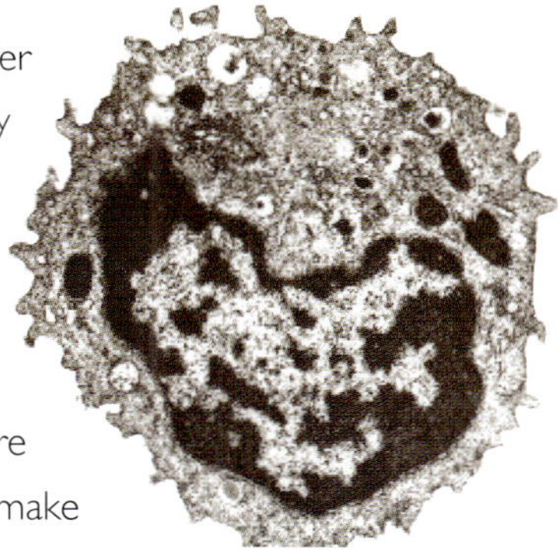

Of all the immune system's soldiers, natural killer cells (NK cells) are the most aggressive. They are the first line of defense against mutant and virus infected cells like Severe Acute Respiratory Syndrome (SARS) or West Nile that are a health threat. They are lymphocytes with no immunological memory and are part of the innate immune system. NK cells make up about 5–16% of the total lymphocyte population. Their specific function is to destroy infected and cancerous cells.

NK cells do not kill indiscriminately. They look for an IFF (Identification: Friend or Foe) banner flown by normal cells. If the NK cell sees this banner, it receives a signal to spare that cell. This signal overrides the NK cell's urge to kill. If this banner is absent on the target cell, the NK cell proceeds with its attack. It attaches to the target and releases a lethal burst of chemicals that penetrate the cell wall. Fluids begin to leak in and out and eventually the cell explodes (lyses).

In addition to their role in the control of infections, NK cells help in the regulation of other aspects of the immune system that affect our overall health. Immunotherapy to help increase NK cell activity is becoming available and will become more widely used as knowledge of the immune system increases.[506]

Colostrum peptides of PRPs act to modulate cytokine activity. NK cells are activated in response to balancing balancing interferons or macrophage-derived cytokines.[124]

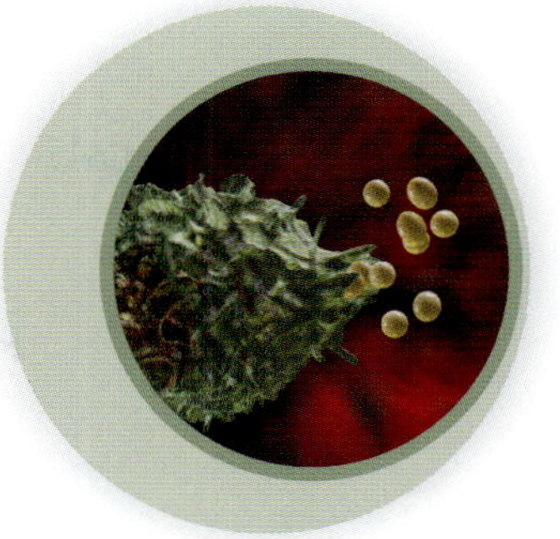

CHAPTER 15

FREQUENTLY ASKED QUESTIONS ABOUT PROLINE-RICH POLYPEPTIDES

Following are many of the common questions asked about PRPs:

How do PRPs work?

PRPs directly support the natural killer (NK) cells of the immune system. Natural killer (NK) cells provide the front line of defense specially equipped to locate and kill disease cells. NK cells attach to the surfaces of foreign substances or their outer cell wall and inject a chemical "grenade" (granule) into the interior. Once inside, the granules explode and destroy the foreign invader within five minutes. The NK cell itself remains intact and moves on to destroy the next immune attacker. Many doctors and clinics are finding PRPs helpful in promoting NK function and activity as well as supporting a healthy immune system for all patients.

The immune system plays a vital role in the quality of our health. Strong, active and optimally functioning NK cells promote optimal health and deter foreign substances from affecting immune function.

How was the active component (PRPs) discovered?

In 1949 Dr. H. Sherwood Lawrence was working on the problem of tuberculosis, which was a major health concern of the time. What he was trying to discover was if any component of the blood could convey a tubercular sensitivity from an exposed recovered donor to a naive recipient. Whole blood transfusions could be used but only between people of the same blood type. Lawrence first separated the blood's immune cells, the lymphocytes or white blood cells, from the whole blood. Then he broke open the lymphocytes and separated the contents of the cells into various size fractions. What he found was that a fraction of small molecules was able to transfer tuberculin sensitivity to a naive recipient. This is what Dr. Lawrence called Proline-rich Polypeptides (PRPs)—the active peptides in PRPs.

Is blood the only source of PRPs?
Originally it was. It was not until the mid-1980s that two researchers came up with the idea that PRPs or infopeptides may also be present in colostrum. The confirmation of this discovery was awarded a patent in 1989. Bovine (cow) colostrum is now the best source of PRPs.

What is the actual definition of infopeptides?
The term applies to a class of small peptides or proteins that circulate in the blood of mammals and accumulate or concentrate in their colostrum, in their milk, and in their blood sera. Infopeptides appear to convey information necessary for appropriate cellular function.

What prompted these scientists to look for PRPs in colostrum?
Those who have worked with cattle know that if a calf is not allowed to nurse from its mother it will most often die within a short time. The calves would die in spite of an abundance of food. Death in these cases was cause by infections brought on by the most common organisms. For whatever reason the immune systems of these calves were not working. Seeing this suggests that there is some kind of immune information being transferred from the mother to her infant. The logical question then became: was it PRPs? The answer was a resounding YES! How does PRPs™ liquid compare with whole colostrum supplements?

Comparing PRPs liquid to a whole colostrum supplement would be like comparing a precious metal to the ore from which it is derived. It is composed of highly concentrated PRPs which offer maximum immune benefit. Whole colostrum contains a much smaller concentration of PRPs.

Can these infopeptides be as effective for adults as for a newborn infant?

Infopeptides need to be processed to be effective for adults. The polypeptides from colostrum are not absorbable (or more properly, not "readable") by adults unless separated and broken up into smaller sizes. One company has successfully accomplished this goal, and refers to its product as PRPs™.

Can we get enough human colostrum to provide enough of the infopeptides?

Bovine colostrum—that is, from cows—provides infopeptides that are fully effective in humans. Good thing, otherwise they would be prohibitively expensive. But does the bovine source of infopeptides really work as well as human?

This answer is yes. Whereas bovine colostrum and lactoferrin are close but not precise matches of their human counterparts, infopeptides from cows may be even closer. Dr. Stephen Levine, a biochemist, says that these polypeptides are so important to animal survival that they may have been genetically conserved through the evolutionary process with virtually no change from species to species, much like vitamin C or melatonin.

The clinical experience with bovine products is sufficiently compelling to imply that the bovine immune system is every bit as "smart" as the human one.

What is meant by the phrase, "No clear relationship between dose and benefit"?

In the studies done to date, it has been noted that the administration of PRPs above the minimum levels necessary for response does not enhance or intensify the benefit.

What do these infopeptides do for adults, anyway?

Early studies suggest that infopeptides are extremely effective as anti-inflammatory agents as well as immune modulators.

What specific types of conditions are likely to respond to PRPs?
A variety of conditions have been helped, including infectious diseases, progressive degenerative disorders, allergic disorders, and even a dozen or so rare diseases.

What types of conditions are least likely to respond to PRPs?

Those least likely to respond are those suffering from the effects of permanent tissue damage or environmental toxins.

How are PRPs administered?
In most cases, oral administration is preferred. Amounts from 1/4 to 1 teaspoon are placed in the mouth, or sprayed in the mouth and held or circulated for a few seconds prior to swallowing.

Topical application is also effective for burns, sutures, and other healing skin conditions.

How much is needed to be effective?
Again, small doses are effective. The usual mode of administration is a teaspoon of liquid or spray in the mouth, for example 2 mls or 3 sprays, held in contact with oral mucosa for a few minutes and then swallowed.

Are PRPs safe?
The safety of PRPs has been demonstrated in physician-monitored safety studies, and in normal use. As with any food, should evidence of intolerance develop, it is recommended that the use of PRPs be discontinued until an adequate assessment of the circumstances can be made. But in all of my research, talking at length to physicians and patients, no one has reported any deleterious side effects.

Should I take PRPs as a preventive?

Not necessarily, but if you feel you have been exposed or may be exposed to unhealthful surroundings, that's the time to take it. The developer of the product explains: "If I take PRPs in the morning, before going to work, and my coworkers are sneezing and coughing, I could be protected for six hours. However, more frequent dosages are recommended if symptoms persist."

Interesting stuff! Interesting concept! You should know that I have been tracking the progress of PRPs with its history of success for problems ranging from acute viral attacks to serious chronic and even life-threatening disorders for a few years.

PRPs appears to have the potential to revolutionize at least three major areas of treatment. PRPs are helpful for:

- Immune dysfunction, including underactive and overactive immune system, from minor to major, including AIDS and autoimmune disorders
- Childhood diarrhea
- Myalgias and muscle pains, including arthritis and fibromyalgia

Keep in mind that PRPs are not a magic bullet against a specific organism or disease. It appears to stimulate your immune system to action. In other words, it is a health maintenance product rather than a medicine.

Although its ability to conquer the first two areas of very serious afflictions is thrilling, I must admit that it is the third that has me reeling with excitement. Is there any among us who doesn't know at least one person suffering from fibromyalgia? At last, I now have a more positive response when so many of you come up to me at meetings, pleading for help because of this debilitating disorder.

Homeostasis requires the coordinated functioning of trillions of cells. Some influence on our cells inclines us toward wellness. This would require communication or advice and perhaps some form of informational media. It just may be that infopeptides are that media, advising every function of every well cell!

There's so much we have yet to understand. No matter. I don't know what the pistons or spark plugs do in my car, but that's no deterrent for me to drive.

Since PRPs are isolated from colostrum, what about milk allergies and lactose intolerance?

Milk allergies are caused by the large milk proteins, primarily casein, and to a lesser extent the immunoglobulins. These proteins are completely removed from the PRPs. Lactose intolerance is most common in Oriental populations; much less so in those of European or African decent. We are conscious of this, but we have noticed that the dose of lactose that a person receives is only 70mg, less than the 80mg needed to promote an allergic result from taking lactose in lactose-intolerant people. Lactose intolerance itself is a food allergen, and because PRPs help modulate the Interleukin levels in the body, this reduces the probability of an allergic response.

How do PRPs compare to the colostrum products that are on the market now?

We looked seriously at hyperimmunized colostrum and eggs. These products are good, but certain issues must be addressed. First, the milk allergy and lactose intolerance issues as we discussed above. Second, the issue of immunoglobulin or antibody effectiveness. The use of cross-species antibody therapy can be effective in the short run. Long-term use, however, is ineffective since the recipient develops antibodies to the foreign antibody thus destroying its effectiveness. Antibody therapy is given intravenously since oral consumption leads to degradation of the antibodies in the stomach.

Are PRPs only good for newborns?

PRPs are good for everyone who has an immune imbalance. The three groups who are most in need of immune modulation are the young, the old, and anyone under stress. Almost all of us fall into one of these categories. We often talk of the baby boom generation. Most of these people are at an age where their immune systems are already becoming weaker. PRPs are a way to boost a lagging immune system and greatly improve one's health. However, pregnant woman or those trying to get pregnant should not take PRPs as this may interfere with the TH1/TH2 cytokine balance.

Have PRPs been scientifically validated?

Since Lawrence's discovery of PRPs in blood in 1949 (which he called transfer factor), there have been over 3000 scientific studies published on PRPs.

What conditions are responsive to PRPs?

PRP preparations have been used to effectively help with a wide range of diseases. These include bacterial, mycobacterial, fungal, parasitic, viral, and cancerous conditions. It is in part because of AIDS, or more specifically our frustration in treating AIDS, that PRPs are experiencing a resurgence of research interest. In fact, a recent international symposium held in Italy was titled: PRPs in the Era of AIDS.

If PRPs are so effective, why hasn't the pharmaceutical industry jumped on PRPs?

In the 1950s antibiotics were the golden child of medicine followed in the '60s by steroids, such as cortisone, for inflammation and the synthetic steroid hormones like ethinyl estrogen and progestin that were used to create the birth control pill.

After an initial delay, PRPs (then known mainly as transfer factor) hit their heyday in the 70s and early 80s. Results, however, were inconsistent as researchers dove in sometimes with more enthusiasm than skill. The key feature that was missing in these investigations was a dependable assay technique for quality control of the product. The quality control issue was not resolved until the mid 1980s. Given that PRPs are not a single entity, pharmaceutical companies had fits trying to purify the material without losing efficacy. This forced fit into the single-entity, single-function drug dogma was disastrous.

The next issue that slowed PRP research is the age-old issue of funding. When AIDS hit the popular press, politicians shifted funding into AIDS research but with the focus on finding the cause and then finding a drug that would cure AIDS. The work of a few dedicated, but underfunded, researchers and the inability of the mainstream medical-pharmaceutical industry have combined to again focus attention on PRPs as one of the few modalities that is effective against diseases of viral origin.

Are there reasons why we haven't seen PRPs as a dietary supplement before now?

Yes, there are two doors that recently have opened that allow PRPs to be effectively marketed now. The first door to open was the passage of DSHEA (Dietary Supplement Health and Education Act) in 1994. The provision for structure-functions claims allows the story of PRPs to be told without jeopardizing its status as a nutritional supplement. The second is technical. PRPs was definitely an idea way ahead of its time, and it had to wait for technology to catch up. The processing methods that allow for large-scale extraction of PRPs have only recently been perfected, and a commercial product has only been available for the past few years.

How does one discuss PRPs in terms of structure-function claims?

Simplistically, PRPs strengthen the immune system. But that is overly simplistic and could be used to describe a number of herbal products and other supplements.

Let me answer the question by first reiterating that PRPs are not just a single entity. PRPs are in fact a complex mixture containing three separate fractions. These three fractions are an INDUCER fraction, an ANTIGEN-SPECIFIC fraction, and a SUPPRESSOR fraction.

Since our immune systems fight the microbe wars for us, let me use a military analogy to explain these three functions. The inducer fraction serves as the drill sergeant of basic training, whipping the immune system into shape but not telling them who to go out and attack. The antigen-specific fraction is like a set of wanted posters identifying critical features of the bad guys. If we were microbes, these specific identifiers would be our fingerprints, mug shots, etc. Similarly a whole set of PRPs are made against a single microbe type. Finally, the suppressor fraction is like the politicians who declare an end to the war and demobilize the troops. Without this final action, a lot of collateral damage would be done, whether in war or within ourselves.

When our immune system does not demobilize or overreacts, we suffer from autoimmune conditions such as multiple sclerosis and allergies. Unlike most immune supplements that provide the building blocks for proper immune function, PRPs function as an immune intelligence network. They pass on immune information and education that focuses the immune system, keeping it on task and effective. This is a whole new concept in immune system strengthening.

Are PRPs FDA approved?

It is approved as a dietary supplement, but not as a drug, according to Dr. Fudenburg (Progress in Drug Research, 1994, 42:378). Foods and dietary supplements are not approved per se by the FDA, and food supplements derived from milk would certainly fall under the category of GRAS (Generally Recognized As Safe).

Are PRPs safe?

YES! Researchers have given huge doses of PRPs to volunteers in an attempt to trigger some sort of adverse reaction. No harmful negative side effects were observed even when massive doses were used. Consuming several glasses of PRPs liquid may promote symptoms associated with lactose intolerance. Also, one should not consume large quantities of anything, even water because it may cause brain swelling and other health problems.

Are there any reports about PRPs helping people with cancer?

Radiation, chemotherapy, and surgery are the commonly used conventional cancer treatments. Both radiation and chemotherapy are highly damaging to fast growing cells in the body, such as intestinal lining cells, the cells of bone marrow, and the cells of the immune system. After such treatments, persons often have to be on very strong antibiotics in order to prevent infections, which presents a whole new set of problems.

The use of PRPs in combination with radiation or chemotherapy protects the immune system by some mechanism which we do not fully understand at the present. In cases of surgical removal of certain tumors the use of PRPs as an adjuvant therapy results in a higher survival rate.

What about colds?

Colds are viral diseases, and PRPs are used most commonly against viral conditions. Studies of PRPs and colds have not been officially done but interestingly, cold relief is a commonly reported side effect of taking PRPs.

Are PRPs safe for infants?

Colostral PRPs were designed by nature for newborns and can be taken safely by infants.

Why are PRPs different from other PRP products or colostrum products?

Within the spectrum of PRP activities, PRPs have a unique enhanced activity for several viruses, including Human Herpes Virus-6 (HHV-6) variants A and B, Epstein-Barr Virus (EBV) and Cytomegalovirus (CMV). This enhanced activity provides for an improved immune response against active HHV-6, EBV and CMV infections. This should lead to a decrease in viral activity and improved immune function since these viruses are known to be immunosuppressive. Colostrum itself does not have this unique activity.

What types of responses are possible with PRPs?

Overall, PRPs have shown very promising responses. In looking at a prototype group of patients with a history of chronic fatigue syndrome (CFS) or fibromyalgia (FM), improvement in symptoms has been seen in approximately 85% of those who have taken both TF560 and TF540 (now available as Immune Care™-64). Common symptoms such as fatigue, diminished activity level, muscle aches, joint aches, and impaired memory function have substantially improved when these patients took both TF560 and TF540. Some patients (approximately 25%) have noted a very dramatic reduction in symptoms, essentially resolution of all symptoms. Immune function appears to improve as well. Laboratory assessment of immune function utilizing the natural killer (NK) cell function assay has shown impressive improvements. 70% to 80% of patients' NK function assays improve from very low baseline levels to normal function values after taking PRPs.

What are the reasons some patients do not respond?

There may be a variety of reasons. The most widely studied herpes viruses have been Herpes simplex virus (HSV-1) and genital herpes (HSV-2). In the extensive literature regarding PRP administration in these patients, there was a definite reduction in overall symptoms and frequency of outbreaks. However, some patients did not respond. Thus, prior PRP studies have shown good responses for a variety of viruses, but responses vary. PRPs rarely result in a 100% response rate. It is intuitive that a similar pattern may be seen with newly developed concentrated PRP products (PRPs). A number of other factors may be involved with suboptimal or inadequate responses, including duration of illness, co-infections, hypercoaguable syndrome, and other chronic medical conditions (e.g., diabetes mellitus and cardiovascular disease).

Adverse side effects of taking PRPs?

The majority of patients have no adverse effects at all. However, some patients may notice a sense of bloating caused by taking more than the 2ml dose. This is caused by the moderate levels of lactose in PRPs (4% w/w of PRPs solution). Moreover, lactose intolerance is a food allergy. By taking a PRP supplement this can balance the specific cytokines responsible for lactose intolerance.

How should one take enhanced PRP products for Human Herpesvirus-6 (HHV-6) and Epstein-Barr Virus (EBV)?

It may be prudent to start at the lower dose and work up over a week or two. We would generally suggest starting at one dose (2ml, or 3 sprays) per day for 5–7 days, then increase to two doses per day for 5–7 days, and then increase to three per day. Slowly escalating the dose may diminish the bloating symptoms. If bloating symptoms are noted, do not increase the dose until the symptoms have resolved. The most effective dose for viral infections appears to be 2ml (3 sprays) six times per day for adults, albeit smaller doses may be effective in some individuals. For autoimmune disorders, three doses per day. For maintenance of a healthy immune system, two doses per day.

SUMMARY OF PRPS

- PRPs were discovered in the 1940s and have been extensively studied for the past fifty years.
- PRPs can transfer cell-mediated immunity (CMI) from an immune donor animal to a non-immune recipient.
- PRPs are manufactured by leukocytes (white blood cells), mainly T lymphocytes.
- The structure of PRPs has not been entirely established, but is a small peptide, probably with a small piece of RNA attached.
- PRPs stimulate cell-mediated immunity (CMI; for a specific antigen), probably via T lymphocytes.
- PRPs is antigen-specific, i.e., for each specific type of infection.
- PRPs can cross species lines and does not cause allergic reactions from one species to another.
- PRPs can be generated from the leukocytes of a donor animal. However, one of the most efficient ways to recover it is from colostrum.
- Once PRPs have been generated, they should be assayed and validated for their immunologic activity, which can be expressed as potency units.
- After PRPs are administered, they can induce internal PRP production by the recipient.
- The ability of an individual to produce internal PRPs varies, in that some do not synthesize internal PRPs very well.
- Most people can respond to externally administered PRPs with initial action within 24 hours.
- PRPs have been found to be extremely safe.
- Since PRPs can stimulate the immune system, they can give rise to flu-like symptoms when one first starts to take it.
- PRPs are most effective in regulating immunity to infections in which cell-mediated immunity (CMI, T cells) is important for controlling the infection.
- PRPs have been shown to increase natural killer (NK) cell activity.

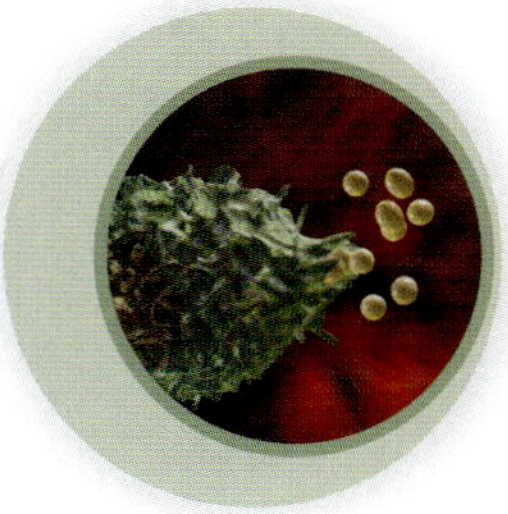

APPENDIX A

BRIEF REVIEW OF THE IMMUNE SYSTEM

The immune response is a defense mechanism by which the body fights infection. It is divided into two functional systems, the ***innate immune system*** and the ***adaptive immune system***. The innate system is the first line of defense by which the host combats infectious agents and pathogenic microbes. This is a non-specific response, which proves effective against most infective agents. In case this primary response is not effective and the invading microbe is led to proliferate the adaptive immune system comes into action. The adaptive immune system produces a specific response in the form of antibodies to the infective agent that normally proves effective in neutralizing that agent. In the case of the innate system resistance (immunity) is not improved by repeated infection. The adaptive immune response involves ***memory*** and gives rise to resistance to repeated exposure to the same infective agent. Childhood diseases such as mumps, measles, and chickenpox produce life-long immunity following an infection.

Most infectious agents enter the body proper via the epithelial surfaces of either the upper respiratory, digestive or genito-urinary tract. Once infectious agents have penetrated the body a variety of physical and chemical defense mechanisms come into play to help protect these tissues from most infections. This involves a specialized set of cells called ***leukocytes*** (white blood cells) and their products that have evolved to help combat infection and disease. Leukocytes fall into two broad categories of cell types: ***phagocytes*** and ***lymphocytes***. Phagocytes form part of the innate immune system and provide non-specific immunity. Included in this category are neutrophils, basophils, eosinophils, monocytes, and macrophages.

Lymphocytes form the adaptive immune system and provide specific immunity. There are two types of lymphocytes ***B cells*** and ***T cells***. The B cells are differentiated in the bone marrow and found mainly in the lymph nodes and spleen. They are the cells that make ***antibodies (immunoglobulins)***. The T cells are differentiated in the thymus and fulfill two major functions. They regulate the activity of the B cells and directly attack infectious agents.

Passive Immunity

During embryonic development the unborn animal's immune system is not sufficiently developed to ward off potentially harmful microbes. Fortunately the fetus is protected from harmful environmental factors by its position in the womb; potentially harmful agents cannot pass the placental barrier. At birth the newborn without a complement of antibodies would find its environment very hostile, being quite susceptible to infection from invading organisms. To alleviate this potentially lethal situation a very interesting phenomenon, known as ***passive immunization***, has evolved. The maternal blood contains a full complement of antibodies to various antigens to which the mother has been exposed during her lifetime. In humans and apes the mother passively immunizes her young ***in utero*** by passage of antibodies through the placenta. In animals where the maternal antibodies are unable to pass the placental barrier (cattle, pigs, and sheep), the young are passively immunized immediately after birth by way of colostrum. In these species the maternal antibodies present in the colostrum are absorbed directly through the gut in the first few days after birth. When newborn cattle, pigs and sheep are deprived of colostrum, a significant increase in mortality rate is observed.[509,510] In a study conducted by the Invermay Agricultural Center it was shown that the post-treatment mortality of triplet lambs was significantly increased from 7.4% to 19.4%. The association of high neonatal survival rates and the successful transfer of colostrum has been reported.[511,512,513]

IgG is the form in which antibodies occur most abundantly. In all species of mammals IgG is passed from the mother to its young, although the actual mechanism of transmission varies species to species. In humans and apes it has been shown that IgG and its complement of antibodies pass across the placental barrier from mother to fetus during the second two-thirds of gestation. This passage appears to be selective in that IgG is transferred but not the other immunoglobulins (IgA, IgM, IgE, IgD). Albumin is also transferred but to a lesser degree. Other plasma proteins are not transferred across the placental barrier. In cattle it appears that the same type of selection occurs in absorption of antibodies through the gut in that there is a preferential passage of IgG but not IgA, IgM, IgD or IgE.

Passive Local Protection

In humans, passive transmission of maternal antibodies takes place prior to birth and occurs ***in utero***. After birth, the antibodies present in human milk function in local passive protection. Once again the predominant immunoglobulin in human breast milk is of the IgA class. In most other animals such as the horse, cow, pig and sheep there is no passive transmission of immunity prior to birth. In these animals passive transmission of maternal antibodies occurs in the first 20–48 hours after birth by way of colostrum. During this time they absorb intact antibodies via the newborn's digestive tract. After these first few days the direct absorption of intact antibodies ceases, and any antibodies present in the colostrum and milk then function in local passive protection of the gastrointestinal (GI) tract.

The importance of this passive local protection is evidenced in the newborn calf where diarrhea and other enteric infections (scours) can prove fatal.[514] It has been reported that the best source of nourishment for the infant mammal is mother's milk.[515] This has largely been attributed to not only the nutritional benefits of milk but also to the presence of milk immunoglobulins providing local passive protection to the GI tract. A very important aspect of this local immune protection is that it is not species specific and as such we as humans, and all other animals, can use bovine colostrum for its various health benefits.

The immune system is made up of two basic parts:

Innate immune system—nonspecific immunity, including barrier defenses (skin, intestinal lining, brain-blood barrier, macrophages, neutrophils, dendritic cells etc.), airway cilia (remove antigens and small particles that are breathed in), mucus, chemicals such as lactoferrin, lactoperoxidase and lysozyme which are potent killers of pathogens, strong acids in the stomach, and so forth[516]

Adaptive immune system—system which consists of immune and scavenger cells (lymphocytes, macrophages, NK [natural killer] cells, mast cells, monocytes and other blood cells) that react to specific antigens

The adaptive immune system furthermore has two response modes:

Humoral Immunity—production of specific antibodies in response to an antigen, mediated by B cells
Cell-Mediated Immunity—production of cytotoxic lymphocytes, activated macrophages and NK cells, and cytokines in response to an antigen, mediated by T cells

Lymphocytes come in several different varieties. B lymphocytes (B cells) are produced in the bone marrow, and T lymphocytes (T cells) are produced in the thymus gland. T cells are further broken down into:

Cytotoxic or killer T cells (CD8)—the cells which actually kill invading pathogens
Helper T cells (CD4+)—cells which direct the immune response through the secretion of cytokines[517,518]
Suppressor T cells—inhibit the production of cytotoxic T cells when no longer needed to prevent excess tissue damage and turn down an adaptive immune response
Memory T cells—retain memory of an encountered antigen so that if encountered again the response time will be much shorter

Helper T cells secrete various cytokines to stimulate the production and differentiation of cytotoxic T cells and B-cells, which produce antibodies. They also attract neutrophils (white blood cells) and stimulate macrophages to engulf and destroy pathogens.

Helper T cells also have subsets:[519,520]

TH1 cells—secrete the cytokines tumor necrosis factor-alpha (TNF-α) and interleukin 12 (IL-12) which control cell-mediated immunity; TH1 activation can inhibit TH2 cell activation

TH2 cells—secrete the cytokines IL-4 and IL-5 which control humoral immunity; TH2 cell activation can inhibit TH1 cell activation

Regulatory TH3 (Tr) cells514—at least three different type of regulatory TH cells exist:

Type 1 (Tr1)—secrete large amounts of IL-10 and low-to-moderate amounts of transforming growth factor-beta (TGF-β), may help terminate TH1-related inflammatory responses

Type 3 (Tr3)—primarily secrete TGF-β, regulates multiple facets of immune response

CD4+CD25+—inhibit immune responses through direct cell-to-cell contact

The diagram on the following page may help clarify how the immune system works as a coordinated system to protect the organism:

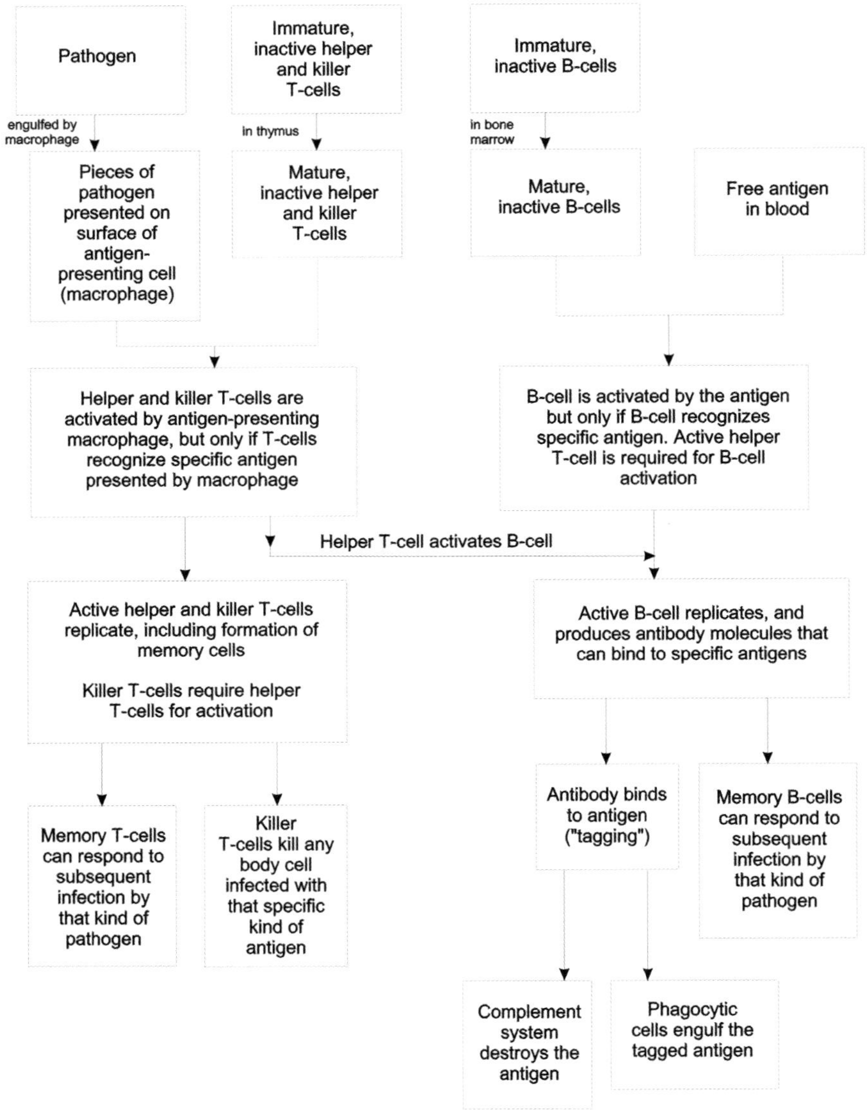
Pathogen
Immature, inactive helper and killer T-cells
Immature, inactive B-cells
engulfed by macrophage
in thymus
in bone marrow
Pieces of pathogen presented on surface of antigen-presenting cell (macrophage)
Mature, inactive helper and killer T-cells
Mature, inactive B-cells
Free antigen in blood
Helper and killer T-cells are activated by antigen-presenting macrophage, but only if T-cells recognize specific antigen presented by macrophage
B-cell is activated by the antigen but only if B-cell recognizes specific antigen. Active helper T-cell is required for B-cell activation
Helper T-cell activates B-cell
Active helper and killer T-cells replicate, including formation of memory cells
Killer T-cells require helper T-cells for activation
Active B-cell replicates, and produces antibody molecules that can bind to specific antigens
Memory T-cells can respond to subsequent infection by that kind of pathogen
Killer T-cells kill any body cell infected with that specific kind of antigen
Antibody binds to antigen ("tagging")
Memory B-cells can respond to subsequent infection by that kind of pathogen
Complement system destroys the antigen
Phagocytic cells engulf the tagged antigen

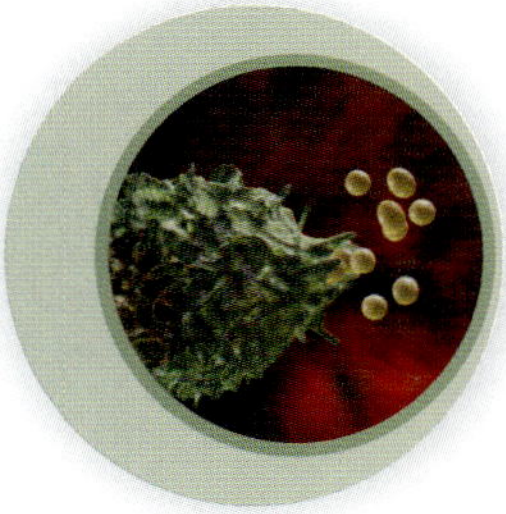

APPENDIX B

TYPICAL SPECIFICATION OF A FIRST MILKING WHOLE COLOSTRUM POWDER

Description and Suggested Applications

Whole colostrum powder produced from raw colostrum collected only from milkings within 16 hours after birth. It should be processed both at low pressures and temperatures and spray or freeze dried using indirect steam to maintain maximum bio-activity. It should be free from antibiotics.

Suggested applications include: immune system enhancement, nutritional supplement, digestive health improvement, protein supplement and alternative treatment for general health.

Major Active Component Analysis

	Specification	Typical	Method
Protein % (Nx6.38) db	45.0 min	50.0	Kheldal
Total Immunoglobulins %	18.0 min	22.0	HPLC (dry basis)
Immunoglobulins (Type G1 & G2) %	15.0 min	18.0	HPLC (dry basis)
Immunoglobulins (Type A) %	2.0 min	2.60	HPLC (dry basis)
Immunoglobulins (Type M) %	0.75 min	1.40	HPLC (dry basis)
Immunoglobulins (Type D) %	0.15 min	0.20	HPLC (dry basis)
Immunoglobulins (Type E) %	0.10 min	0.15	HPLC (dry basis)
Lactoferrin %	0.5 min	0.75	HPLC (dry basis)

Transferrin (mg/g)	3.0 min	4.50	HPLC (dry basis)
Lactoperoxidase-thiocyanate %	0.3 min	0.45	HPLC (dry basis)
Proline-rich Polypeptides (PRPs) %	3.0 min	4.0	HPLC (dry basis)
Insulin Growth Factor (Type 1) μg/g	1.0 min	2.3	ELISA (dry basis)
Insulin Growth Factor (Type 2) ng/g	100 min	140	ELISA (dry basis)
Derived Platelet Growth Factor ng/g	3.5 min	4.2	HPLC (dry basis)
Epidermal Growth Factor μg/g	0.8 min	1.1	ELISA (dry basis)
Fibroblast Platelet Growth Factor ng/g	4.0 min	5.0	ELISA (dry basis)
Transforming Growth Factor Alpha ng/g	15.0 min	22.0	ELISA (dry basis)
Transforming Growth Factor Beta mg/g	0.15 min	0.21	ELISA (dry basis)
Nerve Growth Factor ng/g	8.0 min	11.0	ELISA (dry basis)
Leptin ng/g	35.0 min	50.0	ELISA (dry basis)

Vitamin Analysis*

Vitamin B6 μg/g	10.0 min	15.0	Mass spec. (wet basis)
Vitamin B12 μg/g	0.10 min	0.16	Mass spec. (wet basis)
Vitamin E μg/g	0.15 min	0.20	Mass spec. (wet basis)
Vitamin A μg/g	15.0 min	20.0	Mass spec. (wet basis)
Vitamin C μg/g	0.25 min	0.40	Mass spec. (wet basis)
Vitamin D μg/g	1.00 min	1.20	Mass spec. (wet basis)
Thiamin (Vitamin B1)μg/g	100.0 min	150	Mass spec. (wet basis)
Folic Acid μg/g	2.0 min	2.3	Mass spec. (wet basis)
Pantothenic Acid μg/g	2.0 min	2.3	Mass spec. (wet basis)
Riboflavin (Vitamin B2) μg/g	50.0 min	60.0	Mass spec. (wet basis)
Beta-carotene μg/g	18 min	22	Mass spec. (wet basis)
Glycoconjugates μg/g	2.0 min	2.4	Mass spec. (wet basis)
Glycogen μg/g	40.0 min	56.0	Mass spec. (wet basis)
Retinoic Acid μg/g	5.0 min	8.0	Mass spec. (wet basis)

Analytical and Microbiological Analysis*

	Specification	Typical	Method
Moisture %	5.0 max	4.50	CEM
Protein % (Nx6.38) db	45.0 min	50.0	Kheldal
Ash %	9.0 max	7.0	Mass Spec.

Fat %	24.0 max	22.0	Mojonnier
Lactose %	20.0 max.	16.5	by difference
Energy Content (cal./g)	10.0 max	6.0	
Sediment	B	A	Pad
pH	6.5 < 7.5	7.0	10% sol., 20C
Bulk density	0.25 < 0.35	0.30	grams / cc
Standard Plate Count (col/g)	50,000 max	5,000	Standard**
Yeast and Mold (col/g)	10 max	<10	Standard**
Coliform (col/g)	10 max.	<10	3M Petrifilm
E.Coli (col/g)	10 max.	<1	3M Petrifilm
Staphylococcus aureus	10 max.	<1	3M Petrifilm
Salmonella sp.	Neg. / 25g	Neg.	ELISA
Listeria sp.	Neg. / 25g	Neg.	ELISA

Essential Amino Acid Analysis* (weight/weight basis)(GC/MS)		Non Essential Amino Acid Analysis* (w/w) (GC/MS)	
Isoleucine	1.46%	Arginine	2.30%
Leucine	2.37%	Cystine	1.12%
Histidine	1.46%	Glutanic Acid	9.13%
Methionine	4.08%	Alanine	2.50%
Lysine	4.18%	Tyrosine	4.96%
Threonine	4.03%	Glycine	1.77%
Phenylalanine	2.42%	Proline	5.12%
Valine	2.16%	Aspartic Acid	5.57%
Tryptophan	1.17%	Serine	4.77%

Other Minor Components not Quantified

Beta 2- microglobulin, Enzymes, Haemopexin, Haptoglobin, Orotic Acid, Peroxidase, Xanthine Oxidase Enzyme, Gonadotropin-Releasing Hormone (GnRH), Prolactin, Insulin, Sulfur, Glycoproteins:—(Including Protease and Trypsin Inhibitors), Lactalbumin, MuAltimeric α-Lactalbumin, Cytokines, Lysozymes, Gamma Globulin, β-lactoglobulin, Complement 3 & 4 (C3 & C4), Kappa Casein, Alpha 2-AP glycoprotein, Alpha 1-antitrypsin, Alpha 2-macroglobulin, Orosomucoids, Prealbumin, Albumin, Oligosaccharides, Non

Specific Inhibitors (NSI's), Secretory IgA (SigA), IgA Specific Helper

Mineral Analysis* and Physical Properties

Specification mg/100gm		Typical	Heavy Metals		Properties
Sodium	150 < 300	200	Lead	<1ppm	Solubility: Good
Calcium	150 < 400	250	Mercury	<1ppm	Flavor: Clean & Bland
Potassium	150 < 400	250	Arsenic	<1ppm	Odor: Clean
Magnesium	250 <500	400			Appearance: Free flowing & non-caking
Chromium	30 < 60	40			
Zinc	5 < 20	8			
Chloride	< 100	40			

Packaging, Shipping and Storage

Colostrum powders are hygroscopic and can absorb odors. Temperatures below 75 degrees F, relative humidities below 65% and an odor free environment will extend storage life. Stocks should be used in rotation and preferably within three years.

MATERIAL SAFETY AND DATA SHEET OF A COLOSTRUM POWDER

SECTION 1—COMPOSITION & INFORMATION ON INGREDIENTS

100% Whole Colostrum Powder

SECTION 2—HAZARDS IDENTIFICATIONS

• EMERGENCY OVERVIEW

Off-White. Non-flammable. Non-hazardous to eyes, skin and throat.

POTENTIAL HEALTH EFFECTS

ROUTES OF ENTRY: Eye contact, dermal, inhalation, ingestion

ACUTE EFFECTS OF OVEREXPOSURE:

Eyes—Nuisance dust

Skin—Non-hazardous

Inhalation—Non-hazardous

Ingestion—Non-hazardous

CHRONIC EFFECTS OF OVEREXPOSURE: None known

MEDICAL CONDITIONS AGGRAVATED BY EXPOSURE: None known.

CARCINOGENICITY: NTP: No IARC: No OSHA: No

SECTION 3—FIRST AID MEASURES

EMERGENCY AND FIRST AID PROCEDURES:

Eye Contact—If material comes in contact with the eyes, promptly wash the eyes with water. Get medical attention if any discomfort continues.

Skin Contact—No special precautions; flush with water.

Inhalation—If a person breathes in large amounts of this material, move the exposed person to fresh air at once. Other measures are usually unnecessary.

Ingestion—No special precautions.

SECTION 4—FIRE-FIGHTING MEASURES

Flash Point: N/A AUTO IGNITION TEMP: N/A

FLAMMABLE LIMITS IN AIR LOWER

UPPER % BY VOLUME N/A N/A

Extinguishing Media: Use appropriate media to extinguish source.

SPECIAL FIRE FIGHTING PROCEDURES: N/A

UNUSUAL FIRE AND EXPLOSION HAZARDS: None

HAZARD RATINGS: NFPA 704: Health—0 Fire—0 Reactivity—0

SECTION 5—ACCIDENTAL RELEASE MEASURES

No hazard

SECTION 6—HANDLING & STORAGE

HANDLING AND STORING: Store in a dry area.

SECTION 7—EXPOSURE CONTROL—PERSONAL PROTECTION

ENGINEERING CONTROLS: No requirements

RESPIRATORY EQUIPMENT: No requirements

EYE PROTECTION: No requirements

PROTECTIVE CLOTHING: No requirements

OTHER (SAFETY SHOWERS, EYE WASH STATIONS, ETC.): None

SECTION 8—PHYSICAL & CHEMICAL PROPERTIES

APPEARANCE: Off-White ODOR: N/A

BOILING POINT: N/A

SPECIFIC GRAVITY (water=1): N/A

VAPOR PRESSURE: Negligible

VAPOR DENSITY (air=1): Negligible

SOLUBLE IN WATER: Not soluble EVAPORATION RATE (ether=1): negligible

SECTION 9—STABILITY & REACTIVITY

STABILITY: STABLE X

UNSTABLE

INCOMPATIBILITY: N/A

HAZARDOUS DECOMPOSITION PRODUCTS: N/A

HAZARDOUS POLYMERIZATION: Will not occur

CONDITIONS TO AVOID: N/A

MATERIALS TO AVOID: N/A

SECTION 10—TOXICOLOGY INFORMATION

Bovine Colostrum Powder has no established ingestion limits.

Toxicology reports on Colostrum by the United States regulatory body of National Nutritional Foods Association (NNFA).

SAFETY OF BOVINE COLOSTRUM POWDER DERIVED FROM COLOSTRUM AND ITS TOXICOLOGY

There appear to be no reports of adverse effects due to the use of colostrum or Bovine Colostrum Powder as a dietary supplement. The presence of IGF in colostrum, and the reported increase in serum levels of IGF following colostrum use, if confirmed, do, however, raise some concern about its safety. However the levels of IgF-1 and other growth factors in Bovine Colostrum Powder are undetectable. Please visit http://www.nnfa.org for complete article and references.

Bovine Colostrum Powder is extracted from colostrum. Since colostrum is derived from bovine lacteal sources it Generally Regarded as Safe (GRAS) by the United States Department of Agriculture (USDA).

Bovine Colostrum Powder is approved as a dietary supplement, but not as a drug, according to Dr. Fudenburg in Progress in Drug Research 42:378 (1994). Foods and dietary supplements are not approved per se by the FDA and food supplements derived from milk would certainly fall under the category of Generally Recognized As Safe [GRAS], and because colostrum comes from a bovine milk source it is Generally Recognized As Safe [GRAS].

SECTION 11—ECOLOGICAL INFORMATION

There has not been any specific ecological tests done on this product.

SECTION 12—DISPOSAL CONSIDERATION

Use normal waste disposal procedures that are in compliance with federal, state, and local regulations.

SECTION 13—REGULATORY INFORMATION

DOT PROPER SHIPPING NAME: Not regulated by DOT
DOT HAZARD CLASS: N/A
DOT IDENTIFICATION NUMBER: N/A DOT EMER. RESPONSE GUIDE NO.: N/A

SECTION 14—OTHER INFORMATION

This product does not contain toxic chemicals subject to the reporting requirements of SARA Section 313 of the Emergency Planning and Community Right-To-Know Act of 1986 and of 40 CFR 372.

SARA SECTON 311-312 HAZARD CATEGORIES (40 CFR 370.2):
FIRE: No
SUDDEN RELEASE OF PRESSURE: No
REACTIVE: No
ACUTE: No

TYPICAL PRODUCT SPECIFICATIONS OF A *LIQUID PRPS ISOLATE*

1.0 Characteristics

Item	Item Description		Specification
1.1	Dosage form		Spray
1.2	Route of Administration		Oral
	Appearance		Greenish liquid
1.3	Serving size		.7 ml per spray
1.4	Shelf life		Two years
1.5	Storage conditions		25°C ± 2°C
1.6	Pack size		4.25 oz. (125.7 ml)
1.7	Container:		
	1.7.1	Product container	Bottle 4.25 oz., HDPE, white
	1.7.2	Closure system	.7 ml spray dispenser
	1.7.3	Product carton	9.75 x 8 x 6.25
	1.7.4	Tamper evident features	None
1.8	Insert(s)		None
1.9	Daily dosage		
	1.9.1	Minimum	1 spray
	1.9.2	Maximum	4 sprays

2.0 Active Ingredients per serving

Item	Ingredient	Label Claim		Input w/Over		Over %	Ref/Std
2.1	Bovine Colostrum @ .33 % protein	.434	ml	.434	ml	-	

3.0 Non-Active Ingredients

Item	Ingredient	Input Amount		Ref/Std
3.1	Sodium Benzoate	.0007	Ml	
3.2	Potassium Sorbate	.0007	Ml	
3.3	Natural Vanilla Flavoring	.0035	Ml	
3.4	Make up water	.261	Ml	

4.0 Purity Assays

Item:	Test	Release limits:	Method:
4.1	Heavy Metal		AA/ICP
	4.1.1 Arsenic	< 0.14 µg/kg b.w./day	ICPMMS
	4.1.2 Cadmium	< 0.09 µg/kg b.w./day	ICPMMS
	4.1.3 Lead	< 0.29 µg/kg b.w./day	ICPMMS
	4.1.4 Mercury	< 0.29 µg/kg b.w./day	ICPMMS
4.2	Pesticides	USP Limits	USP
4.4	Solvent Residues	USP Limits	USP
4.5	Identification	NLT 80% or top five matches	FTIR/Visual

5.0 Chemical Assays

Item:	Ingredient:	Release Limits:	Method:
5.1	Protein	NLT 80% of Label (0.3 % protein)	AOAC 991.20.1

6.0 Microbiological Assays

Item:	Test	Release limits:	Method:
6.1	Total plate count	NMT 10 cfu/g	BAM 8th ED.
6.2	E. Coli	Negative	BAM 8th ED.
6.3	Salmonella	Negative	BAM 8th ED.
6.4	Staphylococcus Aureus	Negative	BAM 8th ED.
6.5	Yeast and mold	NMT 1 cfu/g	BAM 8th ED.

MATERIAL SAFETY AND DATA SHEET OF A PRPS ISOLATE

SECTION 1—COMPOSITION & INFORMATION ON INGREDIENTS

Bovine Colostral Whey Permeate liquid dairy product:

Active Components:

Proline Rich Polypeptides (PRPs) (0.3% PRPs solids)

Inactive Components:

Vitamins A, B1, B2, B5, B6, B12, B13, C, E, Folic Acid, Beta-carotene, and Retinoic Acid, Sulphur. (<0.5% vitamin solids)

Lactose sugar (3% sugar solids)

This product contains 96% filtered water.

SECTION 2—HAZARDS IDENTIFICATIONS

• EMERGENCY OVERVIEW

Transparent green liquid. Non-flammable. Non-hazardous to eyes, skin and throat.

POTENTIAL HEALTH EFFECTS

ROUTES OF ENTRY: Eye contact, dermal, inhalation, ingestion

ACUTE EFFECTS OF OVEREXPOSURE:

Eyes—Non-hazardous

Skin—Non-hazardous

Inhalation—Non-hazardous

Ingestion—Non-hazardous

CHRONIC EFFECTS OF OVEREXPOSURE: None known

MEDICAL CONDITIONS AGGRAVATED BY EXPOSURE: None known.

CARCINOGENICITY: NTP: No IARC: No OSHA: No

SECTION 3—FIRST AID MEASURES

EMERGENCY AND FIRST AID PROCEDURES:

Eye Contact—If material comes in contact with the eyes, promptly wash the eyes with water. Get medical attention if any discomfort continues.

Skin Contact—No special precautions; flush with water.

Inhalation—If a person breathes the spray in large amounts of this material, move the exposed person to fresh air at once. Other measures are usually unnecessary.

Ingestion—No special precautions.

SECTION 4—FIRE-FIGHTING MEASURES

Flash Point: N/A AUTO IGNITION TEMP: N/A

FLAMMABLE LIMITS IN AIR LOWER

UPPER

% BY VOLUME N/A N/A

Extinguishing Media: Use appropriate media to extinguish source.

SPECIAL FIRE FIGHTING PROCEDURES: N/A

UNUSUAL FIRE AND EXPLOSION HAZARDS: None

HAZARD RATINGS: NFPA 704: Health—0 Fire—0 Reactivity—0

SECTION 5—ACCIDENTAL RELEASE MEASURES

No hazard

SECTION 6—HANDLING & STORAGE

HANDLING AND STORING: Store in a cool dry area or at standard room temperature and pressure.

SECTION 7—EXPOSURE CONTROL—PERSONAL PROTECTION

ENGINEERING CONTROLS: No requirements

RESPIRATORY EQUIPMENT: No requirements

EYE PROTECTION: No requirements

PROTECTIVE CLOTHING: No requirements

OTHER (SAFETY SHOWERS, EYE WASH STATIONS, ETC.): None

SECTION 8—PHYSICAL & CHEMICAL PROPERTIES

APPEARANCE: Light green transparent liquid: N/A

BOILING POINT: 212F (100degC)

SPECIFIC GRAVITY (water=1): 1

VAPOR PRESSURE: 2.86 kPa at 25degC (standard room temperature)

VAPOR DENSITY (air=1): 1

SOLUBLE IN WATER: It is 96% water.

SECTION 9—STABILITY & REACTIVITY

STABILITY: STABLE X

UNSTABLE

INCOMPATIBILITY: N/A

HAZARDOUS DECOMPOSITION PRODUCTS: N/A

HAZARDOUS POLYMERIZATION: Will not occur

CONDITIONS TO AVOID: N/A

MATERIALS TO AVOID: N.A

SECTION 10—TOXICOLOGY INFORMATION

Colostral Whey Permeate has not established injestion limits,

Toxicology reports on Colostrum by the United States regulatory body of National Nutritional Foods Association (NNFA). There appear to be no reports of adverse effects due to the use of colostrum or colostral whey permeate as a dietary supplement. The presence of IGF in colostrum, and the reported increase in serum levels of IGF following colostrum use, if confirmed, do, however, raise some concern about its safety. However the levels of IgF-1 and other growth factors in Colostral Whey Permeate are undetectable. Please visit http://www.nnfa.org for complete article and references.

Colostral whey permeate is extracted from colostrum. Since colostrum is derived from bovine lacteal sources it Generally Regarded as Safe (GRAS) by the United States Department of Agriculture (USDA).

Colostral Whey Permeate is approved as a dietary supplement, but not as a drug, according to Dr. Fudenburg Prog in Drug Res. 1994, 42, p378. Foods and dietary supplements are not approved per se by the FDA and food supplements derived from milk would certainly fall under the category of Generally Recognized As Safe [GRAS].

SECTION 11—ECOLOGICAL INFORMATION

There has not been any specific ecological tests done on this product. Biological Oxygen Demand (BOD) is 30mg/L, Chemical Oxygen Demand (COD) is 100mg/L.

SECTION 12—DISPOSAL CONSIDERATION

Use normal waste disposal procedures that are in compliance with federal, state, and local regulations.

SECTION 13—REGULATORY INFORMATION

DOT PROPER SHIPPING NAME: Not regulated by DOT

DOT HAZARD CLASS: N/A

DOT IDENTIFICATION NUMBER: N/A DOT EMER. RESPONSE GUIDE NO.: N/A

SECTION 14—OTHER INFORMATION

This product does not contain toxic chemicals subject to the reporting requirements of SARA Section 313 of the Emergency Planning and Community right-To-Know Act of 1986 and of 40 CFR 372.

SARA SECTON 311-312 HAZARD CATEGORIES (40 CFR 370.2):

FIRE: No SUDDEN RELEASE OF PRESSURE: No REACTIVE: No ACUTE: No CHRONIC: No

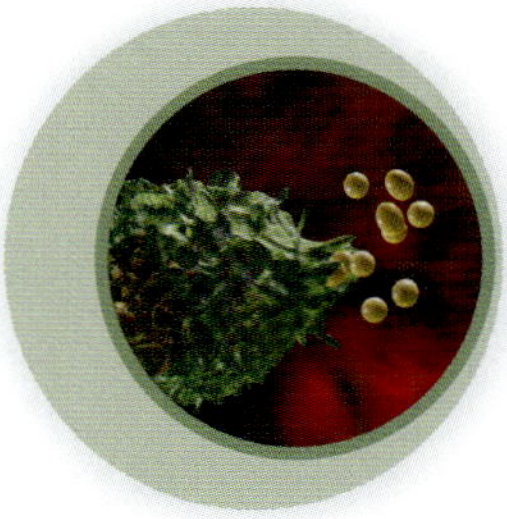

APPENDIX C

INSTITUTE FOR COLOSTRUM RESEARCH

The Institute for Colostrum Research is an organization dedicated to being a central information resource for consumers, health practitioners, and researchers on the subject of colostrum and its components. Located in New Zealand, where the use of colostrum as a nutritional supplement is well established, the center's website is a good source of research articles and general information about colostrum and its uses.

Michail Borissenko, Chief Scientist at the Institute, has graciously allowed us to reprint several articles and a FAQ from their Website, www.colostrumresearch.org.

ICR QUALITY SCALE

Michail Borissenko
Chief Scientist
Institute of Colostrum Research

Background

Colostrum is not only a highly nutritious functional food but also a substance that contains many life supporting and health promoting substances. The significance of colostrum is best illustrated by the fact that most animals require colostrum just after birth to survive. Some of these life supporting and growth promoting substances are as follows: antibodies, immune factors, growth factors, attachment factors, cytokines, oligosaccharides, essential fatty acids, and phospholipids. The remarkable thing about colostrum is that all these substances act synergistically in such a way as to enhance the overall affect of each individual component.

Colostrum has many functions and properties which make it most probably the single most important food in the world. Among these properties are the abilities to fight disease and to promote growth and well-being. Colostrum has also been shown to speed up the recovery process following injury and stress. Other attributes associated with colostrum include anti-aging properties, balanced blood sugar levels, increased performance, increased mental alertness and weight loss—specifically, accelerating the burning of fat.

Overall health begins in the gut, and this is where colostrum's actions begin. The significance of colostrum is self-promoting in that good health has no substitute. Whether young or old, fit or weak, colostrum can be of benefit. Backed by literally thousands of research studies and clinical trials, colostrum has been shown to be an effective means by which overall health can be obtained.

The sales of colostrum for the basic maintenance of good health are rising dramatically. Add to this the increased use of colostrum in the medical, nutrition and nutraceutical markets. This growth is fantastic as colostrum is truly nature's wonder food. It is not only a highly nutritious food but also contains numerous factors which not only help fight disease, but also help to promote growth and the healing process. In short, colostrum helps to promote overall good health and well-being. It does this by removing existing deficiencies, promoting the power of resistance, and supporting the healing process.

With the increase in consumption of colostrum, a dramatic rise in the number of manufacturers, suppliers, and distributors has been observed. Add to this the dramatic rise in various types of formulated colostrum products available to the consumer. Unfortunately, associated with this growth, it has been observed that the quality of some colostrum products are better then others, and more concerning is that many claims by some distributors of colostrum products are confusing, incorrect or clearly misleading.

The Institute of Colostrum Research (ICR) has undertaken to establish criteria by which colostrum products can be evaluated. ICR has undertaken this task to educate the consumer as to how to judge colostrum products from different distributors. In this way the consumer can make a more educated choice as to what colostrum product is best.

What is the ICR Quality Scale? Simply put, it is a method by which one can quantify or measure the quality of a colostrum product. Different manufacturers use various processes to manufacture their colostrum products. They also source their colostrum from different suppliers. In addition, manufacturers vary as to what additives and ingredients they add to their colostrum products. The ICR Quality Scale is designed to measure or quantify the quality of colostrum products.

Key Quality Indicators of colostrum are as follows:

1) Pasteurization
2) Low Temperature Processing
3) Immunoglobulin Values—levels of IgG, IgA, and IgM
4) Growth Factor Values—IGF, TGF, TNF, EGF
5) Immune Factors—lactoferrin, cytokines, lysozyme, lactoperoxidase
6) Environmental factors influencing quality
7) Quality manufacturing
8) Additives
9) Solubility (dispersibility)
10) Science

Pasteurization

This is a crucial step in any commercial dairy process. Do not purchase any colostrum product that has not been pasteurized. There are alternative methods that employ other means of sterilization, but these must meet the same International Standards as pasteurization.

Low Temperature Processing

It is imperative that colostrum be processed in such a way as to avoid prolonged exposure to heat. Pasteurization is necessary and is performed so as to ensure microbiological quality. Typically this is performed at 72°C for a period of 15 seconds. It has been shown that pasteurization has no significant negative effect on the bioactive molecules present in colostrum. The drying process used by some colostrum manufacturers may have a detrimental effect on colostrum quality. Specifically, in the case of spray-drying—which is the most common method of drying colostrum—some manufacturers of colostrum powder may incorporate high heat for prolonged periods. This can be evidenced in the final product in the form of discolored product, poor solubility, very low or no growth factors present, low levels of immunoglobulins and other proteins.

Immunoglobulins

The great majority of colostrum retailers stipulate only Immunoglobulin G (IgG) values. Colostrum is more then just IgG—in fact, IgG is only one of the immunoglobulins. The immunoglobulin fraction present in colostrum consists of IgG, IgA, IgM, IgD, and IgE. Both IgD and IgE are present in very low quantities whereas IgG, IgA, and IgM are found in considerable amounts. Thus commercial sources will optimally give also IgA and IgM, in addition to IgG, values.

Affinity vs Immunoassay

Currently, most manufactures of colostrum determine IgG concentration by using a technique called Protein G HPLC. Protein G can only be used for obtaining IgG values and cannot be used for determining IgA and IgM. Further, Protein G was not designed for determining IgG values but rather for the processing of IgG.

The use of Protein G to determine IgG values was a nice little trick developed by the New Zealand Dairy Research Institute. The basis for using Protein G is that it possesses an affinity to a portion of the IgG molecule (Fc portion). As such this technique can be referred to as an affinity assay.

The commonest and most recognized methods employed to measure specific protein levels are commonly referred to as immunoassays. These types of assays employ specific antibodies that are directed towards the protein (antigen) under investigation. In fact, these antibodies are not only specific but are also monospecific in that they will only react with that specific protein. With the exception of IgG, all the other proteins are quantified using immunoassay.

There are various types of immunoassays, such as radial immunodiffusion (RID), enzyme-linked immunoassay (ELISA), nephelometry, turbidometry, and (RIEP). In some cases these techniques are highly automated (nephelometry), whereas others are labor intensive (ELISA). In some cases immunoassays are available in commercially available kit form (RID and ELISA).

Standardization

Approximately 20 years ago the World Health Organization (WHO) in conjunction with the American Association of Clinical Pathologists (AACP) conducted a study to establish a world standard for human plasma proteins. Unfortunately, at the time of this writing, no such equivalent exists for bovine colostrum proteins. This means there is a lack of standardization involving the quantization of bovine proteins. Though this may seem to be a minor issue, the reality is that it is a major issue indeed. This is especially true when comparing different colostrum products from different manufacturers who use different methods to measure the proteins present.

A major problem associated with assigning specific protein values to colostrum products at present is that there appears to be a very wide variation in what is actually present. Most suppliers of colostrum provide IgG values for their products. At present this is how most colostrum is judged—by its IgG content. A preliminary investigation was conducted comparing Protein G and RID quantization of IgG. In this investigation involving four commercially available RID kits, it was revealed that a variation of up to 40% in quantified IgG value was observed between the kits. This variability is simply not acceptable. Until there is a universally accepted standard for IgG and the other bovine colostrum proteins, the best advise to the consumer is simple— "Let the buyer beware."

Very recently we conducted a comparison study involving four commercially available colostrum products. These products were sent to an independent registered and accredited laboratory in order to have the (IgG) determined. The method of analysis was Protein G HPLC. The quantified values determined by the independent laboratory were then compared to the respective label values of the products. The results ranged from 46.7% lower IgG than stated to 50% more IgG than stated on the label—an overall variability of close to 100%. Once again, simply not good enough!

Growth Factors and Immune Factors

Commercially available immunoassay kits are presently available for the quantization of lactoferrin, lactoperoxidase, lysozyme, interleukins, interferons, insulin-like growth factor, tumor necrosis factor, transforming growth factors and epidermal growth factor. In addition, immunological reagents in the form of primary antibodies reactive to these molecules are also commercially available. Why aren't these growth factors and immune factors routinely assayed in all colostrum products?

Prolonged exposure to heat or over processing can have a detrimental effect on any or possibly all these bioactive molecules. As such it is imperative that to ensure high quality and bioactivity the colostrum must be produced in such a way as to avoid elevated temperatures. Low growth factor levels will indicate that most probably the colostrum was subjected to high heat processing.

Environmental Factors

The environment from which the colostrum is sourced is key to the supply of good quality colostrum. A recent investigation conducted at Otago University in New Zealand revealed that a natural, non-hyperimmunized, commercially available product had significantly higher specific antibody titers to 19 pathogens compared to a commercially available equivalent which was derived from cows actively hyperimmunized (vaccinated) against these same 19 pathogens.

These results are significant in that it appears that natural immunization in the form of chronic low dose exposure via the oral route is far superior to active hyperimmunization. The non-immunized colostrum product in the Otago study was derived from the colostrum or early milk of healthy, untreated, pasture-fed cows.

Additives

Various manufacturers add any one of a number of additives to their colostrum products. The important thing is that the additives not hinder the effectiveness and bioavailability of the colostrum. It is also important that any additive not have a negative or detrimental effect on the colostrum. A case in point is one manufacture who utilizes papain as an additive in one of their colostrum products. Papain is an enzyme derived from the papaya fruit and is typically used as a digestive aid. Unfortunately, this manufacturer obviously doesn't realize that papain is a proteolytic enzyme that digests proteins. In fact, papain is typically used to cleave the IgG molecule in certain research applications. It most certainly also cleaves (partially digests) the other immunoglobulins as well. Its effect on growth factors, immune factors and other bioactive constituents in colostrum? Who knows?

Quality Manufactured Product

Is the colostrum manufactured to the highest standards? To make sure, only government certified colostrum producers and processors should be used. These organizations would have Product Safety Programs in place so as to ensure that all the colostrum they produce is of the highest standard.

Solubility

Solubility is an important issue to consider. This is especially true since poor solubility can reflect poor bioavailability of product. Causes of poor solubility are usually linked with flaws in manufacturing, such as high heat exposure, overprocessing and drying conditions. Is the colostrum powder soluble in water? It should be if it was processed correctly. If it is not, then it most likely is second rate.

Science

Many claims by some distributors of colostrum products are confusing, incorrect or misleading. Does the manufacturer or distributor of the colostrum back their product with proper science? Is the scientific and technical information associated with the product correct? A credible supplier of colostrum products will back up any such information with referenced material.

Further, no responsible supplier of nutraceutical products, such as colostrum, would make any direct health claims. This is especially true as labeling and product information restrictions are quite clear in that only registered drugs (pharmaceuticals) can make any specific health claims. It must be noted that there are a number of lunatic fringe type of companies that are operational in the field, unfortunately. Their marketing is truly aggressive, and their credibility is questionable. Hopefully their existence will be short-lived.

BOVINE LACTOFERRIN

Michail Borissenko
Chief Scientist
Institute of Colostrum Research

Lactoferrin is the best example of a powerful bioactive derivative of colostrum that is close to reaching a bio-pharmaceutical status.[522,523] Several manufacturers around the world are isolating lactoferrin on a commercial scale. It is showing great promise and has recently gained a great deal of international attention based on its broad range of beneficial physiological effects. Lactoferrin is a unique protein that influences cell proliferation and differentiation. It functions as an immune modulator, antimicrobial, antiviral, anticancer, anti-inflammatory, iron carrier, antioxidant and promoter of balanced intestinal flora.

Lactoferrin was first isolated in milk, but it is also found in other secretions such as tears and saliva. Its main biological function relates to its very high affinity for iron. Because of this, lactoferrin is an excellent inhibitor of a wide range of microorganisms that require iron for growth and proliferation. Lactoferrin activates the non-specific immune response by stimulating phagocytosis and complement. Recent scientific evidence has linked lactoferrin with significant potential beneficial effects in the treatment of cancers, specifically in the reduction of tumors.[524,525] Though the actual mechanism of action is yet to be elucidated, lactoferrin has been shown in vitro to suppress colon cancer tumors and also to inhibit lung cancer metastasis.[526] Further, it has also been shown to successfully inhibit hepatitis C virus in patients suffering from chronic infection.[527]

Lactoferrin plays a significant role in cellular defense. This most likely is by modulating macrophage activity and stimulating the proliferation of lymphocytes.[528] A very important function of lactoferrin is modulating the immune response, and colostrum has been shown to be very effective in preventing the immune response from getting out of control. In animal studies it has been shown that orally administered lactoferrin results in an increase in total immunoglobulin levels present in intestinal fluid, thereby stimulating the mucosal immune system.

Lactoferrin has been shown to be effective against a wide variety of microbes and function as both a bacteriostatic (not allowing pathogens to grow) and bactericidal agent (destroying pathogens).[529,530,531,532] The bacteriostatic function is attributed to its ability to remove free iron and thus limit the growth or colonization of pathogens requiring iron in order to proliferate—iron deprivation. The bactericidal function is attributed to lactoferrin's ability to act directly with pathogens and neutralize them.[533] In this manner lactoferrin has been shown to be effective against a wide variety of pathogens including the following pathogens: ***Salmonella, Staphylococcus, Listeria, Campylobacter, Clostridia,*** and ***E. coli*** O157:H7.[534,535] Further, it has been demonstrated that lactoferrin can reduce the severity and duration of enteric infection thus limiting the spread of disease.[536] It is also of interest that Lactoferrin has been shown to act synergistically with antibiotics and antifungal agents, thus increasing their effectiveness.[537,538]

Lactoferrin's action as an antiviral agent has recently come to light.[539,540] The mode of action appears to be that lactoferrin inhibits the binding of virus to the cell wall.[541] Significant beneficial results were observed against HIV, cytomegalovirus, herpes type 1&2, hepatitis C, influenza, and rotavirus.[542,543,544]

Lactoferrin has been shown to help promote the growth of probiotic or good bacteria, such as Bifidobacterium, in the gut. It does this by inhibiting the growth of various pathogenic microbes, thereby ensuring a balance of intestinal flora.

Lactoferrin has a very high affinity for iron. Because of this, lactoferrin is an optimal transporter of iron. In this way, lactoferrin increases the bioavailability of iron. Lactoferrin is a natural antioxidant due its ability to bind iron. As an iron scavenger, lactoferrin prevents the formation of free radicals caused by the oxidation process.[545] Lactoferrin functions to reduce inflammation by regulating potent stimulators of cytokines. Cytokines are substances that are produced by the immune system in response to infection and inflammation. Lactoferrin regulates the immune response, thus limiting inflammation.[546]

GROWTH FACTORS

Michail Borissenko
Chief Scientist
Institute of Colostrum Research

Colostrum is a very complex mixture containing many substances that have yet to be fully appreciated. Among these substances are a group of low molecular weight peptides collectively referred to as growth factors.[547] Growth factors are hormone-like peptides that either act alone or in conjunction with other substances to affect the growth (proliferation) and maturation of various cell types. For example, some growth factors help epidermal cells (skin and digestive tract) grow faster, while other growth factors stimulate muscle and bone cell proliferation and development. Of significant interest is the fact that bovine growth factors found in colostrum are almost identical to that of human in both structure and function. In addition to growth factors, there are also cytokines present in colostrum. Two of these, interferon and interleukin, also demonstrate growth promoting actions.

Growth factors and cytokines present in colostrum and their respective actions include:

Epidermal Growth Factor (EGF)—Stimulates tissue repair and wound healing and maturation of the digestive tract in infants.[548]

Insulin-like Growth Factors 1 & 2 (IGF-1 & IGF-2)—Stimulates muscle and bone cell proliferation and development, associated with the anti-aging process.[549,550]

Fibroblast Growth Factor (FGF)—Stimulates muscle and bone cell proliferation and development

Platelet-Derived Growth Factor (PDGF)—Stimulates the proliferation and development of a wide range of cell types

Transforming Growth Factor (TGF)—Stimulates tissue repair and wound healing

Interleukins—Stimulates the immune response by promoting proliferation and maturation of activated T cells

Interferons—Antiviral, stimulate the immune response by modulating the activity of natural killer cells

Insulin-like growth factor 1 is found in relatively high concentrations in bovine colostrum and is of specific interest in regard to athletic performance and the anti-aging process. Specifically, this growth factor mediates the growth or metabolic effects of growth hormone.[551,552,553,554] On a molecular level, IGF-1 functions to stimulate muscle and bone cell proliferation and development, i.e., helps to build muscle and strong bones.[555] In a recent study it was shown that oral supplementation with bovine colostrum enhances the recovery process following physical exercise or exertion.[556] Thus it allows harder training with improved recovery.[557] Two further studies have shown that bovine colostrum has a positive effect on maximal power output—increases vertical jump performance and improves rowing performance in elite female rowers.[558] It has been demonstrated in laboratory studies that IGF-1 can promote an increase of up to 15% in muscle mass and a 14% increase in strength. Further, it has been shown that IGF-1, through its action on growth hormone, can retard the aging process, including decreasing cardiovascular associated mortality, reducing osteoporosis and improving brain function.[559,560,561,562]

Transforming growth factors and epidermal growth factors are also found in relatively high amounts in bovine colostrum. Both these growth factors stimulate tissue repair and wound healing.[563] Physical exercise and training cause muscle and tissue damage. The degree of damage and time required for repair depends on various factors, such as physical condition, level of stress, dietary and medicinal considerations. Bovine colostrum has been shown to help in this recovery process.[564]

Inflammation is associated with physical exertion and strenuous exercise. Though typically inflammation is centered in the joints, it also observed in the digestive tract and in muscle tissue. There are various anti-inflammatory agents available to treat inflammation. Unfortunately, there are also potential side effects and adverse reactions associated with these compounds. In fact, the adverse side effects associated with certain anti-inflammatory agents limit their use. The most commonly used compounds used to treat inflammation are non-steroidal anti-inflammatory drugs (NSAIDs), such as aspirin or salicylates. Commonly observed side effects associated with these compounds include gastric upset and gastric bleeding. It has been observed that the use of bovine colostrum has been proved effective in the treatment of gastrointestinal disorders caused by aspirin and other non-steroidal anti-inflammatory medications.

DISCLAIMER:
The statements contained herein have not been evaluated by the Food And Drug Administration. It is not intended to diagnose, treat, cure or prevent disease. The statements are for informational purposes only and is it not meant to replace the services or recommendations of a physician or qualified health care practitioner. Those with health problems or pregnancy are specifically advised that they should consult their physician before taking colostrum or any nutritional supplement.

IGF-I AND CANCER—NOT! DAIRY PRODUCTS AND CANCER: THE REAL FACTS

BY ALFRED E. FOX, PH.D.

There has been considerable adverse publicity and confusion recently regarding the relationship between the intake of dairy products, particularly milk, and the development of certain types of human cancer. One of the most outspoken antagonists supporting programs that attack the intake of dairy products is Robert Cohen, who identifies himself as the Executive Director of the Dairy Education Board. In reality, Mr. Cohen is an investigative reporter who has found a cause to champion and uses the Dairy Education Board, an "organization" he founded, as a soapbox. Mr. Cohen has published a book on the subject, ***MILK—The Deadly Poison***, and authors a website (www.notmilk.com) as a means to disseminate his views and those of his supporters.

When one looks at the website of Mr. Cohen, it is evident that although he professes to state only the facts, he has grossly distorted them to suit his own needs. For example, in a supposed factual newsletter written in June 1998, but still used on the website, Mr. Cohen reports that Virgil Hulse, MD, wrote a book entitled ***Mad Cows and Milk Gate*** in which he reported that most of the dairy cows in America have bovine leukemia, bovine immunodeficiency virus or bovine tuberculosis. Mr. Cohen then states "We drink body fluids from diseased animals in the name of good health." Anyone familiar with the dairy industry in America, or who will take the time to properly investigate it, knows that all dairy cows are vaccinated against these diseases and that such vaccinations are mandatory if the dairy farmer intends to sell milk for human consumption. Further, virtually all milk sold in commercial outlets for human consumption is pasteurized at temperatures that would destroy these microorganisms even if they were present.

Mr. Cohen's attack on milk has focused primarily on insulin-like growth factor-1 (IGF-1) wherein he claims that this hormone makes human cancers grow. Throughout the website, he cites scientific articles by reputable authors from prestigious institutions that he claims state that IGF-I is a key factor that promotes the growth of prostate, breast and colon cancers. The website contains an article written by Hans R. Larsen, a chemical engineer, which makes similar misrepresentations of scientific findings. Mr. Larson cites numerous articles and then makes statements about them, such as the following.

"On January 23, 1998, researchers at the Harvard Medical School released a major study providing conclusive evidence that IGF-I is a potent risk factor for prostate cancer."

"In 1995, researchers at the National Institutes of Health reported that IGF-I plays a central role in the progression of many childhood cancers and in the growth of tumors in breast cancer, small cell lung cancer, melanoma, and cancers of the pancreas and prostate."

"In September 1997, an international team of researchers reported the first epidemiological evidence that high IGF-I concentrations are closely linked to an increased risk of prostate cancer. Other researchers provided evidence of IGF-I's link to breast and colon cancers."

These statements are inaccurate misrepresentations of the actual conclusions drawn by the scientific investigators in their publications. The investigators' findings have been distorted to try and lead the reader to the erroneous conclusion that the intake of IGF-I will lead to enhanced tumor development in human cancers. The truth is that no one has ever demonstrated a cause-and-effect relationship between IGF-I and cancer. In fact, when the quoted articles are reviewed, one finds that none of the investigators ever even suggested that IGF-I was a causative agent in tumor development associated with human cancers but instead found that people with certain types of tumors had high levels of IGF-I in their circulation as a manifestation of their disease. The elevated levels of IGF-I seem to occur very early in tumor development and several authors cited by Mr. Larson have actually suggested that measurement of IGF-I in the blood of people may be an early warning indicator that a tumor could be developing in the body. They believe that making such measurements of IGF-I could mean possible earlier diagnosis and treatment. This situation is analogous to the elevated white blood cell count seen in association with appendicitis. The elevated white blood cell count is a manifestation of the condition and an indicator of infection. No reasonable person would say that it caused the appendicitis.

What are the real facts about IGF-1?

Insulin-like growth factor-1 and its closely related counterpart insulin-like growth factor-2 are potent hormones that are found in association with almost all cells in the body. IGF-1 is the best described and most potent of this pair. These molecules are produced by all mammals and in every case have a very similar chemical structure regardless of the species. IGF-1 is essential for normal cell growth and for the development of the fetus in the uterus.[565] Both IGF-1 and growth hormone are required for normal postnatal development,[566] and that is why they are both present in colostrum. The IGFs are structurally very similar to insulin and in fact, in certain diseases the specific receptors for insulin on cells in the body are sometimes incapable of distinguishing between IGF-1 and insulin.

Scientific knowledge about the IGFs, what they do and how they act on cells in the body, has evolved very rapidly during the past few years. It is now known that there are specific receptors on almost all cells in the body capable of interacting with IGF-1 and triggering a series of chemical events within the cell.[567] There are also six different proteins present inside the cell and on cell surfaces that control the actions of IGF-1 on the cell after it binds to a receptor. These are called insulin-like growth factor binding proteins (IGFBPs). In addition, there are at least 87 other related proteins either capable of binding to IGF-1, altering its actions, or influencing the effects of the IGFBPs. These are called insulin-like growth factor binding protein-related proteins (IGFBP-rPs). The entire collection of these proteins is referred to as the insulin-like growth factor binding protein (IGFBP) super family.[568] The key event that triggers the effects of any of these proteins appears to be the interaction of IGF-1 with its specific cell-surface receptor, an event that some of these proteins regulate.

The multitude of available IGF-1binding proteins and related proteins available in the cell is indicative of the many potential effects that the binding of IGF-1 to its specific cell-surface receptor can have on cells. To keep these many effects under control, some of the binding proteins act as checks and balances, allowing the secondary chemical switches in a cell to be turned on and then turning them off when it is appropriate. Therefore IGF-1 is like the captain of a ship. When it binds to its specific receptor, the ship can move forward, but there are all kinds of systems in place to keep it moving at the right speed and in the right direction. The main triggered events include activation of the process by which the cell grows and reproduces itself and maintenance of the metabolic pathways by which the cell converts glucose into glycogen and uses amino acids to create proteins. The actual pathway by which the cell uses glucose and converts it to glycogen is first switched on by the binding of insulin to its specific cell surface receptors. Glycogen is stored in the liver and muscles and is the main source of readily available energy when the muscles are exercised. The IGFBP super family also has a direct role in how the cell uses amino acids to build proteins. As we age, the ability of our body to create an adequate supply of IGF-1 is diminished. Thus, by eating a well-balanced diet and maintaining a constant supply of IGF-1 in our body, we can keep the ship moving at the right speed and in the right direction. And when we exercise, this becomes even more critical since there is an increased demand for glycogen to provide energy to our muscles, and the preference is to build more muscle protein. Even more importantly, as we age, the cells in our body do not reproduce themselves as well, and since IGF-1 is a primary factor in the ability of cells to grow and reproduce, it is highly desirable to have an appropriate level of IGF-1 in the circulation through dietary supplementation to limit the ever increasing rate of cell senescence.

Why is there excess IGF-1 in the circulation in certain types of cancer?

You will recall that Mr. Hans Larsen, writing on behalf of Mr. Robert Cohen, drew the following conclusion in his article on Mr. Cohen's website:

"In 1995, researchers at the National Institutes of Health reported that IGF-1 plays a central role in the progression of many childhood cancers and in the growth of tumors in breast cancer, small cell lung cancer, melanoma, and cancers of the pancreas and prostate."

In actual fact, in the 1995 article cited,[569] these researchers reported that the cell surface receptors for IGF-1 mediate most of the effects of IGF-1, and despite its structural similarity to the insulin receptor, the IGF-1 receptor is mainly involved in the support of growth and sends different types of signals than the insulin receptor. They concluded that the gene encoded for the IGF-1 receptor is expressed by most cells in an organism, which is consistent with the role of IGFs as survival factors, and that the receptor gene is modulated by many physiological and pathological factors, including developmental stage, nutritional status, hormones, growth disorders and malignancy. In 1996,[570] the same researchers reported that the IGF-1 receptors are integral cell membrane proteins that demonstrate important effects on the regulation of cellular processes. The same investigators and others[571] also found that the IGF binding proteins (IGFBPs) were made by cells and could be secreted such that they could accumulate on external cell surfaces. As such, the IGFBPs were found to be involved in regulating cell processes by modulating the interaction of the IGFs with their cell surface receptors. Later it was recognized that certain of the IGFBPs were growth inhibitory molecules and as such, were primary regulators of the effects of IGF-1 interaction with its cell surface receptor on cell growth.[572,573]

Multiple studies have shown that there is an elevated level of IGF-1 in the circulation of patients with certain types of malignancies including, prostate cancer,[574,575,576,577,578] breast cancer,[579,580,581,582,583,584,585,586,587] colorectal cancer,[588] acute lymphoblastic leukemia,[589,590] and non-small cell lung cancer.[591] Many of these studies also reported other associated factors. A group from the Harvard School of Public Health investigated the relationship of intake of dairy products to the risk of prostate cancer and found such patients also had reduced circulating levels of vitamin D, a factor believed to be protective for prostate cancer.[592] In several cases, increased circulating levels of IGF-1 were paralleled by extremely low levels of a particular IGFBP (IGFBP-3) known to be a very potent inhibitor of the cell growth-promoting effects of IGF-1 and IGF-1 receptor interaction.[593,594,595] More recent studies have shown that levels of some of the IGFBP-related proteins that control the inhibitory effects of IGFBP-3 are also altered in certain malignant diseases.[596,597] One study has shown that another IGF-binding protein (IGFBP-6) that is involved in programmed cell death is increased in non-small cell lung cancer.[598] In some studies, associations have been drawn between the levels of certain hormones, increased circulating IGF-1 and cancer risk. In prostate cancer there have been proposed relationships to high levels of testosterone[599] and in breast cancer with the progestins, which seem to interfere with the interaction of IGF-1 and its cell surface receptors.[600,601]

It is difficult to understand how a comprehensive review of the scientific literature would lead one to the conclusion that IGF-1 is responsible for enhanced tumor development in certain types of human cancer. This is particularly true when it is seen that the same increased circulating levels of IGF-1 and modifications of certain controlling protein substances have been found in various nonmalignant diseases. For example, similar alterations in IGF-1 and IGFBP-3 are found in patients with benign prostatic hyperplasia.[602] In both Type 1 and insulin-resistant Type 2 diabetes, patients demonstrate increased circulating levels if IGF-1[603,604,605] and in Type 2 diabetes patients an inverse correlation between levels of insulin and a particular IGFBP (IGFBP-1) has been shown.[606] In another study from the Harvard School of Public Health, it has been shown that men with higher levels of testosterone are more likely to have vertex baldness and in those that additionally have higher than normal blood levels of IGF-1 the odds of vertex baldness is doubled.[607] Published studies have also shown that in growth-retarded individuals the gene encoding for the IGF-1 receptor is defective, and as a result, these individuals have substantially elevated levels of circulating IGF-1.[608]

There is no question that there is an increased circulating level of IGF-1 in patients with prostate, breast, colorectal, lung cancer and some leukemias. The effects of IGF-1 on the cells, which include cell growth, survival and transformation, are mediated through its interaction with IGF-1 receptors on cell surfaces. The interaction of IGF-1 with its receptors is further controlled by the IGFBPs, some of which can independently act on cell processes. The controlling aspects of the IGFBPs are further modulated by many additional regulating substances in both normal and disease processes.[609,610] Studies from the National Institutes of Health have shown that in malignant disease there are more than enough IGF-1 receptors on cell surfaces, but the ability of these receptors to interact with IGF-1 is significantly reduced. They were also able to demonstrate that the most frequently mutated gene in human cancer, p53, lowers the ability of the IGF-1 receptors to bind IGF-1 and function.[611] Studies from Germany reported in September 2000 have added to the understanding of this process.[612] These investigators found that a protein encoded by the human papilloma virus binds to IGFBP-3, which restricts cell growth following the interaction of IGF-1 with the IGF-1 receptor, and enzymatically degrades it. This protein is a product of the p53 gene, and it has long been known that it can immortalize primary human cells and overcome cellular senescence. Therefore the underlying cause for elevated levels of IGF-1 seen in cancer is related to a cascade of events that begin with an alteration of basic genetic information and culminate in an impaired functioning of the IGF-1 receptors on the surface of the cells. In this case, other IGFBP and related proteins that can act independent of IGF-1 interaction with its receptors have apparently redirected cell growth without the involvement of IGF-1. Since IGF-1 does not have operating, functional receptors to interact with, it naturally backs up in the circulation as a manifestation of the disease process.

GLUTATHIONE: A POWERFUL ANTIOXIDANT FOUND IN COLOSTRUM

Michail Borissenko
Chief Scientist
Institute of Colostrum Research

Colostrum is the most significant food in the world. It was designed by nature to protect the newborn. The significance of colostrum and the role it plays is best illustrated in the typical farm animal. Take the horse, cow, sheep, goat, cat, dog—unless these and most other animals receive colostrum in the first day or two of life they have a very significant chance not surviving. This phenomenon is due to a wonderful mechanism by which the mother can pass on her complement of antibodies to her newborn, known as passive transmission of immunity.

Because of this and the role that colostrum plays in the newborn, some other very important actions or properties associated with the biological function of colostrum have been overlooked. One of these properties is the fact that colostrum, in addition to all its other benefits, is a source of a wide range of antioxidants. One such antioxidant, glutathione, has been described as the ultimate antioxidant. It is very well documented that glutathione and its precursors are present in colostrum in relatively high levels. In this capacity, glutathione and glutathione precursors play an important part in colostrum's role in overall health.

Glutathione, also referred to as GSH, is a naturally occurring peptide or small protein which has a primary function as an antioxidant.[613] Linus Pauling was a leading advocate of antioxidants and their respective role in prevention of disease and the promotion of overall good health. Antioxidants, for the most part, are naturally occurring compounds that possess the ability to neutralize unstable free radicals. Unchecked, these free radicals have been linked, at least in part, as the causative agents of a number of disease conditions including cancer, heart disease, stroke, and improper nervous and immune system function.[614,615] A growing number of scientific and medical research studies have shown that antioxidants can deactivate free radicals and thus limit the spread of certain disease states. Basically, antioxidants act as free radical scavengers that remove them from the body before they can cause their harmful effects. Many foods such as fruits, vegetables, grains and oils contain vitamins and minerals that have antioxidant properties. Vitamins A, C and E, carotenoids and flavonoids are probably the best known antioxidants. The growing body of scientific and medical research substantiates the role that glutathione and other antioxidants play in sustaining health and combating disease. This mountain of evidence suggests that by simply increasing one's levels of glutathione, a corresponding increase of overall good health can be envisioned.[616]

The development of cancer and disease is usually a long, slow process. One exception is childhood cancers, which are usually attributed to inherited defective genes. Cancer cells in adults contain a large number of mutations acquired over a lifetime's exposure to environmental carcinogens, toxins and free radicals. These substances damage the body's DNA—the blueprint of life. Antioxidants have been shown to protect DNA from excessive damage and help in its synthesis and repair.[617,618] In fact, the glutathione levels have been described as a predictive factor in determining our life expectancy.

Glutathione regulates the actions of other, less effective antioxidants, such as vitamins C and E.[619] It has been reported that low levels of glutathione are associated with liver and immune system malfunction, heart disease, premature aging and death. Further, it has been reported that glutathione functions in not only detoxification of toxins but also neutralizing carcinogens.

Glutathione has also been described as having potent antiviral and antibacterial properties. Glutathione has also been shown to have a wide variety of functions that help boost the immune system. Lymphocytes (T cells and B cells), so vital in the immune response, have been shown to be dependent on glutathione for proper function. As we age, our levels of glutathione drop. These lower levels of glutathione have been implicated in diseases associated with aging. Finally, glutathione has been shown to enhance athletic performance by increasing muscle strength and weight gain.[620]

As an antioxidant, glutathione helps protect the overall integrity of every cell and tissue against damage caused by free radicals and disease. Acting as a scavenger of free radicals, glutathione helps to protect us from pollutants and other disease-causing agents. Glutathione is a trimer composed of three amino acids—glycine, glutamic acid and cysteine. Though free glutathione is surely of benefit, the main benefit comes from the internalization of its precursors and subsequent assembly and action within the cell. In fact, a recent investigation involving piglets showed that intercellular glutathione production was almost exclusively from dietary consumption of glutathione precursors.[621,622]

There are a number of products available that contain glutathione and its precursors. For the most part they are derived from colostrum, milk, and/or whey. They are typically referred to as whey protein isolates. A number of these products are being marketed as significantly higher in glutathione and its precursors. The fact is that compared to low temperature processed colostrum, these products do not have significantly higher levels of either glutathione, glutathione precursors or other bioactives that are present in properly processed colostrum. In fact, it has been recently reported that the antioxidant activity of bovine colostrum is significantly greater than a number of such products, including whey protein hydrolysates. Figure 1 illustrates the lack of any significant difference between a whey protein glutathione-enriched product and a quality produced colostrum. Note the glutathione precursors, glycine, glutamic acid, and cystine, and the relative values found in the respective products.

Amino Acid	Whey Derived Product	Colostrum 20% Ig's
Glycine	20mg/g protein	18.1 mg/g protein
Glutamic Acid	201	126.3
Cystine	24	16.8
Proteins		
Lactalbumin	9.7%	2%
Lactoglobulin	59.1%	19%
Lactoferrin	0.14%	0.15%
Total Immunoglobulins	24.6%	25%
IGF-1		1000ng/g
IGF-2		250ng/g
TGF–β1		150ng/g
TGF-β2		950ng/g
EGF		250μg/100g
Vitamins		
A		100 IU/100g
B1	1.5—2.0 mg/60g	
B2	1.7—2.2 mg/60g	1.12 mg/100g
B6		0.03 mg/100mg
B12		13.6 μg/100g
C		2.5 mg/100g
D		< .2μg/100g
E		130μg/100g

FIGURE 1. REPORTED COMPOSITION OF A COMMERCIALLY AVAILABLE WHEY PROTEIN ISOLATE WHICH IS REPORTEDLY ENRICHED WITH GLUTATHIONE AND ITS PRECURSORS AND A QUALITY PROCESSED COLOSTRUM PRODUCT.

It is of interest that the whey protein isolate, which is reportedly enriched with glutathione and its precursors, does not contain a significantly greater amount of glutathione precursors than the quality colostrum product. This is also true of other constituents that make up the composition of the respective products. It is also of interest that cysteine has been reported to be a rate-limiting amino acid for the biosynthesis of glutathione. The fact that lactoglobulin and lactalbumin are a rich source of this essential amino acid and that both are found in relatively high amounts in colostrum should also be noted.

Of utmost importance is the simple fact that if there is a substance that can improve quality of life, then this information should be available to and shared by everyone. The scientific and medical evidence generated from producers of whey protein isolate products is significant. However, most, if not all, their claims based on their findings can and for the most part have been attributed to colostrum.

Further, the process of manufacturing whey protein isolate products for the most part includes ultrafiltration or microfiltration of raw material in order to concentrate the various constituents responsible for bioactivity.[623] Typically this requires that this material is subjected to filtration through a 10,000 molecular weight (Daltons) membrane. Thus many small molecular weight molecules are removed from solution. These include many factors that are involved with the healing and recovery process, including growth factors and cytokines which have a wide variety of biological functions. This is indicated by the fact that the manufacturers of whey protein isolates who claim enriched glutathione levels typically do not include growth factor and cytokine levels as part of their respective compositional information.

Colostrum is a magical substance composed of many, many substances that work together in a synergistic manner in such a way that the overall effect of colostrum is greater than the individual components. In regard to whey protein isolate products, they have attributed the action to one constituent—glutathione. This is only part of the answer as many other bioactive molecules are involved—antibodies, immune factors, growth factors, cytokines, etc. In reality, it is an ever changing story with only part of the answer on how colostrum and its derivatives, such as whey protein isolates, actually function and work. The wonderful thing is that they actually do work and that this is backed by scientific and medical evidence.

DISCLAIMER:
The statements contained herein have not been evaluated by the Food And Drug Administration. It is not intended to diagnose, treat, cure or prevent disease. The statements are for informational purposes only and is it not meant to replace the services or recommendations of a physician or qualified health care practitioner. Those with health problems or pregnancy are specifically advised that they should consult their physician before taking colostrum or any nutritional supplement.

COMPLEX LIPIDS

MICHAIL BORISSENKO
Chief Scientist
Institute of Colostrum Research

Introduction

Phospholipids are complex lipids and the predominant structural element of all physiological membranes. Amphipathic lipid compounds are essential components of all biological membranes. Phospholipids are present in every cell of animals and plants. In animals, they are found abundant in the tissues of the brain, heart, liver, muscle, kidneys, and bone marrow. Though phospholipids function primarily as structural elements they are also essential in three very critical areas—the growth, maturation and proper functioning of the cells in the body[624,625].

Phospholipids are either derived from glycerol or sphingosine and are designated either glycerophospholipids or sphingolipids respectively. The predominant form of phospholipids are the glycerophospholids of which phosphatidylcholine (lecithin), phosphatidylserine, phosphatidylethanolamine, and phosphatidylinositol are the predominant species.

Sphingolipids are specific to animal sources and are not found in plants (such as soy). There are two types of sphingolipids: sphingophospholipids and sphingoglycolipids. As the nomenclature implies, the sphingophospholipids are phospholipids with a sphingosine backbone. Sphingoglycolipids also have a sphingosine backbone but instead of containing a phosphate group have a sugar group. Prime examples of sphingophospholipids and sphingoglycolipids are sphingomyelin and gangliosides respectively.

Phospholipids are an excellent source of choline, which has been shown to increase brain function. Phospholipids, in particular phosphatidylserine, have been associated with improved memory. Phospholipid supplementation has been shown to be beneficial in the treatment of Alzheimer's and similar diseases. Phospholipids have also been shown to reduce mood swings and elevate depression. Phospholipids, in particular phosphatidylcholine, have been shown to have a protective effect on the liver, protecting it against damage caused from toxins, including alcohol, drugs and viruses[626].

Sphingomyelin

The sphingolipid sphingomyelin represents 25–33% of the total phospholipids present in milk. Sphingolipids function in variety of physiological roles, from initiating cellular defense, tumor suppression and cholesterol mobilization, to making liposome membranes rigid[627].

Milk-derived sphingomyelin has been shown in in vitro studies using a human cell line to boost cellular production of interferon-beta, which plays an important role in cellular defense against viral infection. The breakdown products of sphingomyelin are sphingosine and ceramide. Sphingosine has been shown to inhibit protein kinase, C an important component in the internalization of growth factors into the cell. Thus it has been theorized that sphingomyelin contains components that act as second messengers which are important in cell growth and regulation. The digestive products of sphingomyelin have also been shown to be highly antimicrobial and be effective in vitro against such pathogens as Salmonella, Campylobacter, Vibrio, Listeria, and pathogenic E. coli.[628]

Along with other phospholipids in milk, sphingomyelin can protect gastric mucosa against injury caused by acid, pepsin or exogenous irritants. Sphingomyelin, along with phosphatidylcholine, is an important source of choline which is important for brain function. Sphingomyelin accounts for approximately 10% of the lipids present in the brain—primarily associated, as their name implies, with the myelin sheathes of nerves.

Considerable research has been undertaken on the functions of phospholipids and, more recently, sphingolipids in health and disease. Recently it has been shown that both sphingolipids and their breakdown products—ceramide and sphingosine—are highly bioactive compounds that have a profound effect on various biological functions in the body. Regulation of cell growth, differentiation, signaling, and programmed cell death (apoptosis) have all been attributed to sphingolipids. Further, sphingolipids have also been implicated in playing a vital role in neuronal development. In animal studies it has been revealed that dietary sphingolipids inhibit colon carcinogenesis.[629]

Studies on mice who were administered with 1,2 dimethlylhydrazine—a powerful tumor inducing agent—revealed that an up to 70% reduction of tumors was observed after being fed milk derived sphingomyelin. With longer feeding, an even greater reduction of tumors was observed. Mice fed as little as 25mg of sphingomylein/100g of diet had a 57% reduction in incidence of colon tumors.[630] Further studies on mice fed milk-derived sphingomyelin, as compared to a control group fed a standard diet, showed a reduction in aberrant colon tumors and most importantly revealed a shift from malignant tumors to ones that were benign[631]. Thus it has been postulated that sphingomyelin-containing foods may have anti-cancer activity. Though no clinical trials have been conducted on humans to date, the results of ***in vitro*** studies using human cancer cells lines show great promise. Sphingomyelin also has been shown to increase the effectiveness of chemotherapy agents in killing cancer cells.

Gangliosides

The sphingoglycolipids, such as gangliosides, are present in substantial amounts in nerve cell membranes. In addition, gangliosides are found in the membranes of white and red blood cells. It is of interest that ganglioside content is diminished in the brains of Alzheimer's patients. Of further interest is the significant and vital role gangliosides play in the brain development of the young[632].

Gangliosides, like sphingomyelin, exhibit a high level of antimicrobial activity in that they are both bactericidal and bacteriostatic to organisms that are frequently associated with causing diarrhea in young mammals. In addition, gangliosides have been shown to protect the intestine against disease.

Phosphatidylserine

Phosphatidylserine (PS) makes up approximately 8% of the total phospholipid in bovine milk. There is substantial evidence that indicates that PS improves memory and improves brain function. PS is most concentrated in the brain where it functions to support many crucial nerve cell functions. It is the primary component of the cell membranes of neurons. In brain disorders such as Alzheimer's, Parkinson's, and multiple sclerosis, there is an association with neuron degeneration and dysfunction[633]. PS has been shown to stimulate the production of a brain messenger chemical (dopamine) that helps regulate memory. PS has also been shown to stimulate protein kinase C production and help modify mood changes arising from stress. In addition, a growing amount of evidence is associated with the beneficial aspects of PS in mood elevation and reducing the symptoms of depression.[634] PS has been shown to have positive effects in treating early Alzheimer's and the onset of premature memory loss due to dementia.[635,636,637,638,639,640]

Phosphatidylethanolamine

Phosphatidylethanolamine (PE), also known as cephalin, makes up approximately

30% of the total phospholipid content of bovine milk. PE comprises the backbone of cell membranes and contributes to the fluidity and structural environment of cells. In regard to the brain and nervous tissue, PE plays an important role in myelin structure and nerve endings in the brain. Phospholipids, particularly PE, have been shown to be beneficial in lowering serum cholesterol levels and thus reducing the risk of heart disease[641].

Phosphatidylcholine

Phosphatidylcholine (PC), also known as Lecithin, makes up approximately 30% of the phospholipid present in bovine milk. Along with sphingomyelin, PC is a major source of choline. Choline is a major neurotransmitter, acetylcholine. Dietary PC has been shown to improve neurological malfunctions such as tremors, ataxis and mood swings. Choline is required to sustain tissue growth, and thus a ready supply of this phospholipid is required for maintenance of good health.

PC is a major building block for all cell membranes, and it supports cellular, tissue and organ function. This is particularly true of the liver with its vast network of cell membranes. Thus the liver is particularly dependent on PC for proper function. In fact, it has been shown in clinical trials that dietary PC has beneficial aspects in helping individuals recover from toxic liver damage. PC has also been shown to protect the liver from damage due to viral infection, medication, alcohol, and nutritional deficiency. It has also been shown to be beneficial in speeding the recovery process resulting from liver damage.

Phosphatidylinositol

Phosphatidylinositol (PI), also known as inositol, comprises approximately 5% of the total phospholipid present in milk. Inositol is necessary for the proper functioning of the brain, nerves and muscle. Inositol is a "lipotropic" substance helping to prevent build-up of fatty deposits in the liver. Inositol is also an essential nutrient for proper growth in newborn children.[642]

Phospholipids Are Natural Emulsifying Agents

Phospholipids, in particular sphingomyelin, are natural emulsifying agents and are used in a wide variety of applications. The ability of sphingomyelin to form very stable micelles and liposomes makes it an ideal candidate in developing delivery systems. These delivery systems can be utilized to increase dispersibility and target specific target dissolution. With the advent of new technologies in isolation and purification of phospholipids, specific phospholipids can now be targeted for end use.

Milk-derived Phospholipids vs Soy Lecithin

The significant difference between plant-based soy lecithin and milk-derived phospholipid is the actual composition of the phospholipids in question. As was mentioned previously, only animal based phospholipid preparations contain sphingomyelin. In addition, milk-derived complex lipids are more similar to human lipids than vegetable sources. Further, the emulsion properties of sphingomyelin are far more superior to that of soy lecithin. The actual phospholipid compositional differences are seen below:

Phospholipid Class	**Soybean***	**Milk***
Phosphatidylcholine	30%	30%
Phosphatidylethanolamine	20%	30%
Phosphatidylserine	3%	10%
Phosphatidylinositol	20%	5%
Sphingomyelin	Not present	25%

*Expressed as total phospholipid present

DISCLAIMER:

The statements contained herein have not been evaluated by the Food And Drug Administration. It is not intended to diagnose, treat, cure or prevent disease. The statements are for informational purposes only and is it not meant to replace the services or recommendations of a physician or qualified health care practitioner. Those with health problems or pregnancy are specifically advised that they should consult their physician before taking colostrum or any nutritional supplement.

LACTOSE INTOLERANCE, DAIRY PRODUCTS, AND COLOSTRUM

MICHAIL BORISSENKO
Chief Scientist
Institute of Colostrum Research

Introduction

The main carbohydrate present in milk is **lactose**. This milk sugar is a disaccharide (two sugars) composed of glucose and galactose subunits. Normally lactose is digested in the small intestine by the enzyme **lactase** into its subunits, and the **glucose** and **galactose** are then absorbed through the intestinal wall into the bloodstream. The enzyme lactase is normally found in high levels in babies, infants, and children, and as such the young generally can consume high levels of foods containing lactose. In the majority of population, excluding Caucasians, as the infant grows, the relative levels of lactase present in the intestine gradually decline to the point where certain adults are not able to digest the lactose properly. This inability to digest lactose has been termed **lactose intolerance** or **lactose maldigestion**.[643] Symptoms of lactose intolerance include bloating, abdominal pain, diarrhea, and flatulence. It is important to note that these symptoms are typically only observed in individuals who are lactose maldigesters and who consume large quantities of lactose containing dairy products. **Research has shown that even lactose maldigesters can easily tolerate 1-2 cups of milk per day, cheese (which contains little if any lactose), yogurt and even colostrum.**[644,645,646]

What Is Lactose Intolerance?

The main carbohydrate present in milk is lactose. In fact, this disaccharide sugar is one of the main components of mammalian milk. It is made up of monosaccharide sugar subunits glucose and galactose linked by a 1,1,4 β-glycosidic bond. In the human small intestine lactose is normally broken down or digested by the enzyme lactase (known also as β-galactosidase) into its monosaccharide sugar subunits and then absorbed through the intestine into the bloodstream.

In humans, intestinal lactase activity changes with age, reaching its peak at birth in the young and remaining high during infancy and early childhood. In a great percentage of the world's population there is then a gradual decline in intestinal lactase activity with age. However, in a small minority of people, mainly individuals of European heritage, high levels of lactase activity remain well into adulthood. These individuals can readily and easily digest large quantities of lactose and are often referred to as being **lactose persistent**.

However, as previously mentioned, the majority of adults in the world have reduced levels of lactase in the small intestine. In these individuals, if they consume more lactose then there is lactase present to digest it, symptoms may appear. The undigested lactose is fermented by the enteric bacteria present in the large intestine to produce lactic acid, short chain fatty acids, carbon dioxide, hydrogen and methane gas. It is this fermentation of the undigested lactose which causes the gastrointestinal symptoms of lactose intolerance.

Lactose Intolerance Defined

Lactose intolerance, also referred to as hypolactasia, can be defined as an inability to tolerate a standard or test dose of lactose without developing diagnostic biochemical changes with or without clinical signs and symptoms of bloating, flatulence, abdominal pain and diarrhea. The standard dose of lactose used to determine lactose intolerance is 50 grams.

Incidence of Lactose Intolerance

The incidence of lactose intolerance varies greatly between races and populations worldwide. However, a majority of adults world wide have a reduction in lactase activity. This appears to be especially true in post-weaning Asian and African populations, Eskimos, Native American Indians and African-Americans. The exceptions in African peoples are the cattle raising populations of Niger and Nigeria. It is quite a different story in European, North American, and Australian populations where the incidence of lactose intolerance is typically observed in less than 30% of adults. The general belief is that lactase persistence is genetically linked and not environmentally triggered.

Lactose in Milk and Dairy Products

The relative levels of lactose in the milk of common species is as follows:

Species	Lactose (grams/liter)
Human	7.0
Cow	4.7
Sheep	4.8
Goat	4.1
Horse	6.2

The lactose present in fermented dairy products is broken down by lactic acid bacteria used in the culture.[647] This accounts for an approximate reduction of 30% present as compared to milk. In other dairy products such as butter, cream, cottage cheese, etc., the lactose is reduced in similar quantity. The great majority of cheese types contain little if any lactose as it is completely broken down to glucose and galactose in the cheese ripening process. The actual level of lactose in some dairy products can be seen as follows:[648,649]

Dairy Product	Lactose (grams/100grams)
Natural Yogurt	3.4
Flavored Yogurt	2.9—4.2
Full Cream	3.1
Half Pasteurized Cream	3.3
UHT Milk	3.7
Coffee Cream	3.8
Butter	0.6
Cottage Cheese	2.2
Cheese (Both Soft & Hard)	0.011—0.085
Whole Milk Powder	40 -45
Colostrum Whole	15
Colostrum Skim	5.9

Minimal Dose of Lactose to Cause Symptoms

The standard dose of 50 grams of lactose, used in the lactose test, will induce symptoms associated with intolerance in most individuals who are lactose maldigesters. The actual minimal dose of lactose required to induce symptoms in lactose intolerant individuals has yet to be determined. However, a double-blind, randomized trial involving 13 healthy individuals determined to be lactose intolerant revealed that no significant symptoms arose when they were administered 0, 2, 6 ,12 and even 20 grams of lactose in 240 ml aqueous solutions.[650]

How Much Colostrum Can Be Tolerated?

Further studies have confirmed these results and established the fact that almost everyone, including individuals who are lactose intolerant, can easily tolerate up to 12 grams of colostrum per day without any negative side effects or symptoms. An important point to make is that this corresponds to 2 cups of milk or 200 grams of skim colostrum powder (400 500mg capsules) per day. It must be obvious that 400 capsules of colostrum a day is an insurmountable amount to ingest, but it does illustrate that even individuals who are lactose intolerant can most likely tolerate the recommended daily 2-4 capsules.

DISCLAIMER:
The statements contained herein have not been evaluated by the Food And Drug Administration. It is not intended to diagnose, treat, cure or prevent disease. The statements are for informational purposes only and is it not meant to replace the services or recommendations of a physician or qualified health care practitioner. Those with health problems or pregnancy are specifically advised that they should consult their physician before taking colostrum or any nutritional supplement.

COLOSTRUM PLUS PROBIOTICS, PREBIOTICS, AND COMPLEX LIPIDS THE IDEAL COMBINATION

Michail Borissenko
Chief Scientist
Institute of Colostrum Research

Introduction

The combination of three very unique substances may just prove to be the making of the world's most unique and most powerful food formulation in the treatment of disease and promotion of good health.

The significance of colostrum in the area of overall health lies in two very important features. First, it is a highly nutritious food. Second. it contains many bioactive substances that have been shown to prevent disease and promote overall good health. Bovine Colostrum supplementation has been shown in clinical trials to help prevent disease in a number of species, including humans.

The idea of ingesting beneficial bacteria to maintain a healthy gastrointestinal microbial balance is nothing new. In fact, it was first proposed some 100 years ago. **Probiotics** are the beneficial bacterial inhabitants of our digestive tract. The term "probiotics" was coined to describe the deliberate ingestion of health promoting microorganisms. In addition, probiotic refers to those microorganisms which may prevent or reduce the effect of an infection caused by a pathogenic (disease-causing) microorganism. These pathogenic effects can range from mild discomfort to severe conditions such as irritable bowel syndrome and even cancer. Probiotics have been shown to neutralize these effects.

A **Prebiotic** is a non-digestible food ingredient that beneficially affects the host by selectively stimulating the growth and/or activity of one or a limited number of bacteria in the colon, thus improving the host's health. They selectively and preferentially stimulate the growth of probiotics. In addition, prebiotics inhibit the binding of pathogenic microbes to the gut wall, thus minimizing their threat.

Phospholipids are complex lipids (fats) and are the predominant structural element of all physiological membranes. Though phospholipids function primarily as structural elements, they are also essential in three very critical areas: the growth, maturation and proper functioning of the cells in the body. Phospholipids are an excellent source of choline, which has been shown to increase brain function. Phospholipids, in particular phosphatidylserine, have been associated with improved memory. Phospholipid supplementation has been shown to be beneficial in the treatment of Alzheimer's and similar diseases. Phospholipids have also been shown to reduce mood swings and elevate depression. Phospholipids, in particular sphingomyelin, are natural emulsifying agents and thus are used in a wide variety of applications. The ability of sphingomyelin to form very stable micelles and liposomes makes it an ideal candidate in developing drug delivery systems. These delivery systems can be utilized to increase dispersibility and target specific target dissolution.

Colostrum

The bioactive molecules in colostrum include such things as immunoglobulins, immune factors, growth factors, and antioxidants. **Immunoglobulins**, also known as **antibodies**, and other **immune factors** act to ward off disease. **Antibodies** are large protein molecules produced by the animal's immune system to combat and neutralize foreign, potentially disease-causing agents (antigens). The interesting feature of antibodies is that they are specific in that there is a separate and specific antibody produced for every type of antigen.

Colostrum is produced by the mammary gland of all mammals. It is also known as pre-milk as it is the first milk produced by the mother following the birth of her young. The significance of colostrum lies in the fact that it is the first food the young animal receives after it is born. As such, colostrum is a highly nutritious food. Of paramount importance is the fact that colostrum is involved in a phenomenon known as passive transmission of immunity. This is a life-supporting function and is best exemplified in farm animals such as the horse, cow, dog, sheep, goat, etc. Unless these animals receive colostrum in the first day or two of life they most likely will die.[651,652] Unlike humans, who are passively immunized in the womb via the placenta, these animals are born without any defense mechanism—immune system—by which they can fight off infection. Colostrum contains antibodies produced by the mother against disease-causing agents she has been exposed to during her lifetime.

At the time of birth, the gut of these animals is not yet sealed, and whole antibody molecule can be absorbed through the gut wall directly into the blood system. By ingesting colostrum, the newborn is able to obtain antibodies from the mother to help them survive until their own immune system is sufficiently developed to fight off disease.[653] After a day or two of life, the gut seals, and the antibodies present in the colostrum and milk function in local immune protection of the gut.[654] This local immune protection is not species specific, and as such we as humans, and all other animals, can use bovine colostrum for its various health benefits.[655]

Antibodies belong to a group of bioactive molecules referred to collectively as immunoglobulins. Antibodies function to hunt down, fight, and destroy disease-causing agents or pathogens. Colostrum supplementation has been shown to be an effective means by which infections of the gastrointestinal tract and other areas can be prevented.[656,657,658,659] It has been shown in clinical trials that colostrum supplementation can be effective in preventing and treating diarrhea (scours) and other infections.[660,661,662,663,664] In a recent study conducted in collaboration with the Department of Microbiology, Otago University, New Zealand, it was revealed that colostrum derived from non-immunized, pasture-fed cows had significant specific antibody potency (titer) against a very wide variety of potentially pathogenic (disease-causing) microbes.[665] Bovine colostrum has been shown in clinical trials to have a safe, protective effect in a variety of species, including humans, dogs, cats, horses, and pigs.

In addition to antibodies, colostrum also contains many other substances which help promote good health in the form of growth, maturation and development. These include growth factors and immune factors. Growth factors include Epidermal Growth Factor (EGF),[666] Transforming Growth Factor (TGF), Insulin-Like Growth Factor (IGF), and Fibroblast Growth Factor (FGF).[667] These factors function primarily in the growth, development, and maturation of cells, organs, nerves, muscle, and tissues. Growth factors are also involved with the healing and recovery process.[668] Immune factors include Lactoferrin, Cytokines, Lysozyme, Lactoperoxidase and Transfer Factor. These factors have a very wide assortment of actions including augmenting the action of antibodies and modulating the actions of the immune system.

The direct benefits of colostrum are numerous, and they include overall good health, prevention of disease, improved performance, reduced healing period, increased recovery, and improved immune protection. These benefits are obvious and can be explained through biochemical pathways and various specific actions of specific components present in colostrum. However, the indirect effects of colostrum are not so clear cut. What is clear is that all the wonderful things in colostrum work together in such a way as to increase the effectiveness of each component.

Probiotics

The main function of the digestive system is to prepare food so it may be available to the body for use in energy, growth, and structural maintenance. The digestive tract accomplishes this by the act of digestion where large, complex molecules of food are broken down into much smaller molecules. This begins with physical digestion where the act of chewing helps to break down food into smaller subunits and continues with chemical digestion with enzymes present in the saliva. As the food enters the stomach, it is further partially digested by acids and enzymes. Final digestion occurs in the intestine by literally billions of microorganisms where it is metabolised and absorbed through the gut wall into the body. These microorganisms are bacteria, and they exist in a very complex and delicate ecosystem consisting of more than 400 species.[669] Many of these billions of microorganisms work synergistically in such a way as to help one another. Though most of these microorganisms are beneficial (friendly or probiotic bacteria) to the host, some may be pathogenic if they are allowed to proliferate. A critical balance needs to exist between the various bacteria in order to maintain a healthy intestine. Health starts with the intestine, and so does disease. This critical balance can be affected due to changes in diet, health status, age, immune status, stress, and even medication. If the result of this imbalance causes a reduction in friendly bacteria, it may lead to intestinal distress which can range from mild discomfort to severe conditions such as irritable bowel syndrome and even cancer.

The idea of ingesting beneficial bacteria to maintain a healthy gastrointestinal microbial balance is nothing new. In fact, it was first proposed by Dr. Elie Metchnikoff some one hundred years ago. Though fermented dairy products have been consumed for centuries, the significance of Dr. Metchnikoff's findings are exemplified by the fact that he was awarded the Nobel Prize in 1908 for his work.

Probiotics are the beneficial bacterial inhabitants of our digestive tract.[670,671,672] The term ***probiotics*** was coined to describe the deliberate ingestion of health promoting microorganisms. In addition, probiotic refers to those microorganisms which may prevent or reduce the effect of an infection caused by a pathogenic organism. The predominant microorganisms associated with these effects are from the genera ***Lactobacillus*** and ***Bifidobacterium***.

Lactobacilli are also distributed throughout the gastrointestinal (GI) and genitourinary (GU) tracts of humans and all other mammals.[673] They play a very important role in the fine balance of the gut micro-ecosystem. The actual distribution of these microorganisms throughout the gut is based on a number of factors: pH, available oxygen, substrates present, presence of secretions, and bacterial interactions. These are regarded as health promoters.

Bifidobacteria are microorganisms of significant importance in the complex balance of the intestinal micro-ecosystem of all mammals. They are found throughout the whole GI and GU tracts. Bifidobacterium is the first to populate the digestive tract of infants and in early life is the dominant microorganism present. With increasing age, this bacteria's presence decreases. Eventually it becomes the third most abundant, accounting for approximately 25% of the total gut flora. The other two genera of bacterium represented are ***Bacteroides*** and ***Eubacterium***. With the onset of old age a significant reduction of bifidobacterium is observed.

It has been recommended that adults should routinely supplement their diet with three of these bacteria, ***Lactobacillus acidophilus***, ***Bifidobacterium bifidum***, and ***Lactobacillus bulgaricus***.[674] In the case of infants it has been recommended that they be supplemented with ***Bifidobacterium infantis***.

Intestinal Health

Enteric (gut) infection is a major cause of infant disease and death worldwide, especially in developing countries. Significant research has shown that probiotics are beneficial in the treatment of many types of diarrhea, including diarrhea associated with antibiotic treatment, traveler's diarrhea, and childhood rotavirus-associated diarrhea.[675,676,677,678] Probiotics have also been shown to preserve intestinal integrity and mediate the effects of inflammatory bowel diseases, including irritable bowel syndrome, colitis, and alcoholic liver disease.[679,680,681] In addition, lactic acid can improve intestinal mobility and relieve constipation, particularly in seniors.

Immune System

Research suggests that probiotics can enhance both the specific and non-specific immune response. This mode of action is most likely the result of activating macrophages, increasing local levels of cytokines, increasing natural killer cell activity, and/or having an effect on the immunoglobulins.

Lactose Intolerance

Lactic acid bacteria, such as ***S. thermophilus***, ***L. bulgarucus*** and other lactobacilli can alleviate symptoms of lactose intolerance. These organisms provide bacterial lactase to the stomach and intestine and thereby digest the lactose.

Allergy

Probiotics have a beneficial effect on mucosal barrier function, thus reducing allergic reaction. They also beneficially affect immune system development. Probiotics, such as Lactobacillus, may help in reducing some of the symptoms of food allergies. In addition, probiotics have a very significant influence on the treatment and management of other allergic conditions, such as atopic eczema, asthma, and hay fever.[682]

Cancer

Research has shown that probiotic consumption may reduce colon cancer risk by reducing the incidence and number of tumors.[683]

Nutrition

Probiotics may improve the digestibility of some dietary nutrients such as protein and fat. Probiotics have also been shown to have a beneficial effect on lowering serum cholesterol levels. Short chain fatty acids such as lactic acid, propionic acid and butyric acid produced by lactic acid bacteria may help in maintaining proper pH and protect against pathological challenge.[684]

Prebiotics

Oligosaccharides function as prebiotic ingredients.[685,686] A prebiotic is a non-digestible food ingredient that beneficially affects the host by selectively stimulating the growth and/or activity of one or a limited number of bacteria in the colon, thus improving the health of the host. In the case of dietary inulin, it is preferentially utilized (hydrolyzed and fermented) in the large intestine by the probiotic bacteria (lactobacilli and bidobacteria), thus promoting intestinal health.

A number of studies have also proven that prebiotics such as inulin actually enhance mineral absorption in the colon. These results contradicted the concerns regarding the potential for soluble dietary fiber to bind metal ions. The inulin-mineral complexes formed are degraded during the hydrolysis and fermentation process, and thus the minerals are made available for enhanced absorbtion in the colon.

Some 13 distinct oligosaccharides have been detected and characterized in bovine milk or colostrum.[687] These compounds comprise up to about 0.1% of bovine milk. Their component simple sugars include glucose, galactose, fructose, N-acetyl glucosamine and sialic acid. They represent a large proportion of the non-protein nitrogen in milk. While the actual mechanism of action and functions of all the oligosaccharides is not known, it is generally accepted that many act to promote lactobacillus growth in the digestive tract. Oligosaccharides also have protective functions against certain potentially harmful bacteria and their toxins. This function is attributed to prebiotics acting as competitive inhibitors for binding sites on the epithelial surfaces of the intestine.

Gastrointestinal Tract Health

Oligosaccharides in the diet are known to enhance the growth of these organisms in the gut. Of particular note is the ability of oligosaccharides to promote the proliferation of bifidobacteria, so they are referred to as bifidogenic or bifidus factors. They achieve this by acting as selective energy or food sources for the beneficial bacteria, but potentially harmful bacteria such as clostridia or Enterobacteriaceae cannot utilize them. For the aforementioned reasons, oligosaccharides are often referred to as prebiotics.

Functional Foods

Oligosaccharides are relatively new functional food ingredients, but the production, range, and range of applications of these complex sugars is rapidly increasing. Currently, the major food applications of oligosaccharides are in beverages, infant formulas, confectionary, yoghurts, dairy desserts, and bakery products.[688] Europe and Japan in particular have experienced rapid increases in consumption of oligosaccharides as functional food ingredients in the last decade.[689,690] This is largely due to the perceived health benefits derived from their consumption. The main claim made for these foods is that they are designed to maintain a good gastrointestinal environment and act to increase intestinal bifidobacteria.

Dietary Fiber

Oligosaccharides are most widely incorporated into food formulations in the form of inulin, oligofructose or fructooligosaccharide.[691] Inulin is derived commercially from the chicory root and is classed as a soluble dietary fiber.[692,693] This dietary fiber classification is based on its specific chemical configuration, which makes it resistant to digestion by mammalian digestive enzymes. The physiological benefits of dietary fiber are well known and widely recognized. These benefits include: relief of digestion, relief of constipation and increased stool volume.[694] Studies have also shown that inulin is non-glycemic in that it improves glucose tolerance and insulin sensitvity. Further, it has been shown to have an affect of lowering serum cholesterol and triglycerides. It has also been shown to have an effect on increasing the HDL/LDL cholesterol (good cholesterol vs. bad cholesterol) ratio, thus having a beneficial affect on overall health.

Complex Lipids

Phospholipids are complex lipids and are the predominant structural element of all physiological membranes.[695] Amphipathic lipid compounds are essential components of all biological membranes. Phospholipids are present in every cell of animals and plants. In animals they are found abundantly in the tissues of the brain, heart, liver, muscle, kidneys, and bone marrow. Though phospholipids function primarily as structural elements, they are also essential in three very critical areas: the growth, maturation and proper functioning of the cells in the body. [696,697]

Phospholipids are either derived from glycerol or sphingosine and are designated either glycerophospholipids or sphingolipids respectively. The predominate form of phospholipids are the glycerophospholids of which phosphatidylcholine (lecithin), phosphatidylserine, phosphatidylethanolamine, and phosphatidylinositol are the predominant species.

Sphingolipids are specific to animal sources and are not found in plants (such as soy). There are two types of sphingolipids: sphingophospholipids and sphingoglycolipids. As the nomenclature implies, the sphingophospholipids are phospholipids with a sphingosine backbone. Sphingoglycolipids also have a sphingosine backbone, but instead of containing a phosphate group have a sugar group. Prime examples of sphingophospholipids and sphingoglycolipids are sphingomylein and gangliosides respectively.[698]

Phospholipids are an excellent source of choline, which has been shown to increase brain function. Phospholipids, in particular phosphotidylserine, have been associated with improved memory. Phospholipid supplementation has been shown to be beneficial in the treatment of Alzheimer's and similar diseases. Phospholipids have also been shown to reduce mood swings and elevate depression. Phospholipids, in particular phosphatidylcholine, have been shown to have a protective effect on the liver – protecting it against damage caused from toxins including alcohol, drugs and viruses.

Sphingomyelin

The sphingolipid sphingomyelin represents 25–33% of the total milk phospholipids in the milk.[699] Sphingolipids function in variety of physiological roles from initiating cellular defense, tumor suppression and cholesterol mobilization to liposome membrane rigidification.

Milk derived sphingomylein has been shown in in vitro studies using a human cell line to boost cellular production of interferon-beta, which plays an important role in cellular defense against viral infection. The breakdown products of sphingomylein are sphingosine and ceramide. Sphingosine has been shown to inhibit protein kinase C, an important component in the internalization of growth factors into the cell. Thus it has been theorized that sphingomylein contains components that act as second messengers which are important in The digestive products of sphingomylein have also been shown to highly antimicrobial. They are effective in vitro against such pathogens as Salmonella, Campylobacter, Vibrio, Listeria, and pathogenic E coli.[700]

Along with other phospholipids in milk, sphingomyelin can protect gastric mucosa against injury caused by acid, pepsin or exogenous irritants. Sphingomyelin, along with phosphatidylcholine, is an important source of choline, which is important for brain function. Sphingomyelin accounts for approximately 10% of the lipids present in the brain.

Considerable research has been undertaken on the functions of phospholipids and, more recently, sphingolipids in health and disease. Recently it has been shown that both sphingolipids and their breakdown products—ceramide and sphingosine—are highly bioactive compounds having a profound effect on various biological functions in the body. Regulation of cell growth, differentiation, signalling, and programmed cell death (apoptosis) have all been attributed to sphingolipids. Further, sphingolipids have also been implicated in playing a vital role in neuronal development. In animal studies it has been revealed that dietary sphingolipids inhibit colon carcinogenesis.[701]

Studies on mice who were administered with 1,2 dimethylhydrazine—a powerful tumor inducing agent—revealed that an up to 70% reduction of tumors was observed after being fed milk derived sphingomyelin. With longer feeding even a greater reduction of tumours was observed. It was revealed that mice fed as little as 25mg of sphingomylein/100g of diet had a 57% reduction in incidence of colon tumors. Further studies on mice fed milk-derived sphingomyelin, as compared to a control group fed a standard diet, showed a reduction in aberrant colon tumors, and most importantly revealed a shift from malignant tumors to ones that were benign.[702] Thus it has been postulated that sphingomyelin-containing foods may have anti-cancer activity. Though no clinical trials have been conducted on humans to date, the results of in vitro studies using human cancer cells lines show great promise. Further, sphingomyelin has been shown to increase the effectiveness of chemotherapy agents in killing cancer cells.[703]

Phosphatidylserine

Phosphatidylserine (PS) makes up approximately 8% of the total phospholipid in bovine milk. There is substantial evidence that indicates that PS improves memory and brain function. PS is most concentrated in the brain where it functions to support many crucial nerve cell functions.[704,705] It is the primary component of neuronal cell membranes. In brain disorders, such as Alzheimer's, Parkinson's and multiple sclerosis, there is an association with neuron degeneration and dysfunction.[706,707,708,709,710,711] Phosphatidylserine has been shown to stimulate the production of a brain messenger chemical (dopamine) that helps regulate memory. PS has also been shown to stimulate protein kinase C production and help modify mood changes arising from stress. In addition, evidence is mounting regarding the beneficial aspects of PS to elevate mood and reduce the symptoms of depression. PS has also been shown to have positive effects in treating early Alzheimer's and the onset of premature memory loss due to dementia.

Phosphatidylethanolamine

Phosphatidylethanolamine (PE), also known as Cephalin, makes up approximately 30% of the total phospholipid content of bovine milk. Phosphatidylethanolamine comprises the backbone of cell membranes and contributes to the fluidity and structural environment of cells.[712] In regard to the brain and nervous tissue, PE plays an important role in myelin structure and nerve endings in the brain. Phospholipids, particularly PE, have been shown to be beneficial in lowering serum cholesterol levels and thus reducing the risk of heart disease.

Phosphatidylcholine

Phosphatidylcholine (PC), also known as Lecithin, makes up approximately 30% of the phospholipid present in bovine milk. Along with sphingomyelin, PC is a major source of choline. Choline is a major neurotransmitter, Acetylcholine. Dietary PC has been shown to improve neurological malfunctions such as tremors, ataxis and mood swings.[713] Choline is required to sustain tissue growth, and thus a ready supply of this phospholipid is required for the maintenance of good health.

PC is a major building block for all cell membranes, and it supports cellular, tissue and organ function. This is particularly true of the liver with its vast network of cell membranes. Thus the liver is particularly dependent on PC for proper function. It has been shown in clinical trials that dietary PC has beneficial aspects in helping individuals recover from toxic liver damage. PC has also been shown to protect the liver from damage due to viral infection, medication, alcohol, and nutritional deficiency. It has also been shown to be beneficial in speeding the recovery process resulting from liver damage.

Phosphatidylinositol

Phosphatidylinositol (PI), also known as Inositol, comprises approximately 5% of the total phospholipid present in milk. Inositol is necessary for the proper functioning of the brain, nerves and muscle. Inositol is a lipotropic substance helping to prevent build-up of fatty deposits in the liver. Inositol is also an essential nutrient for proper growth in newborn children.[714]

Phospholipids—Natural Emulsifying Agents

Phospholipids, in particular sphingomyelin, are natural emulsifying agents and are used in a wide variety of applications. The ability of sphingomylein to form very stable micelles and liposomes makes it an ideal candidate in developing drug delivery systems. These delivery systems can be utilized to increase dispersibility and target specific target dissolution. With the advent of new technologies in the isolation and purification of phospholipids, specific phospholipids can now be targeted for end use.

Milk-derived Phospholipids vs Soy Lecithin

The significant difference between plant-based soy lecithin and milk-derived phospholipid is the actual composition of the phospholipids in question. As was mentioned above, only animal-based phospholipid preparations contain sphingomyelin. In addition, milk-derived complex lipids are more similar to human lipids than vegetable sources. The emulsion properties of sphingomyelin are far superior to that of soy lecithin. The actual phospholipid compositional differences are seen below:

Phospholipid Class	Soybean*	Milk*
Phosphatidylcholine	30%	30%
Phosphatidylethanolamine	20%	30%
Phosphatidylserine	3%	10%
Phosphatidylinositol	20%	5%
Sphingomyelin	Not present	25%

*Expressed as total phospholipid present

PASTEURIZATION

MICHAIL BORISSENKO
Chief Scientist
Institute of Colostrum Research

Named after its inventor, Louis Pasteur, the process of pasteurization is an integral part of the dairy industry. The initial discovery demonstrated that organisms responsible for the spoilage of wine could be inactivated by applying heat. This process has since been applied to milk where it remains the single most important step in the manufacturing of dairy products.

The definition of pasteurization is as follows:

The heating of every particle of milk or milk product to a specific temperature for a specified period of time without allowing recontamination of that milk or milk product during the heat treatment process.[715]

The primary purpose of pasteurization is to destroy potentially pathogenic microbes present in milk thus rendering the milk or milk product safe for human consumption. The secondary purpose of pasteurization is to extend the shelf life of the milk or milk product. It is not only organisms but also enzymes, which are involved with spoilage, that are inactivated by pasteurization.

The Pasteurization Marketing Ordinance (PMO) is a regulatory body founded by the US Public Health Service, in conjunction with the US Food and Drug Agency (FDA) and other agencies and institutions. It is the governing body that states limits and compliance standards for pasteurization in the United States of America. It should be pointed out that this is the accepted world standard in regard to pasteurization. The PMO has given the following statement regarding health reasons for pasteurization:

The public health value of pasteurization is unanimously agreed upon by health officials. Long experience conclusively shows its value in the prevention of disease which

may be transmitted through milk. Pasteurization is the only practical, commercial measure which, if properly applied to all milk, will destroy all milk-borne disease organisms. It has been demonstrated that the time-temperature combinations specified by this ordinance, if applied to every particle of milk, will devitalize all milk-borne pathogens. Compilations of outbreaks of milk-borne disease by the US Public Health Service over many years indicate that the risk of contracting disease from raw milk is approximately 50 times as great as from milk labeled "pasteurized."[716]

The extent to which microorganisms and enzymes are inactivated is directly proportional to the temperature and duration of pasteurization. Thus the higher the temperature and the longer the duration the greater the effect of killing microorganisms and inactivating enzymes.

The two most heat stable pathogens found in fresh milk are ***Mycobacterium tuberculosis*** and ***Coxiella burnetti.*** The first is the bacterium which causes tuberculosis, and the second is the bacterium responsible for Q fever. The minimal temperature and duration requirements for pasteurization of milk are based on thermal death time studies on these two organisms. To ensure the safety of all dairy products, these temperature and time combinations are highly regulated. For milk and colostrum, the temperature and duration of pasteurization has been established by the PMO and is as follows:

Milk Pasteurization—PMO Guidelines

Temperature	**Time**
63°C (145°F)	30 min.
72°C (161F)	15 sec
89°C (191°F)	1.0 sec
90°C (194°F)	0.5 sec
94°C (201°F)	0.1 sec
96°C (204°F)	0.05 sec
100°C (212°F)	0.01 sec

As must be apparent, the higher the temperature utilized, the shorter the time required to destroy all potentially pathogenic microbes. It should be pointed out that for diary products containing 10% or more fat or containing added sweeteners the PMO guidelines stipulate that the specified temperature shall be increased by 3°C (5°F).

The process of pasteurization has undergone many improvements since its inception. In the beginning, milk and other fluids were simply boiled, and unfortunately many of the nutrients and bio-active substances were adversely affected. For a growing number of milk and colostrum manufacturers, the preferred method of sanitizing milk and colostrum is by flash pasteurization, also know as High Temperature Short Time (HTST) pasteurization. By incorporating this method to sanitize or kill microbial contamination, the biological integrity of the milk and colostrum is maintained and any loss of bioactivity is minimized.[717]

Flash pasteurization is performed using a continuous plate and tube or heat exchange system. This counter current method ensures that the temperature of the product is elevated to the exact required temperature, held there for the required time and then swiftly lowered in the shortest possible time. Thus the milk and colostrum is heated to 72 since its inception C in the shortest time possible, held at that temperature for a minimum of 15 seconds and immediately cooled. In this way complete destruction of microbial growth and inactivation of enzymatic activity is achieved. Microbiological testing is performed to assure sanitation and product safety. Of significant importance is the fact that this method ensures that maximal biological activity and nutritional benefits are retained.[718]

The thermal stability of immunoglobulin preparations has long been the focus of many research studies. It has been observed that flash pasteurization incorporating high temperature short time (HTST) —72°C for 15 seconds—has minimal effect on protein denaturization and reduction in bioactivity. The following exemplifies the thermal stability of IgG in flash pasteurization.[719]

Thermal Destruction of Immunoglobulins During Processing of Colostrum

Pasteurization is a critical quality parameter used during the manufacture of dairy products. Data collected during processing has shown that minimal loss due to denaturization of immunoglobulins occurs when colostrum is pasteurized (Table 1.).[720,721,722]

Table 2. D-Value of IgG in Bovine Colostrum

Temperature (°C)	D-Value (sec)
70	13,038
72	6,456
74	3,960
78	1,122
82	414

D-value = time required to inactivate 90% of the IgG

If a second pasteurization step is a requirement of further processing, research has shown that 65°C for 30 minutes has no effect on the activity of IgG. Previous research conducted at 72°C for 15 seconds found a reduction in IgG activity of approximately 0.5-10%. However, this reduction is likely to be dependent on the precise system into which the colostrum is incorporated and the interactions of the components within this system. For example, salt causes IgG to become less susceptible to denaturization and aggregation during heat treatment. Further, in a recent investigation it has been reported that IgG values will be only very slightly affected by HTST pasteurization at 72°C for 15 seconds. In fact, what was observed was an approximate drop of 2% in quantified IgG value which is well within the standard error of the assay used in the measurement.

Further antigen binding studies have shown that the bioactivity of antibodies is little affected by the process of flash pasteurization. In determining D-values, the time required to reduce the antigen binding activity of IgG (antibody) by 90% was determined (Table 2.) [723,724]

Table 2. D-Values IgG Antibody/Antigen Binding in Bovine Colostrum

Temperature (°C)	D-Value (seconds)
69	8504
72	1387
77	285
81	152

D-value = time to inactivate 90% of the IgG antibody binding to antigen

Thus modern dairy technology has developed to the point where the process of pasteurization, though effective in neutralizing any potential microbial health hazard, has very little negative effect on the bioactivity, biofunctionality, and nutritional composition of the various components found in milk and colostrums.

DISCLAIMER:
The statements contained herein have not been evaluated by the Food And Drug Administration. It is not intended to diagnose, treat, cure or prevent disease. The statements are for informational purposes only and is it not meant to replace the services or recommendations of a physician or qualified health care practitioner. Those with health problems or pregnancy are specifically advised that they should consult their physician before taking colostrum or any nutritional supplement.

FREEZE DRYING VS SPRAY DRYING

Michail Borissenko
Chief Scientist
Institute of Colostrum Research

Introduction

The purpose of drying biological material is simple. By removing the moisture from the material, bacteria, yeast and molds cannot grow. Simply, this is a way of preserving food and other biological materials. The basic concept behind food preservation is either to slow down the activity of disease-causing bacteria or to kill the bacteria altogether. Pasteurization is an example of the latter of these two options. In regard to the former, refrigeration and freezing are the most frequently used options. When frozen, bacteria are completely, inactive whereas when refrigerated their action is simply slowed down.[725,726]

In freezing, biological material is preserved in that microorganisms are prevented from multiplying. However, those that survive the freezing process can reanimate in the thawing material and often grow more rapidly than before freezing. To combat this or to reduce this action, the material is typically sterilized by either pasteurization, sterile filtration or irradiation prior to freezing. Preserving agents can also be introduced prior to freezing. The greatest disadvantage of freezing is that the water in the biological material expands and forms ice crystals during the freezing process. The slower the freezing process, the larger the size of crystals formed and the greater the effect on cellular membranes of the material being frozen. Blast or quick-freezing reduces the size of the ice crystals and thus reduces the damage to the cell membranes. Cryoprotective agents can also be introduced prior to freezing in order to minimize the effect on cellular membranes. In the case of pure protein solutions, sugar is typically used for this purpose, whereas in the case of cells (tissue culture), ethylene glycol or DMSO are typically used.[727]

In both spray drying (warm air drying) and freeze drying, water is removed, thereby preserving the biological material because microorganisms and enzymes require moisture to grow, proliferate, and function. In regard to logistics, the removal of water also decreases both the volume and weight of biological material, thereby reducing transport and storage costs.

The principal difference between spray drying (warm air drying) and freeze drying is temperature. Spray drying employs a higher temperature while freeze drying is performed at low temperature. In spray drying, a liquid in the form of a fine spray is passed through a chamber of warm air where the liquid is dehydrated by evaporation. This is a relatively inexpensive process and is ideal when temperature sensitive materials are not involved. In addition, due to the configuration change involved in the spray drying process, solubility of the final dried product can be affected.

However, it should be noted that recent developments in the spray drying process have come to light where reduced temperature drying is now possible. In this way large-scale spray drying of material that would otherwise be damaged is now not only possible but a reality. A case in point is the spray drying of colostrum. In a recent comparability study conducted in collaboration with Otago University, New Zealand, it was revealed that low temperature spray dried colostrum contained the same amounts of IGF-1 as colostrum which was freeze dried.[728] IGF-1 is a small peptide which is very heat sensitive. Thus it has been shown that low heat spray drying can be successfully used to dry biological material. Further, numerous studies have shown that the process of low temperature spray drying does not adversely affect the various bioactives present in colostrum. These studies include a recent investigation run in conjunction with Otago University showed that the low temperature spray drying process does not discernibly affect antibody function. This information corresponds to earlier investigations in which the efficacy of spray dried colostrum was evidenced.[729,730,731]

Freeze drying, on the other hand, is a relatively expensive process and is typically used in the drying of temperature sensitive, high cost materials (e.g. cells, pharmaceuticals). Freeze drying is typically utilized for drying materials that would be adversely effected by drying temperatures above the freezing point. In freeze drying the material is dried in a frozen state under vacuum. The process of sublimation removes the liquid or water in this manner, that is, ice sublimes directly to gas. Because the material is dried in a rigid frozen condition (stabilized state) the resulting integrity of the dried material remains more or less intact and is readily soluble.

Summary

Freezing and drying of biological material are ways of preservation. In spray drying, a powder is formed when a liquid, in the form of a spray, is subjected to warm air. This is a relatively inexpensive method of drying and is ideal when it involves large volumes of material which are not temperature sensitive or easily oxidized. Due to the configurational change involved in this process, solubility of the final product can be effected. In freeze drying, the moisture is removed from the frozen product directly by the process of sublimation. This is a stabilizing process which has little effect on the configuration of the molecule. Thus the integrity of the product is not effected. In the case of biologically active products, such as proteins, which are heat sensitive, freeze drying is the method of choice. However, it should be pointed out that the recently developed technology of low temperature spray drying has been shown to have a minimal effect on the integrity and bioactivity.[732]

ADDITIVES VS ACTIVES

Michail Borissenko
Chief Scientist
Institute of Colostrum Research

Many colostrum manufacturers are adding extra ingredients to their colostrum products. This is being done for a number of reasons. Unfortunately in only a very limited number of cases does this addition actually improve the colostrum product. In fact, in most cases it is simply to add a new gimmick or to reduce the amount of colostrum being used. The only reasonable thing that should be incorporated into colostrum are actives and specifically actives which improve the effectiveness of the product. The addition of sugar will only make the product sweeter and certainly not more effective. In fact, it will make it less effective as the colostrum is being diluted down. Some manufacturers add vitamins and supplements to their colostrum products. Will these improve the effectives of the product? I think not. Some manufacturers add digestive aids such as enzymes. The only thing this will do is most probably act to destroy the effectiveness of the colostrum.

Colostrum was developed by Mother Nature to be the most important food in the world. It has to be as it is the first food a newborn receives when it is born. In short, if it doesn't improve the action of the colostrum or if it doesn't improve the effectiveness of the colostrum, why add it?

ATHLETIC PERFORMANCE AND COLOSTRUM

Michail Borissenko
Chief Scientist
Institute of Colostrum Research

Introduction

The significance of colostrum in the area of athletic performance lies in several very important features, all of which the athlete can take advantage of to reach a higher level of performance, and most probably a better form of life. It is a highly nutritious food and contains many, many bioactive substances which have been shown to prevent disease and promote overall good health. Of specific interest to the athlete is the fact that colostrum supplementation can be an effective way by which the athlete can increase lean body mass, improve muscular strength, increase endurance and capacity, and at the same time speed recovery. What this means to the athlete is simple: they can train harder, longer and recover faster, thereby increasing their respective level of athletic performance. Of significant importance to the athlete is the simple fact that colostrum is perfectly safe and that the International Olympic Committee (IOC) has designated colostrum to be an accepted and safe dietary supplement. Thus it is recognized as perfectly safe and legal by all the sports regulatory bodies.

Overall Health

One very important aspect of performance is overall good health. This is especially true in the case of the athlete who wants to perform at maximal level. The use of bovine colostrum supplementation has been shown in clinical trials to help prevent disease. Most infections and disease conditions start in the gastrointestinal tract, and this is exactly where the benefits of colostrum begin—in the gut.

The bioactive molecules in colostrum include such things as immunoglobulins, immune factors, growth factors, and antioxidants. To begin with, immunoglobulins in the form of antibodies and other immune factors act to ward off disease. Antibodies are large protein molecules produced by the immune system to combat and neutralize foreign, potentially disease-causing agents, or antigens. The interesting feature of antibodies is that they are specific in that there is a separate and specific antibody produced for every type of antigen.

Colostrum is produced by the mammary gland of all mammals. It is also known as pre-milk as it is the first milk produced by the mother following the birth of her young. The significance of colostrum lies in the fact that it is the first food the young animal receives after it is born. As such, colostrum is a highly nutritious food. However, of paramount importance is the fact that colostrum is involved with a phenomena known as passive transmission of immunity. This is a life-supporting function and is best exemplified in farm animals such as the horse, cow, dog, sheep, goat, etc. Unless these animals receive colostrum in the first day or two of life they most likely will die. Unlike humans, who are passively immunized in the womb via the placenta, these animals are born without any defense mechanism (immune system) by which they can fight off infection. Colostrum contains antibodies produced by the mother against all the disease-causing agents she has been exposed to during her lifetime.

At the time of birth the gut of these animals is not yet sealed, and whole antibody molecules can be absorbed through the gut wall directly into the blood system. By ingesting colostrum, the newborn is able to obtain antibodies from the mother to help them survive until their own immune system is sufficiently developed to fight off disease. After a day or two of life the gut seals, and the antibodies present in the colostrum function in local immune protection of the gut. This local immune protection is not species-specific, and as such we as humans, and all other animals, can use bovine colostrum for its various health benefits.[733]

In addition to antibodies, colostrum also contains many other substances which help promote good health in the form of growth, maturation and development. These include growth factors and immune factors. Growth factors include epidermal growth factor (EGF), transforming growth factor (TGF), insulin-like growth factor (IGF), and fibroblast growth factor (FGF). These factors function primarily in the growth, development, and maturation of cells, organs, nerves, muscle, and tissues.[734,735,736] Immune factors include lactoferrin, cytokines, lysozyme, lactoperoxidase, and transfer factor (PRPs). These factors have a very wide range of actions and include augmenting the action of antibodies and modulating the actions of the immune system.

Antibodies belong to a group of bioactive molecules who as a group are referred to collectively as immunoglobulins. Antibodies function to hunt down, fight, and destroy disease-causing agents or pathogens. Colostrum supplementation has been shown to be an effective means by which infections of the gastrointestinal tract and other areas can be prevented.[737] It has been shown in the form of clinical trials that colostrum supplementation can be effective in preventing and treating diarrhea (scours) and other infections.[738,739,740,741,742,743] In a recent investigation conducted in collaboration with the Department of Microbiology, Otago University, New Zealand, it was revealed that colostrum derived from non-immunized pasture fed cows had significant specific antibody potency (titer) to a very wide variety of potentially pathogenic (disease-causing) microbes.[744,745] Bovine colostrum has been shown in clinical trials to have a safe, protective effect in a variety of animals, including humans.[746]

In addition to immunoglobulins, colostrum also contains other immune factors which help ward off disease and promote overall health, including bioactive peptides, lactoferrin, secretory component, lysozyme, lactoperoxidase, cytokines, oligosaccharides, complex lipids, many others. Colostrum also contains growth promoting substances collectively referred to as growth factors which help to accelerate the growth or healing process thus aiding the athlete to train harder and recover faster.

It has recently been discovered that colostrum is a significant source of antioxidants.[747,748,749] One such antioxidant, glutathione, has been described as the ultimate antioxidant. In this capacity glutathione and glutathione precursors play an important part in colostrum's role in overall health. Glutathione, also referred to as GSH, is a naturally occurring peptide or small protein, which has a primary function as an antioxidant.[750,751,752,753] Linus Pauling was a leading advocate of antioxidants and their respective role in prevention of disease and the promotion of overall good health. Antioxidants for the most part are naturally occurring compounds that possess the ability to neutralize unstable free radicals. Unchecked, these free radicals have been linked, at least in part, as the causative agents of a number of disease conditions, including cancer, heart disease, stroke, and improper nervous and immune system function.[754,755] A growing number of scientific and medical research studies have shown that that antioxidants can deactivate free radicals and thus limit the spread of certain disease states. Further, it has been shown that glutathione enhances athletic performance by increasing muscle strength and weight gain.[756]

The direct benefits of colostrum that have been observed to date are numerous and include overall good health, prevention of disease, improved performance, reduced healing time, increased recovery, and improved immune protection. These benefits are obvious and can be explained through biochemical pathways and various specific actions of specific components present in colostrum. However, the indirect effects of colostrum are not so clear cut. What is clear is that all the wonderful things in colostrum work together in such a way as to increase the effectiveness of each component.

Colostrum and Athletic Performance

The beneficial aspects of colostrum on athletic performance is well documented in clinical trials. It has been shown that colostrum supplementation in athletes improves running, jumping, rowing, swimming and cycling performance.[757,758,759,760,761,762] It has also been shown that colostrum supplementation has a positive effect during periods of heavy training and improves physical work capacity. Of major significance is the fact that the athletes who received colostrum supplementation experienced a greater capacity for endurance. Thus the athletes who received colostrum were shown to run further, jump higher and longer, cycle and row faster and longer. Further, they where shown to recover faster as compared to the placebo group. In an investigation into the effects of bovine colostrum supplementation on body composition in association with exercise, it was revealed that the colostrum group experienced a significant increase in lean body mass as compared to the placebo group. Thus the results to the athlete must be obvious—colostrum supplementation can increase lean body mass, improve muscular strength, increase endurance and capacity, and at the same time speed recovery. What this means to the athlete is simple—they can train harder, longer, and recover faster, thereby increasing their respective level of athletic performance.[763]

How Does It Work?

It has long been established that both milk and colostrum contain peptide growth factors, which stimulate growth and differentiation of mammalian cells. The predominant growth factor activity is typically concentrated in the colostral phase. A number of growth factors have been described in bovine colostrum. These include insulin-like growth factor (IGF-1, IGF-2), transforming growth factor (TGF-β1 and TGF-β2), and epidermal growth factor (EGF).

Insulin-like growth factor-1 (IGF-1) is found in relatively high concentrations in colostrum and is of specific interest in regard to athletic performance.[764] Specifically, this growth factor mediates the growth or metabolic effects of growth hormone.[765] On a molecular level, IGF-1 functions to stimulate muscle and bone cell proliferation and development, i.e., helps to build muscle and strong bones.[766,767,768] In a recent study it was shown that oral supplementation with bovine colostrum enhances the recovery process following physical exercise or exertion. Thus it allows for harder training with improved recovery. Two further studies have shown that bovine colostrum has positive effect on maximal power output—increases vertical jump performance and improves rowing performance in elite female rowers.[769,770,771]

Improves Recovery

Physical exercise and training cause muscle damage. Recovery from this damage is necessary or subsequent exertion will be limited. Bovine colostrum has been shown to help in this recovery process. It has been demonstrated in laboratory studies that IGF-1 can promote an increase of up to 15% in muscle mass and a 14% increase in strength.

Oxidative stress in the form of training and exercise contributes to muscle fatigue. Glutathione and its precursors, present in colostrum, have been shown to increase the capacity of exercise prior to the onset of fatigue. There is an ever increasing amount of evidence that suggests free radicals play a very important role in muscle damage and inflammation.[772] Glutathione is a powerful antioxidant and as such a powerful scavenger of free radicals.[773]

In a study involving Olympic skiers it was shown that athletes taking colostrum were less fatigued and showed improved performance compared to their counterparts who were given a placebo. Creatine kinase is a critical enzyme involved with muscle metabolism and has been shown to be a marker of muscle cell damage. Elevated circulating (blood) creatine levels are often associated with significant muscle damage. In this study, the athletes who consumed colostrum had, following exercise, approximately half the circulating creatine levels of the control group.[774]

Speeds Healing

Transforming growth factor and epidermal growth factor are also found in relatively high amounts in colostrum. Both these growth factors stimulate tissue repair and wound healing. Digestive disorders are associated with a number of contributing factors: stress, medications, infectious agents, diet , and, in the case of the athlete, overtraining. The use of bovine colostrum has been proven effective in the treatment of gastrointestinal disorders caused by aspirin and other nonsteroidal anti-inflammatory drugs (NSAIDs).

Anti-Inflammatory Properties

Associated with physical exertion and strenuous exercise is inflammation. In fact, at the Sydney Olympics the second most common medication taken by the athletes were anti-inflammatories, being only surpassed by vitamins. Though typically this inflammation is centered in the joints, it is also observed in the digestive tract. In colostrum and milk there are two principle molecules (proteins) that have been implicated as natural anti-inflammatory agents: lactoferrin and secretory component of the secretory IgA molecule. Both proteins are abundant in bovine colostrum.

Inflammation is a complex localized event in response to either injury, an invasive foreign substance (pathogen), or in some instances to internally produced substances (e.g., rheumatoid arthritis). This is a protective adaptation that serves to isolate, destroy, and rid the infected area of both the injurious agent and the injured tissue. Prostaglandins and leukotrines play an important role in mediating the process of inflammation by increasing histamine-mediated vascular permeability. It is predominantly this action which causes the discomfort associated with inflammation.

The common anti-inflammatory analgesic and antipyretic drugs, such as corticosteroids, aspirin and indomethacin, inhibit prostaglandin and/or leukotrine synthesis. In fact, most, if not all, of the anti-phlogistic actions of steroidal and non-steroidal anti-inflammatory drugs' action involve the inhibition of prostaglandin synthesis. The anti-inflammatory effect of aspirin and indomethacin is inhibition of cyclooxygenase, whereas those of corticosteroids are thought to inhibit the release of fatty acids from phospholipids either by inhibition of phospholipase-A2 or by interfering with the release of membrane phospholipids.[775,776] It has been shown by in vitro studies that the secretory component of secretory IgA inhibits phospholipase-A2 activity and therefore prostaglandin and leukotrine synthesis by limiting the release of arachidonic acid.[777]

The fact that colostrum is a natural food that has no contraindications or negative side effects suggests that it is an ideal supplement to be used to counter inflammation. The adverse side effects associated with certain anti-inflammatory agents limits their use. In the case of corticosteroids, the potential side effects include the elevation of blood pressure, water and salt retention, increased calcium and potassium excretion, gastric upset and possibly peptic ulceration. In addition, the use of these compounds may also aggravate diabetes mellitus. The non-steroidal anti-inflammatory compounds (salicylates) are synthetic biochemical substances that can be toxic at high doses. The possible side effects associated with these substances include gastric upset and gastric bleeding, prolonged clotting time, and hepatic injury. Though the number of various anti-inflammatory agents is great, so are the potential side effects and adverse reactions associated with these compounds. It is in this regard where colostrum has also been shown to be of direct benefit. NSAIDs are very effective agents for treatment of inflammation, but unfortunately they cause gastric injury. Colostrum has been shown to be beneficial in the prevention and treatment of gastrointestinal injury caused by NSAIDs.[778,779] Further, colostrum has been shown to be beneficial in treating not only ulcerative conditions but also other diseases of the gut.[780]

Supplementation

It has recently been reported that for top class Olympic athletes the variation in their respective performance of as little as 1% can be the difference between winning and losing. Colostrum, in conjunction with proper nutrition and training, can just be that little extra edge that not only helps the athlete perform better but also keep them healthier.

In a recent survey involving 463 sports coaches in the USA, it was revealed that 87% of the coaches believe that "dietary supplements are a safe and effective means of improving performance." It was also reported that some 80% of these coaches routinely advised their athletes on nutrition and some 40% recommended specific products.[781] Dietary supplementation has long been associated with sport and athletic performance. The increasing number of research and clinical information on the benefits of colostrum is substantiating the fact that colostrum supplementation enhances athletic performance.[782]

Colostrum and the International Olympic Committee

Colostrum is a completely natural substance that has been used as a food for hundreds of years. Everything in colostrum is also found in milk, although at a much lower level. As such colostrum has been labeled by the IOC as being a "strong" milk, and the IOC does not consider colostrum to be a prohibited substance. Further, bovine colostrum supplements are not on the banned drug lists of the IOC or any other sports governing body.[783,784,785,786,787]

Safety of Colostrum

The efficacy and safety of colostrum supplementation in humans and animals has long been established in clinical trials. Currently there are a growing number of either colostrum or colostrum derived products available that are registered for therapeutic use. There are no known contraindications to use of bovine colostrum supplements in athletes. As with all supplements, individuals who are pregnant, lactating, or who have an intolerance to dairy products should consult with their health professional.

In Summary

Colostrum is a very complex mixture containing many bioactive substances that have yet to fully appreciated. Among these substances so far identified are immunoglobulins, growth factors, immune factors and antioxidants. An important feature, which must be pointed out, is the synergistic actions of a highly complex mixture like colostrum. The general belief is that this synergism is paramount for the true benefits of colostrum to be experienced. In regard to the athlete, it has been shown that colostrum is an effective, safe, and legal supplement which can have a very positive influence on performance.

DISCLAIMER:
The statements contained herein have not been evaluated by the Food And Drug Administration. It is not intended to diagnose, treat, cure or prevent disease. The statements are for informational purposes only and is it not meant to replace the services or recommendations of a physician or qualified health care practitioner. Those with health problems or pregnancy are specifically advised that they should consult their physician before taking colostrum or any nutritional supplement.

COLOSTRUM VS CREATINE

MICHAIL BORISSENKO
Chief Scientist
Institute of Colostrum Research

Colostrum

Colostrum, also known as pre-milk, is a natural product and is produced by the soon-to-be mother just before and for several days following the birth of her young. It is the first food available to the newborn

The use of bovine colostrum for its associated health benefits, though known for centuries, has only recently gained much attention.

The significance of colostrum in the area of **athletic performance** lies in several very important features, all of which the athlete can take advantage of to reach a **higher level of performance**, and most probably a better form of life. First, it is a highly nutritious food, and second, it contains many bioactive substances which have been shown to prevent disease and promote overall good health. Of specific interest to the athlete is the fact that colostrum supplementation can be an effective way by which the athlete can increase **lean body mass, improve muscular strength, increase endurance and capacity, and at the same time speed recovery**. What this means to the athlete is simple—he or she can train harder, longer, and recover faster thereby increasing his or her respective level of athletic performance. Of significant importance to the athlete is the simple fact that **colostrum is perfectly safe and has no known side effects**. Further is the fact that the International Olympic Committee (IOC) has designated colostrum to be an accepted and safe dietary supplement. Thus it is recognized as perfectly safe and legal by all the sports regulatory bodies.

At the cellular level, colostrum contains many bioactive substances which function in a variety of ways. The direct benefits of colostrum that have been observed to date are numerous, and they include overall good health, prevention of disease, improved performance, reduced healing period, increased recovery, and improved immune protection. These benefits are obvious and can be explained through biochemical pathways and various specific actions of specific components present in colostrum. However, the indirect effects of colostrum are not so clear cut. What is clear is that all the wonderful things in colostrum work together in such a way as to increase the effectiveness of each component.

Creatine

Creatine is also a natural substance and is a normal constituent of our normal diet. It is found in meat, fish, and poultry. Most of the creatine—up 95%—is found in skeletal muscle. Creatine is produced naturally by the body in the liver, kidneys and pancreas from the amino acids arginine, glycine and methionine. The benefits of creatine in regard to athletic performance lay in its role in muscle contraction. Creatine plays a critical role in the replenishment of anaerobic energy stores in muscle. Muscle contraction requires energy, and this is derived from adenosine triphosphate (ATP). As this energy is being used up, it needs to be replenished or regenerated, and this comes from phosphocreatine stored in the muscle. In order for this to happen, creatine must be available to replenish phosphocreatine stores. This is especially true during intense, short duration exercise. There is a growing amount of evidence which indicates that creatine supplementation may help to increase phosphocreatine stores, thus delaying the onset of exhaustion during heavy exercise. There is also evidence that creatine supplementation helps to improve the recovery process and thereby reduce recovery time required between training sessions. Thus in regard to athletic performance, creatine supplementation may give those individuals in activities involving intense, short bursts an edge.

It should be noted that there are certain side effects associated with creatine supplementation, and certain precautions should be observed. It has been noted that a weight gain of 1-2 kg is typically seen when initiating creatine supplementation. This has been attributed to an increase in fluid stores. It has also been reported that creatine supplementation is associated with muscle cramps and tightness—most probably also due to the increase in water retention.

Creatine in its pure form is permitted in sport and poses no problems in healthy individuals. It should be pointed out that no large long term studies have been performed to evaluate the safety of creatine. However, creatine is not a food but rather a preparation and as such may contain impurities. As such the IOC has indicated that athletes should seek a written guarantee of the supplement's purity from the respective manufacturer to ensure that the material does not contain any harmful and possibly banned substances.

M. Borissenko
3 February, 2002

NEW RESEARCH

A Comparison of IgG and IgG1 Activity in an Early Milk Concentrate from Non-Immunized Cows and a Milk from Hyperimmunized Animals.

McConnell, M. A., Buchan, G. A. A., Borissenko, M. V., Brooks, H. J. L.
Food Research International 34:255-261 (2001)

A recent investigation was conducted in collaboration with Otago University, Department of Microbiology. In this study we compared the antibody specificity of a hyperimmune milk product with that of a colostrum product derived from non-immunized, pasture-fed cows. Specific antibody titers (concentration) to a panel of 19 of the same 22 pathogenic bacteria and yeast that were used as immunizing antigens, were determined by immunoassay. Three of the pathogens used as immunizing antigens were not available due to regulatory import restraints by the New Zealand Ministry of Agriculture and Fisheries (MAF). The following specific antibodies to the following microbes were identified:

PATHOGEN	DISEASE CONDITION
Bacillus cereus	Food poisoning, mastitis
Campylobacter jejuni	Food poisoning
Candida albicans	Thrush, yeast infection
Clostridium difficile	Food poisoning
Escherichia coli	Commensal bacteria
Escherichia coli 0157:H7	Food poisoning
Haemophilus influenzae	Bacterial meningitis, can be fatal
Helicobacter pylori	Stomach ulcers
Klebsiella pneumoniae	Pneumonia, urinary tract infection
Listeria monocytogenes	Food poisoning, can be fatal
Propionibacterium acnes	Acne
Salmonella enteritidis	Food poisoning, can be fatal
Salmonella typhimurium	Food poisoning, can be fatal
Staphylococcus aureus	Pneumonia, osteomyelitis, carditis,
	Meningitis, arthritis, toxic shock syndrome,
	Antibiotic Resistant—MRSA
Staphylococcus epidermidis	Multiple antibiotic resistance (MAR)
Streptococcus agalactiae	Mastitis, bacteremia, meningitis, pneumonia,
	can be fatal
Streptococcus mutans	Periodontal disease, tooth decay,
	Arteriosclerosis, endocarditis
Streptococcus pyogenes	Strep throat, flesh-eating bacteria, myositis,
	toxic shock syndrome, rheumatic fever,
	kidney disease
Yersinia enterocolitica	Food poisoning, septicemia, can be fatal

The results indicated that both the hyperimmunized milk and the non-immunized High IgG colostrum possessed high levels of specific IgG antibodies to all the 19 pathogens tested. It was also indicated that compared to the hyperimmunized product, High IgG colostrum is at least equipotent and is of greater specific antibody titer to that of hyperimmunized equivalent. As compared to the hyperimmunized product, High IgG colostrum consistently exhibited significantly higher titers to all 19 pathogens tested. Even when based on equivalent IgG concentration, High IgG colostrum had a higher level of specific antibody titer to all the pathogens tested.

The significance of these findings lies in the fact that this was a comparative study involving both a natural pasture fed colostrum versus a hyperimmunized equivalent. The results suggest that pasture fed grazing and environmental factors far outweigh the benefits of active hyperimmunization. It is of further interest that the specific antibody titer, even at equivalent IgG concentration, was significantly higher in the non-immunized pasture fed colostrum. Add to this all the other bioactives found in colostrum—immune factors, growth factors, hormones, etc. It is true that for the most part these bioactives are also present in milk, but only in minute amounts. Thus from the information given it appears obvious that the High IgG colostrum product is a far superior product to that of a commercially available hyperimmunized equivalent.

LEPTIN

Michail Borissenko
Chief Scientist
Institute of Colostrum Research

Derived from the Greek word, ***leptos***, meaning thin, leptin is a naturally occurring peptide hormone which is involved with body composition through metabolic regulation, appetite control, and even reproduction. First discovered in 1994, leptin has been hailed as the cure-all and end-all in regard to the prevention and treatment of obesity principally because of its actions in regulating energy expenditure, food intake, and storage of fat.

There is a very close association between obesity and Type-2 diabetes, a potentially serious disease affecting some 15 million individuals in America alone. Type-2 diabetes is characterized by the body's inability to properly use sugar. If left unchecked, diabetes can cause a variety of conditions associated with deteriorating health, including blindness, heart disease, kidney disease, and even death. It has been estimated that in America obesity affects some 58 million and contributes to between 280,000 and 325,000 deaths per year. Because of this, researchers have been trying to unravel the mystery of leptin since its discovery.

Leptin is a small protein (16,000 Daltons) produced by the ob (obese) gene. It was found that mice that have had the ob gene knocked out, missing, or defective produced no leptin. It was also observed that these same animals had voracious appetites and ate continually, becoming grossly obese, sterile, and diabetic. When leptin was administered to these animals by injection, they stopped overeating and rapidly lost weight. These animals also experienced a lowering of percentage body fat, serum insulin, and glucose levels. In addition, their metabolic rate, body temperature and activity levels were increased subsequent to administration of leptin. Even non-obese, normal weight mice injected with leptin lost body weight. It has been reported that this phenomenon was due at least in part to a reduction in fat synthesis and an increase in the burning of fat. It was postulated that leptin is a neurotransmitter that turns the appetite signal off in the brain.

Naturally this attracted enormous excitement throughout the world, the reasoning being that obese people simply do not have enough leptin and thus get fat. Would it not be wonderful if by simply administering leptin and increasing the body's leptin levels obesity could be treated and prevented? The significance and the commercial potential of such a discovery is illustrated by the fact that the California based biotechnology company, Amgen, spent $70 million (US) to obtain the commercial rights to the ob gene and its product, leptin.

However, in clinical trials with leptin on obese humans, the observed results were not so clear-cut. Only a small percentage of obese humans have the mutant ob gene, so most obese individuals produce leptin. In fact, it has been suggested that only some 5% of the obese population can truly be considered leptin-deficient and as such can benefit from leptin therapy alone. Even more surprising is that obese individuals typically produce 20 to 30 times higher levels of leptin as compared to lean individuals. Researchers thus speculated that the obese human body was insensitive to leptin's signal, and thus no trigger or signal to the human brain to stop eating.[788]

Leptin is produced by adipose or fat cells. In the normal rodent model with a properly functioning ob gene, leptin is produced when the fat cells have stored enough fat. The leptin then travels through the blood to the brain where it signals the brain that the body has stored a healthy amount of body fat. The brain then signals the body to down regulate (reduce) food intake in order to maintain normal body mass. Rodents which possess the defective ob gene do not produce leptin when they have ingested sufficient enough food, some of which is stored as fat. Thus they have no leptin to signal the brain to stop eating, so they stay hungry and continue to eat and eat and eat. Various studies have shown that leptin acts as a signal of satiety (fullness) to the brain, thus stimulating feeding behavior. One important study revealed that there exists a leptin receptor at the blood-brain barrier of humans that mediates saturable, specific, and temperature-dependent binding and thus internalization of leptin into the brain.[789]

Like all hormones, leptin must first bind to its receptor so it can be internalized and perform its function. It has been theorized that at least some obese individuals have defective leptin receptors, and thus the brain does not hear the signal to stop eating. It has been hypothesized that obesity in humans is associated with leptin resistance. The results from an investigation to determine whether leptin resistance is related to leptin binding by a serum component other than the leptin binding protein showed that affinity and binding of leptin to the leptin binding protein was specific and that no binding was observed for growth hormone, insulin, IGF-1 or 2, LH, FSH, TGF-beta1, IL-6 or leukemia inhibiting factor. It was also demonstrated that the leptin/leptin binding protein complex had a molecular weight of approximately 450 kDa. Further, it was determined that an inverse relationship exists between concentration of serum leptin and quantity of leptin binding protein. This information provided further evidence that binding of leptin to the leptin binding protein does indeed influence the biological function of leptin. Genetically obese rodents who have mutations of leptin or the leptin receptor are defective in leptin signaling and thus become obese and develop diabetes. In these animals, the circulating levels of both leptin mRNA and leptin receptor mRNA are increased some 20-fold. This gives further evidence that there exists a biofeedback mechanism that controls the leptin concentration in the circulation.

Many hormones circulate bound to proteins found in the blood serum. The belief is that these binding proteins (BP) modulate ligand bioavailability and bioactivity. In a recent study it was revealed that two such proteins are found in humans and three in rodents.[790] Of specific interest is the fact that in humans, free leptin in serum increases proportionally with increase in Body Mass Index (BMI). In lean rodents and humans, a large proportion of circulating leptin was found to be bound to the leptin binding proteins. However, in normal non-ob obese rodents and humans, the predominant form of leptin is in the free form, i.e., not bound to the leptin binding protein. It was also shown that both obese rodents and obese humans lack or have a much reduced expression of leptin binding protein.[791] Thus it has been postulated that leptin binding protein may modulate the bioactivity, transport and clearance of leptin.[792,793]

It has been reported that a lowering of serum leptin levels was associated with dieting and reduction of body fat in obese humans. It has also been reported that serum leptin levels correlated with Body Mass Index (BI) in lean and obese humans with weight loss due to food restriction.[794] In a six month clinical weight reduction trial involving 38 healthy obese women it was found that the average weight loss for this group was 8.4 kg with corresponding plasma leptin decrease of 22.3% under baseline.[795]

Significant increase in circulating leptin levels has been observed in glucose tolerance test (OGTT) experiments on obese individuals.[796] Interestingly enough, no such increase was observed in normal non-obese subjects. It has also been shown that leptin gene expression and thus secretion is increased by insulin but blocked by inhibitors of glucose metabolism. This indicates that leptin synthesis is modulated by insulin and is mediated through glucose uptake and metabolism.[797] Thus it has been postulated that a decrease in glucose metabolism may be responsible for the fact that dieting and fasting decrease serum leptin levels, and in turn increased glucose metabolism is responsible for an associated increase in circulating leptin after resuming food intake. It therefore appears that insulin and leptin interact in a biofeedback system by which insulin up regulates (increases) leptin expression (secretion) which in turn down regulates insulin secretion.

It is also of interest that in mice circulating leptin levels rise some 20-40 fold during pregnancy. Pregnant mutant mice that have the ob/ob gene have no detectable circulating leptin. However, normal mice have very high levels of circulating high molecular weight leptin complex of leptin bound to the leptin binding protein. This may indicate that there is over expression of the leptin binding protein in pregnancy.[798] These studies revealed that the placenta is a source of leptin, leptin receptor and leptin binding protein.[799] Leptin and leptin receptor have also been identified in colostrum and milk where it has a role in neonatal development, especially in regard to energy metabolism, digestive function, thermogenesis, and regulation of growth.[800] Leptin is involved in the development of gastrointestinal tract structure and function (motility and absorption) in the newborn.[801]

The appetite controlling effects alone cannot explain the metabolic response elicited by leptin. A recent study involving the underlying mechanism of leptin's metabolic actions showed that leptin represses the expression and activity of hepatic stearoyl-CoA desaturase-1 (SCD-1).[802] This enzyme is involved with biosynthesis and catalysis of monounsaturated fatty acids. Leptin thus acts at the cellular level and affects the actual mechanism by which fat is stored.

It is becoming obvious that leptin in the treatment of obesity and eating disorders is far from simple. In the first place, it appears that only 5% of the total obese population is actually deficient in leptin. Therefore leptin therapy on its own may be of little use to the other 95% of obese individuals. Also, most obese individuals in fact over produce leptin. It is clear that not only leptin but also leptin binding protein and leptin brain receptor and their respective expression are all linked with obesity in humans.

As previously stated, only some 5% of the obese population can possibly benefit from leptin therapy. In fact, a recent 6 month study involving 54 normal or lean individuals and 73 obese patients showed that exogenenous leptin may affect weight loss. The objective of this study was to determine the relationship between the increased dosage of recombinant human leptin administered daily subcutaneously and weight loss in both obese and lean adults. The lean subjects consumed their normal staple diet while the obese patients were placed on a restricted caloric diet. The results of this study indicate that weight loss was increased with increasing dose of leptin. It should mentioned that at the highest dose more than 95% of the weight loss was due to loss of fat with eight of the patients on the highest doses losing an average of 8.5 kg in weight as compared to the placebo group (36 patients) who lost an average of 2 kg each.[803] It appears that exogenous leptin injected subcutaneously daily may indeed induce fat and weight loss in some obese subjects with only minor side effects.[804] The major drawback of this treatment is that leptin, due to its peptide nature, has to be injected daily in high doses to be even slightly effective for only a small percentage of obese people.[805]

The annual expenditure on weight loss programs in America has been estimated to be approximately $35 billion (US). Of the total 58 million obese Americans it has been estimated that approximately 5% of these individuals are actually deficient in leptin. Thus exogenous leptin therapy could potentially help some 2.9 million obese individuals in America. Though the results to date are far from conclusive, they are promising and warrant further study into the actual mechanism and role leptin, leptin receptor and leptin binding protein play in obesity.[806]

It should be pointed out that recently a number of dietary supplement manufacturers have jumped on the leptin bandwagon and are actively advertising that their leptin-containing elixirs taken orally will cause fat "to literally melt away." The current method of leptin exogenous delivery is by subcutaneous daily injection, and little if any clinical evidence currently exists indicating the efficacy of orally ingested leptin in weight loss. To date, little, if any, information is available regarding the efficacy of using bovine leptin in the treatment and or prevention of obesity in humans.

DISCLAIMER:
The statements contained herein have not been evaluated by the Food And Drug Administration. It is not intended to diagnose, treat, cure or prevent disease. The statements are for informational purposes only and is it not meant to replace the services or recommendations of a physician or qualified health care practitioner. Those with health problems or pregnancy are specifically advised that they should consult their physician before taking colostrum or any nutritional supplement.

FAQs from the Institute for Colostrum Research Website

MICHAIL BORISSENKO
Chief Scientist
Institute of Colostrum Research

Albumin in Colostrum

There are two types of albumin in both milk and colostrum: lactalbumin; and milk albumin. In colostrum they represent approximately 2% of total solids.

Animals and Colostrum – Can They All Benefit?

It's kind of like the Oscar Mayer hot dog jingle—everyone can benefit from taking colostrum, including pets. In fact, I have come across papers on the use of bovine colostrum in the treatment of birds, elephants, mice, even fish.

Arthritis and Colostrum

There are actually two types of arthritis—osteoarthritis and rheumatoid arthritis. In the case of osteoarthritis, this is caused by the actual grinding down of the cartilage due to use, or rather overuse. It is perfectly normal and comes with getting older. Having played rugby, etc, as a youth doesn't help. The other form, rheumatoid arthritis, is an autoimmune disease in which the bodies own immune system attacks the joints and can afflict anyone at any age.

I suspect that you are referring to the former, osteoarthritis. The biggest problem here is inflammation and pain come hand in hand. The degradation of the cartilage causes inflammation, which in turn causes the pain. Now, how can colostrum help? Well, first off, colostrum contains several very keen natural antiinflammatory agents, and these function to reduce and possibly stop the swelling. Secretory IgA and lactoferrin are the bioactives in colostrum which have this anti-inflammatory action. Secondly, there are numerous drugs out on the market which act as anti-inflammatory agents, and this includes aspirin. As a general heading, these drugs fall under the heading non-steroidal anti-inflammatory drugs (NSAIDs). These NSAID drugs, for the most part, are very good in their action to inhibit the resulting inflammation associated with osteoarthritis. The problem is that for the most part NSAIDs also effect the stomach and the rest of the gut in a very adverse way. Basically they eat the gut, causing ulceration, etc, when used for long periods of time. Guess what? Colostrum has been shown to help prevent and treat the damage done to the stomach and gut by NSAIDs.

Apolipoprotein Levels and Colostrum

Briefly, there are actually two major types of cholesterol—one is good, and one is bad. The bad form of cholesterol is called Low Density Lipoprotein (LDL), also known as Apolipoprotein B-100. This is the one that binds onto the walls of blood vessels and causes causes atheriosclerosis or heart disease. The good form of cholesterol is High Density Lipoprotein (HDL), also known as Apolipoprotein A1, and it functions in preventing the LDL from binding to the vessel wall.

Optimally, you want a high ratio of HDL vs LDL. What colostrum does is reduce LDL levels and increase HDL levels. That is very good. The mechanisms involved include insulin-like growth factor-1 (IGF-1), antioxidants (such as glutathione) present in colostrum, and cytokines, also present in colostrum. Colostrum growth factors promote the repair and regeneration of heart muscle and the regeneration of new blood vessels for collateral coronary circulation.

Athletic Performance and Colostrum

The significance of colostrum in the area of athletic performance lies in several very important features—all of which the athlete can take advantage of to reach a higher level of performance, and most probably a better form of life. First, it is a highly nutritious food, and secondly it contains many, many bioactive substances which have been shown to prevent disease and promote overall good health. Of specific interest to the athlete is the fact that colostrum supplementation can be an effective way by which the athlete can increase lean body mass, improve muscular strength, increase endurance and capacity, and at the same time speed recovery. What this means to the athlete is simple: they can train harder, longer, and recover faster, thereby increasing their respective level of athletic performance. Of significant importance to the athlete is the simple fact that colostrum is perfectly safe, and further is the fact that the International Olympic Committee (IOC) has designated colostrum to be an accepted and safe dietary supplement. Thus it is recognized as perfectly safe and legal by all the sports regulatory bodies.

Atopic Skin Allergy and Colostrum

In regard to skin allergies, colostrum contains a very interesting bioactive known as Proline-rich Polypeptide (PRP), also called Colostrinin or transfer factor. This is a very interesting modulator (controller) of the allergic response. Briefly, this substance has been shown to reduce the allergic reaction. You may also try applying colostrum topically to the allergic area. Use any cream as a base and simply dissolve some colostrum in it.

Atopic Dermatitis and Colostrum

Also known as atopic eczema. The word "atopic" refers to a tendency for excess inflammation in the skin, lining of the nose, and lungs.

It may be of interest that this condition often runs in families in which family members are affected with allergies such as hay fever and asthma. In approximately 20% of the cases only a single family member may be affected by this condition. It should be noted atopic dermatitis is very common throughout the world and approximately 10% of infants and 3% of all people in the USA are affected. The most common cause of this condition is allergy, and it may involve environmental conditions, though rarely food allergy.

In regard to colostrum, it may possibly be of benefit, and this is due to a component in colostrum called colostrinin, also referred to as Proline-rich Polypeptides, or PRP for short. Very briefly, colostrinin are small polypeptides which have regulatory activity—stimulating or suppressing the immune response. In the case of allergies, the immune system is over-stimulated, hyper-stimulated. PRP has been shown to reduce the stimulation and thus help alleviate the symptom.

When my kids had dermatitis, I just added some colostrum (1 capsule) to the nappie cream we were using at the time and applied it topically. The results were magic. Virtually overnight the redness, etc, disappeared. You also might try giving the child half a capsule in their bottle. However, as always, it may pay to discuss options with a trained health professional, such as dermatologist. This is especially true as it is not our position to give medical advice. You also might want to check the following website for more details on eczema: www.eczema-assn.org.

Babies—Is Colostrum Safe to Feed Babies

The area of infant formula is a very sensitive one and involves controversy—breastfeeding vs bottle feeding. It is also tightly regulated, and as such I would suggest due caution be observed in this respect and a disclaimer be included. In regard to the feeding of colostrum to infants and babies—though numerous clinical trials have been conducted involving colostrum in the treatment and prevention of enteric infection, it is still classed as a dietary food supplement. As with any dietary food supplement, it is generally agreed that in regard to feeding colostrum to babies, especially ones less than 6 months old, individuals consult with their healthcare professionals first.

There are numerous cow's milk infant formulas currently being used wordwide to not only feed babies under the age of 12 months but from the time of birth, and I thus must question the nurses' motives. I think everyone will agree that breastfeeding is best, but not all mothers are able. Infant formula is an option, and colostrum will most probably improve the associated health benefits if this option is taken. Infant formula companies such as Nutricia, Nestle, Wyeth, and Mead have been investigating just this for some time, the biggest hurdle being manufacturing costs.

The final decision to use or not to use colostrum lies with the parents. We can supply the scientific and medical evidence to them or their chosen representative, but the final decision is theirs. The fact is that colostrum does work!

Babies—Feeding Colostrum to Babies

Colostrum is an ideal supplemental food for the infant in that it supplements the digestive tract with various things that protect against disease. Disease starts in the gut, and so does health. However, in the case of a infant please discuss this with your health care professional if there are any concerns.

Barley, Alkaline pH, and Colostrum

I really cannot see how an increase in pH will effect weight loss, unless somehow you expect to increase the pH of the lower intestine thereby affecting the digestive processes of the friendly bacteria there. Thus no digestion and no absorbtion of food, and what you eat goes right down the toilet. You would certainly need to ingest a lot of barley for that. Why not try sensible diet with exercise. supplemented by colostrum? I think this will serve you better.

From the chemical point of view, barley is simply grass. Yes, it is an insoluble fiber and might work as a prebiotic. Stick with the colostrum, but if you so desire, by all means mix it with colostrum.

Benefits of Colostrum—How Long Before I See Them After Starting

Colostrum is a wonderful thing produced by mother nature for the primary purpose of supporting the newborn. It does this by helping the newborn to fight disease (passive transmission of immunity) and promote development and maturation of various tissues. Further, as the first food the newborn receives, colostrum is very nutritious. For us humans its main function is that it promotes overall good health—you don't get sick. This is very hard to measure. The degree of our health is often masked by our level of fitness, diet, lack of excercise, lack of sleep, alcohol intake, etc. A friend of mine just turned 50 years old, and he told me that he felt great—like a teenager with a hangover.

We as humans come in all kinds of sizes and shapes, and because of this, the time it takes for the various benefits of colostrum to take hold varies. Further, these positive effects may appear subliminally without us noticing them. One classic question I get is, "After taking colostrum for several weeks I noticed my muscles were sore." This typically comes from a sedentary person who after taking colostrum becomes more active and as it turns out starts using muscles they haven't used in years. The best way to determine if the beneficial effects of colostrum are being achieved is to measure them by objective determination. This can be done by keeping a diary and rating how you feel on a daily basis, say, 1-10 (with 1 being close to to death and 10 being the first time you fell in love). I think you will shortly find that with colostrum you will be achieving the higher numbers.

In regard to weight loss, I want to emphasize that colostrum is not the magic bullet in losing weight. You can't simply take colostrum and watch the fat melt away. Colostrum, however, augmented with proper diet and exercise, can help you burn fat and build lean body mass, which has been shown in clinical trials.

Body Building and Colostrum

First, I have written a paper I recently wrote on Athletic Performance and Colostrum. It basically explains how colostrum works as an aid in athletic performance, its safety and its acceptance by the International Olympic Committe (IOC) as an acceptable dietary supplement.

Briefly, in conjunction with proper diet and exercise, colostrum has been shown to help build lean muscle mass and reduce body fat. It has also been shown by way of clinical trials to help improve athletic performance. This is accomplished in two main ways. First, by maintainence of overall good health, second, by improving capacity to train harder, and third, by improving the recovery and healing process. Thus the athlete can train longer, harder and recover faster.

One important substance implicated in these actions is insulin-like growth factor-1 (IGF-1), a substance normally found in our bodies, in milk and colostrum, also in red meat. The use of pure or recombinant (gentically engineered) IGF-1 is banned by the IOC, as is the use of pure Growth Hormone. The reasoning is that this material can be injected intramuscularly (IM) for local action. However, since normal milk, colostrum and even red meat contain IGF-1, its use as a dietary supplement or food cannot be banned. In fact, our bodies produce IGF-1 on their own, and it has been shown that exercise will increase our circulating IGF-1 levels. The normal IGF-1 level for the human adult is approximately 15-500 ug/l in blood. With 6 liters of blood, the human adult will thus have approximately up to 3000ug (3mg) of IGF-1. Colostrum contains approximately 1ug/g of IGF-1 or 1/3000 of what our bodies normally have already. In addition, I would like to point out that IGF-1 is not an anabolic steroid hormone but is a growth factor. How it functions is two-fold: it helps in our utilization of foods; and it controls the metabolic effects of growth hormone which is also normally present in our bodies. In this capacity it helps to build strong muscles and bone.

Breastfeeding

Please consult with your health care provider, but we can quote science and what has been shown to be true in clinical studies. Primarily there is the fact that colostrum has been shown in clinical trials to prevent enteric disease—diseases of the gut. The leading cause of infant disease, as in adults, is gut infection. This is where colostrum can help. There are no contraindications involving colostrum as far as I am aware. It is very simple, really—colostrum will help you stay free of disease, and in turn your baby will be free of disease. I know this is a very simple concept, but it is actually is true.

BSE AND COLOSTRUM

Safety of Milk

The WHO Consultation of 2-3 April 1996 concluded that milk and milk products were safe. This statement was based on unsuccessful attempts to transmit the agent from cows clinically affected by BSE by inoculation of their milk into mice by intracerebral or intraperitoneal routes or by feeding milk.

More recent data from a suckler herd study in the UK further support the conclusions concerning the safety of milk. No BSE cases out of 132 offspring born to BSE-infected cows have occurred so far (minimum age was 20 months in August 1996).

The present Consultation concurs with the view that milk is safe.

CATEGORY III Low infectivity

Peripheral nerves, nasal mucosa, thymus, bone marrow, liver, lung, pancreas.

CATEGORY IV No detectable infectivity

Skeletal muscle, heart, mammary gland,milk, blood clot, serum, faeces, kidney, thyroid, salivary gland, saliva, ovary, uterus, testis, seminal testis, foetal tissue, [colostrum, bile, bone, cartilaginous tissue, connective tissue, hair, skin, urine]*.

*Tissues in brackets were not titrated in the original studies, but relative infectivity is indicated by other data on spongiform encephalopathies.

Cancer and Colostrum

Regarding colostrum and pancreatic cancer, the article below may be useful.

From the ***American Journal Of Natural Medicine:***

"The 1985 Steven Rosenberg book, ***Quiet Strides in the War on Cancer***, first popularized the benefits of cytokines in the treatment of cancer. Since that time, the same cytokines found in colostrum (interleukins 1, 6, 10, gamma-interferon, and lymphokines) have been the single most researched protocols in scientific research for the cure for cancer.

"Colostrum lactalbumin has been found to be able to cause the selective death (apoptosis) of cancer cells, leaving the surrounding noncancerous tissues unaffected. Lactoferrin has similarly been reported to possess anticancer activity.

"The mix of immune and growth factors in colostrum can inhibit the spread of cancer cells. If viruses are involved in either the initiation or the spread of cancer, colostrum could prove to be one of the best ways to prevent the disease in the first place."

Cancer (Leukemia) and Colostrum

In regard to your enquiry regarding leukemia and how colostrum can help, I should initially state that leukemia is a serious medical condition, and it is advised that the individual's healthcare professional should be consulted.

First, leukemia is a type of cancer, of which there are several types. Colostrum can most probably help in some areas, such as following chemotherapy, reducing the incidence of infection caused by secondary or opportunistic pathogens. Case in point is the use of colostrum for the prevention of fungal infection (Candida or yeast) following bone marrow transplant. Finally, in promoting overall health, disease starts in the gut, and colostrum acts to imunosupplement the gut, that is, protect the gut from infection.

Cancer and Colostrum

The IGF-1 controversy is really overplayed to the point of being ridiculous. It is based on the fact that IGF-1 on the molecular level helps make certain cell types divide faster. All normal cells require growth factors for proper cell division. However, when a cell undergoes mutagenesis and becomes cancerous, it loses this requirement for growth factors in cell division.

Insulin-like Growth Factor-1 (IGF-1) is a normal constituent in the milk and colostrum of all mammalian species, including humans. It is also found in the blood, saliva, urine, skeletal muscle and other areas of the body. An adult healthy male will typically have approximately 1-3 million nanograms (0.000000001–0.000000003 grams) of IGF circulating through their blood system. In order to replenish these circulating levels and maintain this concentration, the body produces approximately 1 million ng of IGF daily.

The food we eat and drink is the main source of exogenous or external IGF, and this comes from dairy products, meat, poultry (chicken and eggs) & fish. The IGF-1 concentration found in bovine milk is approximately 500 ng per 100 milliliter (ml) while bovine colostrum contains approximately 30,000 ng per 100 ml.

Produced by the liver and other tissues, IGF-1 plays a very important role in a wide range of actions within the body. This includes various transport processes such as ion transport, RNA and DNA synthesis, protein and lipid metabolism, and glucose and amino acid (food) uptake by cells. IGF-1 is also involved with cell division and differentiation in that it is stimulates muscle and bone cell development. It is because of these actions it was postulated that IGF-1 could play a significant role in various sporting activities. This includes building lean body mass while functioning in improving the healing process. A significant body of clinical evidence suggests that IGF-1 can, among other things, help the athlete train harder, longer, and recover faster. In these studies IGF-1 has been shown to help increase lean body mass (muscle) and burn fat.

Relatively recently the field of biotechnology has developed the technology to produce sufficient quantities of recombinant human IGF-1 to make it economically viable to make pure recombinant human IGF-1 available to the public. It is because of this the International Olympic Committee has designated IGF-1 a banned substance and has placed it on their list of Prohibited Substances. This material is typically administered intramuscularly where there is a local mode of action. On this topic very little information is available but sure to grow. In regard to Growth Hormone (GH), it appears that its inclusion on the Banned Substances list is justified as it has clearly been shown that its use significantly increases circulating IGF-1 levels in test subjects. In fact ,it has been shown that the administration of growth hormone by injection can elevate IGF-1 levels by up to 700%.

In regard to the ingestion of naturally occurring foods containing IGF-1, however, the information is well established, and all the evidence indicates that the ingestion of colostrum and or milk will not increase circulating IGF-1 or GH levels. One very early study investigating the effects of colostrum supplementation on athletic performance did suggest that ingestion of colostrum may cause a negligible increase in serum IGF-1 levels. However, in this same study it was also reported that this change in IGF-1 level could also be attributed to the exercise itself. Heavy resistance exercise has been shown to increase circulating IGF-1 levels by up to 25%. It should also be reported that the same researcher who originally reported a possible increase due to colostrum now supports the fact that the ingestion of colostrum has no significant effect on circulating IGF-1 levels.

Clinical trials involving athletes using as much as 60 grams of colostrum per day (60 times the normal dose) showed that no significant increase in IGF-1 and GH levels, as compared to the control group. Typically a good quality colostrum contains approximately 1,000 to 2,000 ng of IGF-1 per gram powder. These 60 grams of colostrum powder corresponded to 60,000 to 120,000 ng of IGF-1 being taken daily. Thus the ingestion of colostrum containing the equivalent of as much as approximately 10% of the total circulating level of IGF-1 had no effect on elevating existing levels.

Further, it has been shown that diet has a very important role in regulating circulating IGF levels. In fact, it has been determined that processed starchy foods, such as white bread and junk food, elevate IGF levels. If IGF did indeed cause cancer, then physical exercise must also be regarded as a potential cancer risk—I don't think so! Further, could it be that an athlete who consumes high amounts of junk food be at the highest risk of developing cancers? I really don't think so! The controversy may continue, but common sense must prevail. Does colostrum and IGF cause cancer? Definitely no!

Just to kill this thing once and for all I should also point out that there are a number of papers giving evidence how substances in milk and colostrum actually help prevent cancers.

Candida (Yeast Infection) and Colostrum

New Zealand colostrum has been shown to possess very high levels of specific antibody to a wide variety of microbes, and this includes Candida. We have shown that this colostrum will actually inhibit growth of Candida.

Children and Colostrum

Children, like adults, can benefit from colostrum. The age at which one gives colostrum to children is up to the parents. It should be pointed out that there is a registered therapeutic based on colostrum and designed for prevention of rotavirus infection that is designed for children. It should also be noted that there are no known ill side effects associated with colostrum, and it is generally recommended that colostrum is safe to give children over the age of 6 months. This is not a recommendation but rather a rule of thumb as in some countries this age limit does vary. Further, if there is any doubt whatsoever, please consult with a healthcare professional.

Colostrum—What Is It?

The significance of colostrum in the area of overall health lies in two very important features. Firstly, it is a highly nutritious food, and secondly, it contains many bioactive substances that have been shown to prevent disease and promote overall good health. The use of Bovine Colostrum supplementation has been shown in clinical trials to help prevent disease in a number of species, including us humans.

The bioactive molecules in colostrum include such things as immunoglobulins, immune factors, growth factors, and antioxidants. To begin with, immunoglobulins in the form of antibodies and other immune factors act to ward off disease. Antibodies are large protein molecules produced by the animal's immune system to combat and neutralize foreign, potentially disease-causing agents (antigens). The interesting feature of antibodies is that they are specific in that there is a separate and specific antibody produced for every type of antigen. During our lifetime we continually add to the complement of antibodies that are formed in response to the various infectious agents we are exposed to. Antibodies are found in the blood and many other bodily fluids, such as saliva, colostrum and milk.

Colostrum is produced by the mammary gland of all mammals. It is also known as pre-milk as it is the first milk produced by the mother following the birth of her young. The significance of colostrum lies in the fact that it is the first food the young animal receives after it is born. As such, colostrum is a highly nutritious food. However, of paramount importance is the fact that colostrum is involved in a phenomenon known as "passive transmission of immunity." This is a life-supporting function and is best exemplified in farm animals such as the horse, cow, dog, sheep, goat, etc. Unless these animals receive colostrum in the first day or two of life they most likely will die. Unlike humans, who are passively immunized in the womb prior to birth via the placenta, these animals are born without any defense mechanism—immune system—by which they can fight off infection. Colostrum contains antibodies produced by the mother against the disease-causing agents she has been exposed to throughout her lifetime.

At the time of birth, the gut of these animals is not yet sealed, and the whole antibody molecule can be absorbed through the gut wall directly into the blood system. By ingesting colostrum the newborn is able to obtain antibodies from the mother to help them survive until their own immune system is sufficiently developed to fight off disease. After a day or two of life the gut seals, and the antibodies present in the colostrum and milk function in local immune protection of the gut. This local immune protection is not species-specific, and as such we as humans, and all other animals, can use bovine colostrum for its various health benefits.

Antibodies belong to a group of bioactive molecules who as a group are referred to collectively as immunoglobulins. Antibodies function to hunt down, fight, and destroy disease-causing agents or pathogens. Colostrum supplementation has been shown to be an effective means by which infections of the gastrointestinal tract (gut) and other areas can be prevented. It has been shown in clinical trials that colostrum supplementation can be effective in preventing and treating diarrhea (scours) and other infections. In a recent investigation conducted in collaboration with the Department of Microbiology, Otago University, New Zealand, it was revealed that colostrum derived from non-immunized New Zealand pasture fed cows had significant specific antibody potency (titer) to a very wide variety of potentially pathogenic (disease-causing) microbes. Bovine colostrum has been shown in clinical trials to have a safe protective effect in a variety of species, including humans, dogs, cats, horses, and pigs.

In addition to immunoglobulins or antibodies, colostrum also contains other immune factors which help ward off disease and promote overall health—including bioactive peptides, lactoferrin, secretory component, transferrin, lysozyme, lactoperoxidase, cytokines, oligosaccharides, complex lipids, and many others. Colostrum also contains growth promoting substances collectively referred to as growth factors which help to accelerate the growth or healing process.

Colostrum, in addition to antibodies, also contains many other substances which help promote good health in the form of growth, maturation and development. These include growth factors and immune factors. Growth factors include epidermal growth factor (EGF), trophoblast growth factor (TGF), insulin-like growth factor (IGF), and fibroblast growth factor (FGF). These factors function primarily in the growth, development, and maturation of cells, organs, nerves, muscle, and tissues. Growth factors are also involved with the healing and recovery process. Immune factors include lactoferrin, transferrin, cytokines, lysozyme, lactoperoxidase, and transfer factor (PRP). These factors have a very wide assortment of actions and include augmentation (helping) of the action of antibodies and modulation (controlling) of the actions of the immune system.

The direct benefits of colostrum that have been observed to date are numerous, and they include overall good health, prevention of disease, improved performance, reduced healing period, increased recovery, and improved immune protection. These benefits are obvious and can be explained through biochemical pathways and various specific actions of specific components present in colostrum. However, the indirect effects of colostrum are not so clear cut. What is clear is that all the wonderful things in colostrum work together in such a way as to increase the effectiveness of each component.

Compositional Changes in Colostrum Over Time

Yes, the composition of colostrum does change over time. Colostrum is produced for the first 5 days following birth, as defined by the US FDA and NZ MAF. It is highest in concentration in the first milking and then diminishes rather rapidly to form transitional milk, then final regular milk. For example, in the first milking the IgG value is approximately 45mg/ml, dropping to approximately 10 mg/ml at 48 hours and then finally to approximately 0.5mg/ml for regular milk. In New Zealand, colostrum is typically collected in the first six (6) to eight (8) milking only.

Chronic Fatigue Syndrome and Colostrum

Thank your for your enquiry regarding colostrum and salmonella poisoning and Irritable Bowel Syndrome (IBS). One of the most common occurrences following course of antibiotic treatment is secondary infection caused by opportunistic microbes, such as Candida (yeast), etc. The antibiotics typically kill not only the causative agent of the original infection but also the good bacteria which populate the gut, lactobacillus, bifidobacteria, etc. These good bacteria, also known as probiotics, help keep the gut in check. They have numerous functions, including antimicrobial properties. Thus the natural environment of the gut is disturbed and the opportunistic microbes are allowed to colonize. This can lead to chronic infections of the gastrointestinal tract. Irritable Bowel Syndrome, leaky gut syndrome, fibromyaglia, and other disease states have been attributed to this type of chronic infection. This is exactly where colostrum can possibly be of help. Colostrum functions to immunosupplement the gut and thus can help in fighting the infection.

Diabetes and Colostrum

I would like to point out that we do not give any medical advice and suggest that you consult your healthcare provider for medical advice. Also I need to point out that colostrum, at the moment, is still considered by the Ministry of Health to be a food supplement, and as such, no claims can be made as to its use in the treatment or prevention of any disease.

Untreated diabetes can cause extremely high blood sugar levels which, if left untreated, can place great strains on other organs. As such this should be treated seriously. If you suspect you have diabetes, then it would be most wise and prudent to consult with your health care professional.

Type 2 diabetes or non-insulin dependent diabetes typically appears in adults over 40 years of age and is linked to diet. Obesity or overweight is most often linked with this condition. Most individuals with Type 2 diabetes can regulate their condition by proper diet and exercise. Type I diabetes is insulin dependent.

In regard to colostrum, I would like to quote Dr David Henderson in his book, ***Colostrum: Nature's Healing Miracle***: "Colostrum contains growth factors that help your body better utilize the food you eat and burn more fat. These growth factors (in particular, IGF-I or insulin-like growth factor I) are normally produced by the body, but their numbers can be severely reduced be aging, lack of exercise, exposure to environmental toxins, and poor nutrition. Colostrum restores the body's level of IGF-I which, along exercise and a nutritious diet, can result in better destabilization ("burning") of fat, increased rate of growth of muscle mass, better strength and endurance-leading to a leaner, healthier body and appearance."

Further he states that, "Insulin-Like Growth Factor I and 2 (IGF-I and IGF-2) are the most abundant growth factors in bovine colostrum. These proteins affect how the body uses fat, protein, and sugar."

Dosage for Children

Colostrum has been shown in clinical trials to prevent disease in not only adults but also children. Children should half the daily adult dose. In other words, adults 2 capsules per day, children I capsule, and infants half a capsule per day. My kids won't take capsules, so I either give them chewables or dissolve the powder in a drink or even sprinkle on top of ice cream. It should be noted that this is only a rough guideline.

Daily Recommended Dosage of Colostrum

As of yet there is no recommended daily allowance (RDA) for colostrum. As I am sure you aware, there are a wide variety of colostrum products in the marketplace worldwide. These products vary in composition, potency, and quality, and as such it would be very difficult to assign one therapuetic daily dose for all of them. Most manufacturers suggest 1 to 2 grams per day for maintainence of overall good health and up to 10 grams per day for therapuetic dose if under stress or ill. The high doses of up to and surpassing 60 grams a day are for specific purposes, such as extreme sport performance where the test subjects in several clinical trials received 60 grams of colostrum a day—this equates to 120 capsules. It has been determined that 2 grams of colostrum per kilogram body weight can be taken very safely. This would correspond to a person weighing 110 lbs (50kg) can safely take 100 grams (200 capsules) safely every day.

Colostrum is a wonderful thing. It helps to keep us in good health, and it helps our bodies to keep in balance. To take advantage of all the benefits of colostrum requires that it be taken every day. Most probably 1 gram a day for an adult is the minimum while the maximal amount to take to achieve desired effect depends on what outcome is desired, and to a point what one can afford. In regard to how much colostrum to take for specific desired outcomes, you might want to do a search of the ICR website for outcome, disease state, action, etc, and look for clinical trial information. This will give you the amount of colostrum that was administered.

Dosage—Why on an Empty Stomach?

The theory behind taking colostrum on an empty stomach is that this method of delivery will maximize the beneficial effects of colostrum. Whether you take it on an empty stomach with a glass of water or any other way, the most important thing is to take it every day. Build a routine so you take it every day to achieve the benefits, as an ounce of prevention is worth a pound of cure.

Drug Interactions with Colostrum

In regard to drug interaction and negative effects, no drug interaction are known. This is because colostrum is a food. However, it is always advised that individuals taking medication prescribed by a physician first seek medical advive. Further in a just completed clinical trial in which I was involved, we showed that the use of colostrum improved the survival rate of young piglets during a course of antibiotic treatment.

Epilepsy—Can Colostrum Help ?

I have done a pretty thorough search and could not come up with any research involving the use of colostrum and epilepsy directly. But what I have come out with is various things in colostrum which may have a beneficial effect for people with epilepsy. For example, antioxidants may be of help and colostrum contains the ultimate antioxidant, glutathione. Folic acid present in colostrum has been shown to help protect the brain from disease and degenerative disorders. Cystine, glutamic acid and other amino acids present in colostrum could be beneficial. Phospholids present in some colostrum products are known as brain food. Growth factors have been shown to protect and repair adult brain. A group of small peptides (PRPs) found in relatively high amounts in colostrum has been shown to have a very beneficial effect in Alzeimer's patients. Colostrum contains two proteins that have anti-inflammatory function, lactoferrin and secretory IgA. Anti-inflammatory agents have shown to be beneficial in slowing the onset of brain disorders.

In short, there are alot of things in colostrum that may help and probably also important they certainly won't hurt. Further, colostrum will certainly help with overall good health and it will promote well being. Colostrum has been shown in clinical trials to prevent disease. This alone should be a good reason to give it a go! However, as in all conditons which involve medical intervention, it is suggested that you consult with your healthcare provider.

Fat—Why is Fat Removed From Colostrum?

In regard to fat removal, most colostrum is reduced in fat from 4% down to 2%. Though stability may be increased, the major reasoning is processing—whole fat colostrum tends to clog pasteurizers, UF units, etc. Also the growth factors are found in the skim portion, not the fat. The reduction from 4% down to 2% does not lower the complex lipids content significantly.

Freeze Drying versus Spraying Colostrum Products

For the most part colostrum powder is manufactured by spray drying. This is true worldwide of not only colostrum powders but also other milk powders. Freeze drying (lyophilization) is a more gentle form of drying but very costly—something like 30X more costly than spray drying. In addition, economies of scale limit the use of freeze drying as only relatively small volumes can be dried effectively using this technique. Probably the most important point, however, is the fact that dairy processing technology has developed to such a point that the spray drying process can now be performed at reduced temperature and any damage caused by heat is minimal.

Can a Child Suffering G6PD Consume Colostrum?

G6PD stands for glucose 6 phosphate dehydrogenase, which is an enzyme present in the red blood cells in the blood. Individuals suffering from this illness are deficient in this enzyme. G6PD deficiency is one of the most common human enzyme deficiency syndromes affecting some 400 million people wordwide.

Red blood cells carry oxygen in the body, and the enzyme G6PD in normal individuals protects the red blood cells from natural oxygen chemicals that may build up in response to infection, medications or even certain foods. If there is a build up of these chemicals, it can cause destruction of these cells and lead to hemolytic anemia. Medications that should be withheld from individuals suffering from G6PD deficiency include asprin. Though colostrum has no known ill side effects, I think it would still be most wise and prudent for this individual's physician to be consulted first.

Just to make a point, this condition is a very tricky one considering that diet and even aspirin can effect treatment. Further, vitamin K is also implicated in causing anemia in individuals suffering from this disorder, and colostrum is relatively high in vitamin K. Once again, it would be most wise and prudent that the individual's health provider be consulted.

Growth Hormone vs Colostrum

Growth Hormone has definite anti-aging properties, but one thing the manufacturers of these products do not mention are the side effects. First all, GH needs to be injected intramuscularly for it to work or otherwise it will be quickly metabolized by the liver and made inactive. Second, no long-term health studies have been conducted on its use. Third, GH does act to build muscle and lean body mass, but it does cause an increase in organ and bone weight—not a good thing. Fourth, GH administration needs to very controlled as too much can cause gigantism (Acromegaly). You can always tell when body builders or weight lifters are on GH as they usually have wide gaps in between their teeth—the skull has grown! Colostrum, however, has been shown to be a safe alternative.

The good news is colostrum is nature's perfect answer to hGH. Extensive research shows that colostrum is unique because it is the only substance that offers anti-aging hormones in perfect balance, the way nature intended. According to Zoltan Rona, MD, (***Bovine Colostrum, Immunity and the Aging Process*, Nature's Impact**), when colostrum is taken as a supplement, "skin appears more youthful, age and 'liver' spots disappear, bone mass and density increases and sexual function is improved and restored." In other words, it appears colostrum works similarly to hGH with none of the known dangerous side effects.

Guillian-Barre & Colostrum

First of all, I hope you can appreciate the seriousness of this disease state and that we do not provide medical advice—your physician is best suited for that. What we would like to do is give you some scientific information on the subject.

Guillian-Barre syndrome is a relatively rare dissorder in which the body's own immune system attacks the peripheral nervous system. It frequently follows viral infection. The incidence of this disorder is approximately 1-2 cases per 100,000 with most patients recovering with no or minimal long-term effects. However, in some cases this disorder can be very serious and can cause total paralysis and the need for ventilatory assist. Death occurs in less than 5% of the cases.

In approximately 70% of the cases, Guillian-Barre is preceded by a mild respiratory or digestive tract infection. One organism in particular has been singled out as being associated with development of Guillian-Barre—***Campylobacter jejuni***. It is of interest that this microbe has become the leading cause of enteric (gastric) infection in the developed world. It has been theorized that Guillian-Barre arises as result of the immune system producing antibodies to the surface coating proteins (antigen) of ***C. jejuni***.

In other words, the infecting ***C. jejuni*** stimulates the immune system to produce antibodies to help fight the infection, and these antibodies are directed to the surface coating proteins. The unfortunate thing is that these surface coating proteins are very similiar in structure, composition, and configuration to the myelin sheath surrounding the axons of nerve cells. Thus the antibodies initially directed towards ***C. jejuni*** also attack the individual's own nervous system. Guillian-Barre is called an autoimmune disease, and the extent and duration of the syndrome is most probably due the extent and duration of the initial exposure to ***C. jejuni*** infection. Once stimulated to produce antibodies, the immune system continues production as long as the antigen is present. In this case, the antigen becomes the individual's own nervous system, and thus Guillian-Barre can be a chronic illness.

The use of plasmaphoresis and high immunoglobulin therapy has been shown to reduce the severity and duration of Guillian-Barre. Principly this method of treatment involves injection of pooled human plasma and involves the passive transmission of systemic immunity, the reasoning being that a pool of human plasma would have a complement of antibodies to a wide variety of microbes, including *C. jejuni*. Given early on, this extra boost of antibody can thus nuetralize and reduce the level of infection and minimize the body's own autoimmune response mechanism, thus reducing the severity of the disease. It is important to note that this is passive transmission of immunity which in this case functions systemically.

In regard to bovine colostrumm the following information may be of interest. I was involved in a study conducted at Otago University in which we investigated the presence and potency of specific antibodies to a wide variety of microbes. The results indicated that New Zealand colostrum contains very high levels of specific antibody to *C. jejuni*. This is attributed to the fact that the enviromental conditions here combined with our dairy farming practice of free range pasture feeding allows the cows to be exposed to a very large variety of microbes.

Bovine colostrum has been shown in clinical trials to help prevent and treat enteric (gastrointestinal) infections. This includes Campylobacter infection.

Health Benefits of Colostrum

In regard to the health benefits associated with colostrum, there are many. Immune factors in the form of antibodies, lactoferrin and others that help in the immunosupplementation of the gut, growth factors which help in the healing and recovery process, prebotics in the form of oligosaccharides which help promote the growth of beneficial bacteria (probiotics), antioxidants in the form of glutathione and others that not only help in preventing disease but also have certain anti-aging properties. In other words, many things that have many beneficial properties.

Heart Medications and Colostrum

In regard to anyone under the present care of a health professional, it would be both wise and prudent to have them consult on what is best for their respective patient. This is especially true in cases such as high blood pressure and heart disease. Only the prescibing physician knows the whole story including the underlying causes of the symptoms. All that said, colostrum may possibly be of help, and this would probably be due to insulin-like growth factor-1 (IGF-1), which has been shown to help burn fat and build lean body mass, also to have a beneficial apsect in regard to helping the lowering of bad cholesterol (LDL) and raising the good cholesterol levels (HDL). Also IGF-1 has been shown to stabilize elevated blood sugar levels. Phospholipids have been shown to have a beneficial effect on lowering blood pressure also.

Herxheimer Reaction and Colostrum

I have heard of a few people experiencing a Herxheimer reaction when first starting with colostrum. Herxheimer reaction is basically detoxification and is sometimes associated with soreness. It is important to note that this occurs in only a very few people and is short-lived. It is very important to drink a glass of fresh and clean water when one experiences this type of adverse reaction, to help prevent toxins to being redeposited body tissue.

High Blood Pressure and Colostrum

If anything, colostrum should help in lowering blood pressure. Colostrum contains many things that contribute to lowering blood pressure—phospholipids and IGF in particular. Phospholipids have been shown to lower blood cholesterol levels while IGF has been shown to lower and stabilize blood sugar levels.

Colostrum and Horses

The significance of colostrum in the area of the competing horse lies in several very important features, all of which one can take advantage of to reach a higher level of performance, and most probably afford the animal a better quality of life. First, it is a highly nutritious food, and second, it contains many, many bioactive substances which have been shown to prevent disease and promote over-all good health. Of specific interest to the trainer is the fact that colostrum supplementation can be an effective way by which the performance horse can increase lean body mass, improve muscular strength, increase endurance and capacity, and at the same time speed recovery. What this means to the horse is simple—they can train harder, longer, and recover faster thereby increasing their respective level of performance. Of significant importance to the athlete is the simple fact that colostrum is perfectly safe and further is the fact that the International Olympic Committee (IOC) has designated colostrum to be an accepted and safe dietary supplement. Thus it is recognized as perfectly safe and, legal by all the sports and racing regulatory bodies.

Insulin-like Growth Factor (IGF) and Weight Loss

The primary substance in colostrum associated with weight loss is insulin-like growth factor (IGF). IGF is found in relatively high concentrations in bovine colostrum. IGF regulates the metabolic effects of Growth Hormone, which is naturally produced by the body. In so doing, IGF functions to increase lean body mass (muscle) and the burning of fat. As its name indicates, IGF is very similiar in structure and function to insulin and is thus involved with regulating or balancing blood sugar levels. Of utmost importance, however, is the fact that simply taking colostrum doesn't mean you will lose fat. Colostrum augmented with proper diet and excercise will, however, most surely help you loose the flab.

Johnie's Disease and Colostrum

In regard to Johnies disease or Mycobacterium paratuberculosis, this is in fact a bad news kind of disease—no cure, major problem in USA. Fortunately not transmittable to humans. In regard to testing for Johnies disease, the New Zealand dairy industry regularly tests for the presence of the disease. In addition the method of pasteurization in New Zealand ensures that this pathogen is destroyed

Lactating Mothers

As with all supplements, medications, and even diet, individuals who are either lactating or pregnant should advise their healthcare provider.

Lactose Intolerance and Colostrum

Thank you very much for your recent enquiry regarding colostrum and lactose intolerance. Unfortunately to date we haven't been able to remove lactose from colostrum. However, colostrum is reduced in lactose, and the amount present in a daily colostrum is negligible. In fact, the amount of lactose present in 2 capsules (1gram) of colostrum would be equivalent to approximately 1.5 ml of milk.

Did you know that even individuals who are lactose intolerant can for the most part tolerate 240ml of milk per day quite nicely? Did you know that hard cheeses have virtually no lactose as it is degraded during the aging process? The same is true of most yogurts. So if you tolerate hard cheese or lactose, colostrum should present no problem at all. However, if in doubt, by all means consult with your healthcare provider. Also you might want to try the old police trick by just placing a very little bit (~10mg) on the tongue to see how it goes.

Lactose intolerance is a food allergy, and creates an imbalance in specific cytokines in the body. The peptides or PRPs in colostrums actually normalize or modulate the levels of cytokines in the body, so the body does not recognize the lactose as a food allergin.

Does the Addition of Lipid Have a Negative Effect on Colostrum?

In regard to lipid, I suspect you are referring to complex lipids in the form of phospholipids, sphingolipids, and glycolipids which are added to the Alpha Lipid colostrum. Quite the opposite, these complex lipids actually add to the biofunctionality of Alpha Lipid colostrum. The phospholipid forms are phosphatidylserine (PS), phosphatidylcholine (PC), phosphatidylethanolamine (PE). The sphingolipid is in the sphingomylein form while the glycolipid is in the ganglioside GD3 form. The unique benefits these complex lipids add to Alpha Lipid colostrum include added bioavailability due to the delivery system so that all the colostrum is available. Furthermore, the complex lipids function in improving brain function, improve memory, and elevate mood. They have also been shown to help in protection of the gut and aid in liver function.

Colostrum and Lupus

Systemic lupus erythematosus (SLE) is an autoimmune disease which primarily attacks women of childbearing age. It should be pointed out that this is potentially a very serious condition, and as such, individuals who suffer from this disease should consult with their healthcare professional prior to taking any supplement or medication. In lupus the immune system is over-reactive and produces antibodies that attack the patient's own tissues. Lupus can effect many different parts of the body, including joints, organs, heart, nervous system, and blood vessels. Patients that take a PRP supplement for a few weeks may have there Antinuclear Antibody Test (ANA) readings stabilized.

SLE is associated with Antiphospholipid Syndrome (APS), a condition associated also with recurrent miscarriage, coronary disease, preeclampsia, and many other conditions. In APS the individuals produce antibodies to their own phospholipids—the primary structural element of all membranes. Current treatment includes the use of immunosuppresants, NSAIDs, aspirin, and prednisone.

In SLE the patient's immune system is over-stimulated in producing autoantibodies. Colostrinin, also known as Proline-rich Polypeptides (PRPs), is an immunomodulator (regulates the immune response) present in colostrum. Thus colostrinin may be of value in slowing down the production of autoantibodies. Also the autoantibodies that are being produced are directed towards phospholipids. As such, the ingestion of phospholipids, such as Alpha Lipid colostrum, may be of value in that the antiphospholipids may bind to the free phospholid instead of membranes. Further, colostrum has been shown to reverse the damage caused to the gastrointestinal tract by NSAIDs.

Mineral Content of Colostrum?

Thank you very much for your enquiry regarding mineral content of colostrum. I hope you can appreciate that the absolute value for each mineral will most likely vary based on end product—skim vs whole vs whey, etc. The general values in a powder are as follows:

Sodium ~ 3.44mg/1000mg
Phosphorus ~ 4.94mg/1000mg
Magnesium ~ 1.19mg/1000mg
Potassium ~ 8.39mg/1000mg

Pregnant Dogs & Cats

Thank you for your recent enquiry regarding feeding colostrum to pregnant dogs and cats. First, colostrum is a food and has been shown to be free of any known side effects. Second, colostrum has been shown in clinical trials to help prevent disease and promote overall good health. This being the case, why not? If you have any doubts, then please consult with your veterinarian—I am sure he or she will concur.

Radiculopathy and Colostrum

I have attached some information regarding this condition just in case for your information. The direct effect of colostrum in regard to this condition is most probably minimal. However, the indirect effects may be of interest, especially as colostrum contains natural anti-inflammatory agents which may be of benefit. Please discuss this with your physician. Colostrum is a natural food that possesses many health benefits—all of which contribute to overall health

Taste of Colostrum

One thing to remember is the sense of taste and smell are very powerful and sensitive indicators—if it smells bad and tastes bad it most probably is indeed bad. On the other hand, colostrum powder, unless it contains a flavor additive, should have little taste.

Urticaria and Colostrum

Thank you for your enquiry regarding urticaria and colostrum. Urticaria, commonly called hives, is an inflammation of the surface layers of the skin. It is commonly characterized by small, itchy white or red welts. Urticaria is commonly caused by an allergic reaction. However, the allergen or causitive agent has not been identified.

In regard to colostrum, it may possibly be of benefit, and this is due to a component in colostrum called Proline-rich Polypeptides, or PRP for short. Very briefly, PRPs are small polypeptides which have regulatory activity—stimulating or suppressing the immune response. In the case of allergies, the immune system is over-stimulated and PRP has been shown to reduce the stimulation and thus help alleviate the symptom.

Whey Type Products vs Colostrum

The IgG type products are for the most part derived from the whey of milk and not from colostrum. In that sense they are isolates and as such usually are lacking in certain bioactives found in whole colostrum, such as growth factors, cytokines, immune factors, etc.

Both milk and colostrum can be seperated into whey and curd. By removing the curd you increase the concentration of things like IgG or immunoglobulins. However, some other very important bioactives are either lost in the curd or they are simply not present in milk.

The major differences in milk vs colostrum:

Colostrum / Milk
IgG 50mg/ml 0.6 mg/ml
IgA 6 mg/ml 0.06 mg/ml
IgM 7 mg/ml 0.07 mg/ml

Protein 50%/30%

The major difference is the simple fact that all the bioactives in colostrum act in such a way as to make the overall effect or benefit greater than the sum of the individual components. This is called a symbiotic effect. The milk-derived whey IgG products simply do not possess this.

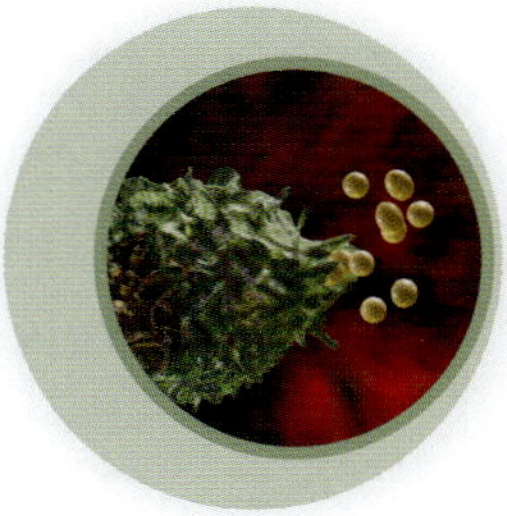

APPENDIX D

CAN COLOSTRUM ASSIST AIDS PATIENTS?

A commentary by Thomas E. Stone, ND, CNHP

In 1995, an article in ***Scientific American*** concluded that ***traditional*** disease fighting methods were not effective in fighting the HIV virus—otherwise known as AIDS.[807] Instead, this author recommended that we focus on finding ways of stimulating the immune system and reducing the viral load. Colostrum can be very effective in both of these ways. Colostrum stimulates and strengthens a weakened immune system and those who take it on a regular basis have a heightened ability to resist and fight infection—exactly what the AIDS patient needs. Colostrum activates or "turns on" the immune system in the newborn and it can do the same thing for the AIDS patient—or anyone, for that matter. It contains over 40 different immune factors which work in harmony to support a stronger defense mechanism. This is so critical for the AIDS patient, who dies —not from the HIV virus—but from secondary infections which the immune system is no longer able to control.

One of the immune components in colostrum falls into a category called ***immunoglobulins***. These are "functional antibodies," ready to combat a host of bacterial pathogens. In this way, colostrum can actually be a sort of secondary immune system for the AIDS patient.

Colostrum and colostral components can also be effective in reducing viral populations. A 1995 study conducted in the Netherlands indicated that the immune factor, lactoferrin, is one of the best ways to reduce viral levels in the body. It inhibited the HIV virus of certain body cells and was able to completely block Cytomegalovirus infection. This same study concluded that bovine (cow) lactoferrin was up to 2.5 times more effective than human lactoferrin.[808] Several other immune factors contained in colostrum have been shown to have antiviral activity as well.[809]

One of the most serious problems with AIDS is something called "wasting." It is brought on by chronic diarrhea and results in a loss of vital nutrients and fluids. It also depletes the supply of intestinal antibodies, leaving the patient even more vulnerable to dangerous pathogens.[810,811,812] A 1992 study showed that out of 37 immunodeficient patients with chronic diarrhea, 72% experienced significant improvement with the use of immunoglobulins from colostrum.[813] Another study stated that colostral immunoglobulins have been able to treat diarrhea-causing infections associated with AIDS where no other treatment was effective.[814]

Wasting occurs when the AIDS-infected body begins burning muscle for fuel. Here again, colostrum can help. The growth factors, contained in colostrum, also play a big role in supporting AIDS patients. Treatment with IGF-1 and growth hormone (GH), both contained in colostrum, produce an increase in muscle mass, preventing the severe weight loss associated with wasting.[815] If colostrum were used for no other reason than to reduce the diarrhea-induced wasting and to prevent the loss of muscle mass, it would greatly enhance quality of life for those who suffer from AIDS. However, in my experience, colostrum can do so much more than this.

Eight months ago I treated a patient with full-blown AIDS, who had been sincerely searching and doing everything in his power to regain his health. When I initially met with him, he had a T cell count in the high teens, despite the fact that he had been following a strict health regime for a matter of months. With megadoses of colostrum (60 capsules/day) and a herb called Maca, we eliminated many of the other things he was doing. He continued to eat healthfully and take ample amounts of green juices. Within two weeks, both he and his medical doctors were shocked to find that his T cell count had risen to 350! His doctor even insisted on a retest to verify these results. Now, eight months later, he has been declared HIV-free, and doctors are saying that they must have misdiagnosed him in the first place. This man is so dedicated to helping other people that he now owns a health food store and is sharing his knowledge with hosts of other people.

A ***desire*** to get well is a critical factor in healing. This man was totally dedicated and when he found the additional nutritional help of colostrum, he made fast progress. Can colostrum assist AIDS patients? In a variety of ways, the answer is a resounding, Yes!

GLOSSARY

Adaptive immune system—the defensive system of the body that produces specific antibodies to a particular antigen.

Apoptosis—programmed cell death. It is the normal process by which unneeded cells in the body are removed, such as the resculpting of body tissues during development.

Autoimmunity—a pathologic condition in which the body makes antibodies against its own tissues.

B-lymphocytes (B cells)—a type of lymphocyte produced in bone marrow and that is mainly responsible for producing antibodies (immunoglobulins). They are also known as Plasma Cells.

Cell-mediated (Th1) immunity—immune defense mediated by cells such as cytotoxic lymphocytes, natural killer cells and macrophages to fight infections and cancer.

Chemokines—small cytokines that mobilize and activate white blood cells, usually by acting as a chemoattractant to attract cells of the immune system to the site of an infection.

Colostrum—the first milk, or pre-milk, produced a mammalian mother following the birth of her newborn. Technically it is only the milk in the mammary glands at the time of birth. It is a normally a thin, yellowish fluid.

Cytokines—regulatory proteins that regulate many bodily processes, including reproduction, growth and development, homeostasis, blood clotting, and the immune response. They generally fall into six groups: interleukins, colony-stimulating factors, interferons, tumor necrosis factor, growth factors and chemokines. They can be produced by a variety of cells.

Dendritic cells—antigen presenting leukocytes (white blood cells) of the immune system. Found primarily in the skin, mucosa and lymphoid tissues, they function to initiate the immune response by activating lymphocytes and secreting cytokines.

Humoral (Th2) immunity—immune defense mediated by antibodies secreted by B lymphocytes to fight infections and toxins.

Immunoglobulins—also known as antibodies, immunoglobulins are the principal components of the adaptive immune system which has the capacity to make antibodies to specific antigens (proteins recognized as foreign by the body). Mammals have five basic types of immunoglobulins: immunoglobulin G (IgG), responsible for systemic immunity to a specific antigen; IgA, responsible for localized immunity to antigens, such as in the gut; IgM, basically five IgG molecules bound together, IgM is the first immunoglobulin produced during an infection; IgE, involved in the allergic reaction in response to the allergen (protein that sets off the allergic response); IgD, binds to the surface of B lymphocytes and appears to play a role in antigen recognition.

Innate immune system—the first line defense system of the body that provides non-specific defense against invaders, such as bacteria, viruses, protozoa and tumor cells. Consists of both cells (NK cells, mast cells, eosinophils, basophils, neutrophils, macrophages, dendritic cells) and proteins (lactoferrin, lysozyme, lactoperoxidase)

Lymphocytes—a type of white blood cell that composes the main cells of the immune system. They are of different types, some which produce antibodies (B cells), some which locate and identify antigens in the body (helper T cells), some which attack and kill pathogens (NK cells and cytotoxic T cells), some which inhibit the activity of other immune cells in order to shut off the immune response and avoid damage to healthy tissue (suppressor and regulator T cells), and some which retain a memory of encountered antigens to speed the response time in case of reinfection (memory T cells).

Macrophages—scavenger cells of body tissue spaces that phagocytize (eat) foreign material, such as bacteria, protozoa, viruses and tumor cells. They are formed when blood monocytes migrate into the tissue spaces.

Mast cells—cells of the innate immune system that are found in connective tissues and mucous membranes. They release histamine and heparin when activated, part of the inflammatory response.

Monocytes—phagocytic cells of the blood which remove foreign material, such as bacteria, viruses, protozoa and tumor cells, from the bloodstream. When they leave the bloodstream and enter the tissue spaces they are known as macrophages.

Natural killer (NK) cells—lymphocytes whose primary function is to kill cells in the body infected by viruses or other pathogens or neoplastic (cancer) cells.

Peptides—short strings of amino acids with no tertiary (three-dimensional) structure. Polypeptides are longer strings of amino acids but still with no tertiary structure.

Phagocytes—literally "eating cell" in Greek, these are scavenger cells, like macrophages and monocytes, which ingest foreign material in the body. The material is then broken down and either assimilated or discarded.

Plasma Cells—see B cells.

Proline-rich Polypeptides (PRPs)—short strings of amino acids that lack the tertiary (three-dimensional) structure of proteins. They act as intercellular signaling molecules. In the case of the PRPs found in colostrum, they act to modulate the activity of the immune system, either stimulating it in the case of an underperforming system, as may be found in the case of a severe infection, or inhibiting it in the case of an overperforming system, such as is found in allergies and autoimmune conditions.

Proteins—large, often very complex molecules composed of amino acids and usually having intricate tertiary (three dimensional) structures. Most of the functions in the body are carried out by proteins, and most structural components of the body are composed of proteins.

Signal transduction—the process by which a message is passed from cell to other cells through the use of signaling molecules, usually peptides or polypeptides, that interact with specific receptors on the surfaces of the target cells, setting off a chain of intracellular events that typically result in a specific protein being produced by the cell.

T lymphocytes (T cells)—lymphocytes which are produced in bone marrow but mature in the Thymus gland, located in the neck. There are a number of subsets of T cells:

- Helper T cells—lymphocytes that act to regulate the immune response by secreting cytokines when activated. They are further broken down into Th_1, Th_2, Th_{17} and other subsets depending on the types of cytokines they produce.
- Cytotoxic T cells—also known as CD8+ T cells, these lymphocytes actively seek out and kill virally infected cells and tumor cells, as well as tumor rejection.
- Suppressor T cells—lymphocytes which suppress the immune response to prevent damage to healthy tissues once the infection is controlled or neutralized. They are thought to be formed through interaction of cytotoxic T cells with helper T cells.
- Memory T cells—lymphocytes that provide a memory of antigens previously encountered and capable of quickly multiplying in the event of reinfection.
- Regulatory T cells—lymphocytes which act to suppress the immune response toward the end of the immune reaction. They are very similar to suppressor T cells but have a different origin.
- Natural Killer (NK) T cells—lymphocytes which form a bridge between the adaptive immune system and the innate immune system. They are

activated by recognizing a certain type of antigen, after which they perform as cytotoxic cells.

- γδ (***gamma delta***) T cells—a small subset of T lymphocytes which tend to concentrate in the gut mucosa. They seem to be able to respond to whole proteins rather than peptides presented by antigen-presenting cells. They appear to be part of the first line of defense against infection.

INDEX

REFERENCES

Chapter 2 Notes

1 Sally Fallon, Planet Thrive. planetthrive.com

2 Heinerman J. Fascinating Colostrum: An Ancient Food for Modern Times. (1999)

3 The Temple of Hathor at Serabit el-Khadim. Egyptianhealing.com.

4 Lotte Hughes, Historian of the Maasai, University of Oxford, 2002.

5 Isaiah 7:15.

6 Wickes IG. **A history of infant feeding. Part I. Primitive peoples: ancient works: renaissance writers.** *Archives of Disease in Childhood* 28:151-158 (1953).

7 Salmon M. **The Cultural Significance of Breastfeeding and Infant Care in Early Modern England and America.** *Journal of Social History* Winter, 1994.

8 Fox PF, McSweeney PLH. **Dairy Chemistry and Biochemistry.** Springer, 1998, p. 90.

9 Ehrlich P. **Über Immunität durch Verebung und Säugung.** *Zeitschrift fur Hygiene und Infektionskrankheiten* 12:183 (1892)

10 Ehrlich P, Hubener W. **Über die Verebung der Immunität bei Tetanus.** *Zeitschrift fur Hygiene und Infektionskrankheiten* 18:51 (1894)

11 Ehrlich P, Wasserman A. **Über die Gewinnung Diphtherie-Antitoxine aus Blutserum und Milch immunsirte Thiere.** *Zeitschrift fur Hygiene und Infektionskrankheiten* 8:239 (1894)

12 Metchnikoff E. **The New Hygiene: Three Lectures on the Prevention of Infectious Diseases.** W.T. Keener, Chicago (1906)

13 Sabin AB. **Antipoliomyelitic substance in milk from human beings and certain cows.** *Journal of Diseases of Children*, 80:866 (1950)

14 Sabin AB, Fieldsteel AH. **Antipoliomyelitic activity of human and bovine colostrum and milk.** *Pediatrics* 29(1):105-115 (1962)

Chapter 4 Notes

15 Prosser C, Stelwagen K, Cummins R, Guerin P, Gill N, Milne C. **Reduction in heat induced gastrointestinal hyperpermeability in rats by bovine colostrum and goat milk powders.** *Journal of Applied Physiology* 96:650-654 (2004).

16 Gastrointestinal Inflammation and Repair Group, Imperial College, London. Unpublished research. In an in vitro experimental study, colostrum stimulated intestinal cell growth and reestablished a healthy epithelial layer following injury. In an in vivo experimental study, colostrum powder was also shown to reduce gastric injury (2003).

17 Carver JD, Barness LA. **Trophic factors for the gastrointestinal tract.** *Clinical Perinatology* 23(2):265-285 (1996).

18 Playford RJ, Woodman AC, Clark P, Watanapa P, Vesey D, Deprez PH, Williamson RC, Calam J. **Effect of luminal growth factor preservation on intestinal growth.** *Lancet* 341(8849):843-848 (1993).

19 Playford RJ, Floyd DN, Macdonald CE, et al. **Bovine colostrum is a health food supplement which prevents NSAID induced gut damage.** *Gut* 44:653-658 (1999).

20 Korhonen H, Suvaoja EL, Ahola-Luttilia H, Sivela S, Kopola S, Husu J, Kosunen TU. **Bactericidal effect of bovine normal and immune serum, colostrum and milk against *Helicobacter pylori*.** *Journal of Applied Bacteriology* 78:655-662 (1995).

21 Bitzan MM, Gold BD, Philpott DJ, Huesca M, Sherman PM, Karch H, Lissner R, Lingwood CA, Karmali MA. **Inhibition of *Helicobacter pylori* and *Helicobacter mustelae* binding to lipid receptors by bovine colostrum.** *Journal of Infectious Diseases* 177:955-961 (1998).

22 Bühler C, Hammon H, Rossi GL, Blum JW. **Small intestinal morphology in eight-day-old calves fed colostrum for different durations or only milk replacer and treated with long-R3-insulin-like growth factor I and growth hormone.** *Journal of Animal Science* 76:758-765 (1998).

23 Pluske JR, Morel PCH. **Increasing weaner pig productivity in New Zealand pig herds.** Unpublished research (1999). Piglets fed a liquid supplement with colostrum powder had a marked increase in villi height in the lumen of the small intestine, indicating greater digestion and absorption of nutrients. There were also an increased number of immune cells in the villi, indicating enhanced immune competency.

24 Blättler U, Hammon HM, Morel C, Philipona C, Rauprich A, Rome V, Huerou-Luron I, Guilloteau P, Blum JW. **Feeding colostrum, its composition and feeding duration variably modify proliferation and morphology of the intestine and digestive enzyme activities of neonatal calves.** *Journal of Nutrition* 131(4):1256-1263 (2001).

25 Deitch EA. **The Role of Intestinal Barrier Failure and Bacterial Translocation in the Development of Systemic Infection and Multiple Organ Failure.** *Archives of Surgery* 125:403-404 (1990).

26 Galland L. **Leaky Gut Syndrome: Breaking the Vicious Cycle.** *Townsend Letter for Doctors.* 145(6):63-68 (1995).

27 Galland L, Barrie S. **Intestinal Dysbiosis and the Causes of Disease.** www.healthy.net/asp/templates/Article.asp?Id=423

28 Rooney PL, Jenkins RT, Buchanan WW. **A Short Review of the Relationship Between Intestinal Permeability and Inflammatory Joint Disease.** *Clinical and Experimental Rheumatology* 8(1):75-83 (1990).

29 Jackson PG, Lessof MH, Baker RWR, Ferrett J, MacDonald DM. **Intestinal Permeability in Patients with Eczema and Food Allergy.** *Lancet* 1(8233):1285-6 (1981).

30 Altekruse SF, Bauer N, Chanlongbutra A, DeSagun R, Naugle A, Schlosser W, Umholtz R, White P. ***Salmonella enteritidis* in broiler chickens, United States, 2000-2005.** *Emerging Infectious Diseases* 12(12):1848-1852 (2006).

31 http://www.wrongdiagnosis.com/f/food_poisoning/death-types.htm

32 Ho PC, Lawton JW. **Human colostral cells: phagocytosis and killing of *E. coli* and *C. albicans*.** *Journal of Pediatrics* 93(6):910-915 (1978).

33 Kim K, Pickering LK, DuPont HL, Sullivan N, Wilkins T. **In vitro and in vivo neutralizing activity of human colostrum and milk against purified toxins A and B of *Clostridium difficile*.** *Journal of Infectious Diseases* 150(1):57-62 (1984).

34 Tacket CO, Binion SB, Bostwick E, Losonsky G, Roy MJ, Edelman R. **Efficacy of bovine milk immunoglobulin concentrate in preventing illness after *Shigella flexneri* challenge.** *American Journal of Tropical Medicine and Hygiene* 47(3):276-283 (1992).

35 Watson C, Alp NJ. **Role of *Chlamydia pneumoniae* in atherosclerosis.** *Clinical Science* 114(8):509-531 (2008).

36 Tortora GJ, Funke BD, Case CL. **Microbiology: an Introduction.** 8th edition, pp 485-488. Pearson Education, 2004.

37 Baglioni T, Fioretti C. **[Serum immunoglobulins in colostrum and cow's milk studied by the immunoelectrophoretic method]** *Archivio Veterinario Italiano* 18(6):419-427 (1967). Both IgG and IgM identified in bovine colostrum using immunoelectrophoresis.

38 Mickelson KN, Moriarty KM. **Immunoglobulin levels in human colostrum and milk.** *Journal of Pediatric Gastroenterology and Nutrition* 1(3):381-384 (1982). Levels of sIgA, IgG and IgM were determined in human colostrum and milk. A mean concentration of 32 g/L was found for sIgA (1.5-83.7 g/L), 1.13 g/L for IgM and 0.53 g/L for IgG. While total amounts declined with time postpartum, relative proportions remained the same.

39 Korhonen H, Marnila P, Gill HS. **Bovine milk antibodies for health.** *British Journal of Nutrition* 84(Suppl.1):S135-S146 (2000). Bovine colostrum provides safe, effective protection against many pathogens.

40 Korhonen H, Syvaoja EL, Ahola-Luttila H, Sivela S, Kopola S, Husu J, Kosunen TU. **Bactericidal effect of bovine normal and immune serum, colostrum and milk against *Helicobacter pylori*.** *Journal of Applied Bacteriology* 78(6):655-662 (1995). Helicobacter pylori is a major cause of gastritis and ulcers in humans. Serum and colostrum from non-immunized Friesian cows were found to be highly bactericidal against *H. pylori*. Post-colostral milk did not show any bactericidal effect against *H. pylori*.

41 Funatogawa K, Ide T, Kirikae F, Saruta K, Nakano M, Kirikae T. **Use of immunoglobulin enriched bovine colostrum against oral challenge with enterohemorrhagic *Eschericia coli* O157:H7 in mice.** *Microbiology and Immunology* 46(11):761-766 (2002). Colostrum can prevent infection against food-borne pathogens by preventing them

from binding to the intestinal lining.

42 Widiasih DA, Matsuda I, Omoe K, Hu DL, Sugii S, Shinagawa K. **Passive transfer of antibodies to Shiga toxin-producing *Eschericia coli* O26, O111 and O157 antigens in neonatal calves by feeding colostrum.** *Journal of Veterinary Medicine* 66(2):213-215 (2004). Feeding colostrum to calves provided protection against Shiga toxin-producing *E. Coli*, a particularly deadly strain of *E. coli*.

43 Elahi S, Buchanan RM, Babiuk LA, Gerdts V. **Maternal immunity provides protection against pertussis in newborn piglets.** *Infection and Immunity* 74(5):2619-2627 (2006).

44 Majumdar AS, Ghose AC. **Protective properties of anti-cholera antibodies in human colostrum.** *Infection and Immunity* 36:962-965 (1982). Colostrum was able to prevent infection with cholera. Colostrum samples from India, where cholera is common, had much higher levels of anti-cholera IgA than those from Sweden, where cholera is rare.

45 Stephan W, Dichtelmuller H, Lissner R. **Antibodies from colostrum in oral immunotherapy.** *Journal of Clinical Chemistry and Clinical Biochemistry* 28:19-23 (1990). An immunoglobulin preparation from pooled bovine colostrum was found to be very effective in treating severe diarrhea, such as often found in AIDS patients.

46 Solomons, NW. **Modulation of the immune system and the response against pathogens with bovine colostrum concentrates.** *European Journal of Clinical Nutrition* 56(Suppl.3):524-528 (2002). The ability of colostrum to protect infants against pathogens, specifically those which cause gastroenteritis and severe diarrhea, makes it an ideal, cheap, safe and effective means of protecting children in those parts of the world where medical assistance is lacking or substandard and could save thousands of lives each year.

47 Rump JA, Arndt R, Arnold A, Bendick C, Dichtelmuller H, Franke M, Helm EB, Jager H, Kampmann B, Kolb P. **Treatment of diarrhea in human immunodeficiency virus-infected patients with immunoglobulins from bovine colostrum.** *Clinical Investigator* 70:588-594 (1992). Immunoglobulins from bovine colostrum were very effective in treating chronic diarrhea in AIDS patients from a variety of causes. Colostral immunoglobulins are highly resistant to digestion in the gastrointestinal tract.

48 Brüssow H, Hilpert H, Walther I, Sidoti J, Mietens C, Bachmann P. **Bovine milk immunoglobulins for passive immunity to infantile rotavirus gastroenteritis.** *Journal of Clinical Microbiology* 25(6):982-986 (1987). Protection against rotavirus, a dangerous pathogen which can cause serious, even fatal diarrhea in infants, can be passed orally through milk or colostrum safely and effectively.

49 Acosta-Altamirano G, Rocha-Ramirez LM, Reyes-Montes R, Cote V, Santos, JI. **Anti-amoebic properties of human colostrum.** *Advances in Experimental Medicine and Biology* 216B:1347-1352 (1987). In addition to its effectiveness against bacterial, viral and fungal infections, colostrum also provides protection against amoebic pathogens.

50 van Hooijdonk, AC, Kussendrager, KD, Steijns, JM. **In vivo antimicrobial and antiviral activity of components in bovine milk and colostrum involved in non-specific**

defense. *British Journal of Nutrition* 84(Suppl.1):S127-S134 (2000). Lactoferrin and lactoperoxidase, both present in colostrum in large amounts, provide non-specific defense against a broad spectrum of pathogens, including bacteria and viruses. This is significant both for the protection of commercially important animals as well as humans.

51 Andersson Y, Lindquist S, Lagerqvist C, Hernell O. **Lactoferrin is responsible for the fungistatic effect of human milk.** *Early Human Development* 59:95-105 (2000). Lactoferrin, through its iron-binding ability, is very effective against fungal infections with *Candida* and other fungi.

52 Qiu J, Hendrixson DR, Baker EN, Murphy TF, St Geme JW III, Plaut AG. **Human milk lactoferrin inactivates two putative colonization factors expressed by *Haemophilus influenzae*.** *Proceedings of the National Academy of Sciences USA* 95:12641-12646 (1998). Lactoferrin prevents colonization of *Haemophilus influenzae*, the primary cause of otitis media and other respiratory infections in children, by inactivating two colonization factors expressed by the bacteria.

53 Ellison RT III, Giehl TJ. **Killing of gram-negative bacteria by lactoferrin and lysozyme.** *Journal of Clinical Investigation* 88(4):1080-1091 (1991). Lactoferrin and lysozyme act together to kill gram-negative bacteria, such as *Vibrio cholerae* (cholera), *Salmonella typhimurium* (food poisoning) and *Eschericia coli*. The lactoferrin attaches to and destroys the cell wall of the bacteria, allowing the lysozyme to enter and lyse (burst) the organisms.

54 Samaranayake YH, Samaranayake LP, Pow EH, Beena VT, Yeung KW. **Antifungal effects of lysozyme and lactoferrin against genetically similar, sequential *Candida albicans* isolates from a human immunodeficiency virus-infected Southern Chinese cohort.** *Journal of Clinical Microbiology* 39(9):3296-3302 (2001). Lactoferrin plus lysozyme is very effective in killing nearly all oral strains of *Candida*, which is of particular importance to AIDS sufferers who are often unable to fight off *Candida* overgrowths, such as thrush.

55 Harmsen MC, Swart PJ, de Bethune MP, Pauwels R, De Clercq E, The TH, Meijer DK. **Antiviral effects of plasma and milk proteins: lactoferrin shows potent activity against both human immunodeficiency virus and human cytomegalovirus replication in vitro.** *Journal of Infectious Diseases*172(2):380-388 (1995). Lactoferrin can protect against infection by HIV and human cytomegalovirus by blocking entrance into the body.

56 Berkhout B, van Wamel JL, Beljaars L, Meijer DK, Visser S, Floris R. **Characterization of the anti-HIV effects of native lactoferrin and other milk proteins and protein-derived peptides.** *Antiviral Research* 55(2):341-355 (2002). Bovine lactoferrin as well as peptides derived from lactoferrin block the entry process of HIV into cells.

57 Hara K, Ikeda M, Saito S, Matsumoto S, Numata K, Kato N, Tanaka K, Sekihara H. **Lactoferrin inhibits hepatitis B virus infection in cultured human hepatocytes.** *Hepatology Research* 24(3):228 (2002). Bovine lactoferrin prevents infection of cultured human

liver cells with hepatitis B virus, while transferrin, casein and lactalbumin had no effect.

58 Ikeda M, Sugiyama K, Tanaka T, Tanaka K, Sekihara H, Shimotohno K, Kato N. **Lactoferrin markedly inhibits hepatitis C virus infection in cultured human hepatocytes.** *Biochemistry and Biophysics Research Communications* 245(2):549-553 (1998). Bovine lactoferrin inhibits the infection of cultured human liver cells by hepatitis C virus while transferrin does not.

59 Superti F, Ammendolia MG, Valenti P, Seganti L. **Anti-rotaviral activity of milk proteins: lactoferrin prevents rotavirus infection in the enterocyte-like cell line HT-29.** *Medical Microbiology and Immunology (Berlin)* 186(2-3):83-91 (1997). Antiviral activity against rotavirus of alpha lactalbumin, beta lactoglobulin, apo-lactoferrin (iron-free) and iron saturated lactoferrin were compared to that of mucin, which has known anti-rotaviral activity. Beta lactoglobulin and both forms of lactoferrin showed anti-rotaviral activity with the strongest response elicited by apo-lactoferrin, which hinders viral attachment to cells by binding directly to the viruses. It also markedly inhibits viral antigen synthesis in the viral adhesion stage.

60 Brinkworth G, Buckley J. **Concentrated bovine colostrums protein supplimention reduces the incidence of self-reported symptoms of upper respiratory tract infections in adult males.** *European Journal of Nutrition* 42:228–232 (2003).

61 van der Strate BW, Beljaars L, Molema G, Harmsen MC, Meijer DK. **Antiviral activities of lactoferrin.** *Antiviral Research* 52(3):225-239 (2001). Lactoferrin is effective against both DNA and RNA viruses, including rotavirus, respiratory syncytial virus, herpes virus and HIV, both by blocking cellular receptors and by directly binding to the viruses.

62 Marchetti M, Pisani S, Antonini G, Valenti P, Seganti L, Orsi N. **Metal complexes of bovine lactoferrin inhibit in vitro replication of herpes simplex virus type 1 and 2.** *Biometals* 11(2):89-94 (1998). Bovine lactoferrin saturated with iron, manganese or zinc proved strongly inhibitory to viral replication of herpes simplex virus types 1 and 2 in cell cultures (Vero).

63 Gahr M, Speer CP, Damerau B, Sawatzki G. **Influence of lactoferrin on the function of human polymorphonuclear leukocytes and monocytes.** *Journal of Leukocyte Biology* 49(5):427-433 (1991). White blood cells (polymorphonuclear leucocytes) exposed to lactoferrin from bovine colostrum exhibit increased motility and produce more superoxide (a powerful antioxidant).

64 Shau H, Kim A, Golub SH. **Modulation of natural killer and lymphokine-activated killer cell cytotoxicity by lactoferrin.** *Journal of Leukocyte Biology* 51(4):343-349 (1992). Lactoferrin strongly augments the cytotoxic functions of natural killer (NK) cells and lymphokine-activated killer (LK) cells. Newborn infants have low NK and LK activity so lactoferrin may 'turn on' these cells in the infant.

65 Hashizume S, Kuroda K, Murakami H. **Identification of lactoferrin as an essential growth factor for human lymphocytic cell lines in serum-free medium.** *Biochimica*

et Biophysica Acta 763(4):377-382 (1983). Lactoferrin is an essential growth factor for lymphocytes. It has higher growth stimulatory activity than transferrin. Bovine lactoferrin was found to be as effective as human.

66 Reiter B. **The lactoperoxidase-thiocyanate-hydrogen peroxide antibacterium system.** *Ciba Foundation Symposia* 65:285-294 (1978).

67 Kussendrager KD, van Hooijdonk AC. **Lactoperoxidase: physico-chemical properties, occurrence, mechanism of action and applications.** *British Journal of Nutrition* 84(Suppl 1):S19-S25 (2000). The lactoperoxidase system acts as an antimicrobial defense in bodily secretions such as tears, saliva and milk.

68 Stelwagen K, Carpenter E, Haigh B, Hodgkinson A, Wheeler TT. **Immune Components of Bovine Colostrum and Milk.** *Journal of Animal Science* epub ahead of print (2008). Human and bovine colostrum contain cytokines and antimicrobial proteins and peptides, including lactoferrin, defensins and cathelicidins.

69 Gopal PK, Gill HS. **Oligosaccharides and glycoconjugates in bovine milk and colostrum.** *British Journal of Nutrition* 84(Suppl.1):S69-S74 (2000). One way colostrum helps protect against infections is through the oligosaccharides and glycoconjugates it contains. These are complex sugars which compete for binding sites in the GI tract with pathogens.

70 Newburg DS. **Human milk glycoconjugates that inhibit pathogens.** *Current Medical Chemistry* 6(2):117-127 (1999). The protection offered by human milk may not be limited to just secretory IgA. However, milk and colostrum contain numerous complex carbohydrates, including glycoproteins, glycolipids, glycosaminoglycans, mucins and oligosaccharides. These complex carbohydrate glycoconjugates and oligosaccharides as synthesized by the many glycosyltransferases found in the mammary gland. Those with homology to cell surface glycoconjugate pathogen may inhibit pathogen binding by competing for binding sites. One of the fucosyloliogosaccharides inhibits *E. coli* toxin. Another inhibits infection by *Campylobacter jejuni.* Milk oligosaccharides inhibit the binding of *Streptococcus pneumoniae* and enteropathogenic *E. coli.* Lactadherin inhibits rotavirus. A mannosylated glycopeptide inhibits binding by enterohemorrhagic *E. coli.* A glycosaminoglycan prevents binding of gp120 (a form of HIV) to CD4, the first step in HIV infection. Milk mucin inhibits binding of S-fimbriated *E. coli.* Ganglioside GM1 reduces diarrhea due to cholera toxin and *E. coli* labile toxin. Glycosphingolipid Gb3 binds to shiga toxin.

71 Korhonen H, Marnila P, Gill HS. **Milk immunoglobulins and complement factors.** *British Journal of Nutrition* 84(Suppl.1):S75-S80 (2000). Bovine colostrum contains three main classes of immunoglobulin IgG (IgG1 75% and IgG2), IgM and IgA, plus hemolytic and bactericidal complement. Complement is a complex group of proteins which act in concert with antibodies to inactivate and/or kill pathogens.

72 Nakajima S, Baba AS, Tamura N. **Complement system in human colostrum:**

presence of nine complement components and factors of alternative pathway in human colostrum. *International Archives of Allergy and Applied Immunology* 54(5):428-433 (1977). All nine components of the complement system (C1-C9) have been found in human colostrum.

73 Armogida SA, Yannaras NM, Melton AL, Srivastava MD. **Identification and quantification of innate immune system mediators in human breast milk.** *Allergy and Asthma Proceedings* 25(5):297-304 (2004). Mediators of the innate immune system were found in human colostrum and milk, including defensins, cathelicidins, and toll-like receptors.

74 LeBouder E, Rey-Nores JE, Rushmere NK, Grigorov M, Lawn SD, Affolter M, Griffin GE, Ferrara P, Schiffrin EJ, Morgan BP, Labeta MO. **Soluble forms of Toll-like receptor (TLR)-2 capable of modulating TLR2 signaling are present in human plasma and breast milk.** *Journal of Immunology* 171(12):6680-6689 (2003). Failure of the innate immune response to bacterial infection can lead to septic shock and death. Toll-like receptors play a crucial role in the innate immune response and is found in human colostrum and milk.

75 Pasare C, Medzhitov R. **Toll-like receptors: linking innate and adaptive immunity.** *Microbes and Infection* 6(15):1382-1387 (2004). Toll-like receptors (TLRs) are the principal means of detection and response to microbial infections, including bacteria, viruses, fungi and protozoa. Initial recognition by the TLRs sets off a complex series of signaling events that sets off the immune response to the infection.

76 Janusz M, Lisowski J. **Proline-rich Polypeptide (PRPs) – an immunomodulatory peptide from ovine colostrum.** *Archivum Immunologiae et Therapiae Experimentalis* 41:275-279 (1993). A unique, non-species specific polypeptide which plays an immunomodulatory role in the immune system. It can induce the differentiation of thymocytes into functional T cells as well as increase the permeability of skin blood vessels. What makes it unique is that a second exposure to the polypeptide reverses the changes induced by first exposure.

77 Julius MH, Janusz M, Lisowski J. **A colostral protein that induces the growth and differentiation of resting B lymphocytes.** *Journal of Immunology* 140:1366-1371 (1988). Colostrinin has also been shown to induce the growth and differentiation of resting B lymphocytes. T and B lymphocytes are the two main types of lymphocytes involved in the immune response.

78 Sirota L, Straussberg R, Notti I, Bessler H. **Effect of human colostrum on interleukin-2 production and natural killer cell activity.** *Archive of Diseases in Childhood: Fetal and Neonatal Edition* 72(3):F99-102 (1995). Colostrum stimulates or inhibits the production of IL-2 depending on its concentration. It also inhibits the activity of natural killer cells, but the production of IL-2 reverses this effect. This is thought to be another way that colostrum modulates the immune system response.

79 Shau H, Kim A, Golub SH. **Modulation of natural killer and lymphokine-activated killer cell cytotoxicity by lactoferrin.** *Journal of Leukocyte Biology* 51(4):343-349 (1992). Lactoferrin strongly augments the cytotoxic functions of natural killer (NK) cells and lymphokine-activated killer (LK) cells. Newborn infants have low NK and LK activity so lactoferrin may 'turn on' these cells in the infant.

80 Pihoker C, Gilliam L, Hampe C, Lernmark A. **Auto-antibodies in Diabetes.** *Diabetes* 54:S52-S61 (2005).

81 McDevitt H. **Characteristics of Autoimmunity in Type 1 Diabetes and Type 1.5 Overlap With Type 2 Diabetes.** *Diabetes* 54:S4-S10 (2005).

82 Boitard C, Efendic S, Ferrannini E, Henquin J, Steiner D, Cerasi E. **A Tale of Two Cousins: Type 1 and Type 2 Diabetes.** *Diabetes* 54:S1-S3 (2005).

83 Tuomi T. **What Do They Have in Common? Type 1 and Type 2 Diabetes. Section 1: Aspects of Pathophysiology.** *Diabetes* 54:S40-S45 (2005).

84 Knip M, Veijola R, Virtanen S, Hyöty H, Vaarala O, Åkerblom H. **Environmental Triggers and Determinants of Type 1 Diabetes.** *Diabetes* 54:S125-S136 (2005).

85 Devaraj S, Glaser N, Griffen S, Wang-Polagruto J, Miguelino E, Jialal I. **Increased Monocytic Activity and Biomarkers of Inflammation in Patients With Type 1 Diabetes.** *Diabetes* 55:774-779 (2006).

86 Dohm GL, Elton CW, Raju MS, Mooney ND, DiMarchi R, Pories WJ, Flickinger EG, Atkinson SM Jr, Caro JF. **IGF-I– Stimulated Glucose Transport in Human Skeletal Muscle and IGF-I Resistance in Obesity and NIDDM.** *Diabetes* 39(9):1028-1032 (1990).

87 **A New Way to Fight Diabetes.** *Newsweek* November 15, 1993

88 Pennisi. **Immune Therapy Stems Diabetes Progress.** *Science News* 145:37, January 15, 1995.

89 Dutta RC. **Peptide immunomodulators versus infection; an analysis.** *Immunology Letters.* 83(3):153-61 (2002). Immune stimulators have been found to be useful in helping to fight off infections, while immunosuppressors have been found useful in autoimmune conditions and transplants.

90 Hughes RA. **Immunological treatment of multiple sclerosis.** *Journal of Neurology* 230(2):73-80 (1983). Transfer factor (PRP) slowed the progression of the disease whereas interferon and levamisole did not.

91 Nitsch, A, Nitsch, FP. **Clinical Use of Bovine Colostrum.** *Journal of Orthomolecular Medicine* 13(2) (1998). Low molecular weight components of colostrum (PRPs) were used in a clinical study for the treatment of rheumatoid arthritis with promising results.

92 Kruzel M, Bacsi A, Choudhury B, Sur S, Boldogh I. **Lactoferrin decreases pollen antigen-induced allergic airway inflammation in a murine model of asthma.** *Immunology* 119(2):159-66 (2006). Pollen grains contain reduced nicotinamide adenine dinucleotide phosphate (NADPH) oxidases and in contact with mucosal surfaces generate

superoxide anion (O2*-). In the presence of iron, O2*- may be converted to more reactive oxygen radicals, such as to H2O2 and/or *OH, which may augment antigen-induced airway inflammation. LF lowered the increase in cellular reactive oxygen species (ROS) levels in bronchial epithelial cells. The results suggest the utility of LF in human allergic inflammatory disorders.

93 Tsai WJ, Liu HW, Yen JH, Chen JR, Lin SF, Chen TP. **Lactoferrin in rheumatoid arthritis and systemic lupus erythematous.** *Gaoxiong Y Xue Ke Xue Za Zhi* 7(1):22-26 (1991).

94 Hraba T, Wieczorek Z, Janusz M, Lisowski J, Zimecki M. **Effect of Proline-rich Polypeptide on experimental autoimmune response to erythrocytes.** *Archivum immunologiae et therapiae experimentalis (Warszava)* 34(4):437-443 (1986).

95 Zimecki M, Hraba T, Janusz M, Lisowski J, Wieczorek Z. **Effect of a Proline-rich Polypeptide (PRP) on the development of hemolytic anemia and survival of New Zealand black (NZB) mice.** *Archivum immunologiae et therapiae experimentalis (Warszava)* 39(5-6):461-461 (1991).

96 Murdoch C, Finn A. **Chemokine receptors and their role in inflammation and infectious diseases.** *Blood* 95(10):3032-3042 (2000).

97 Christopherson KW, Hromas RA. **Endothelial chemokines in autoimmune disease.** *Current Pharmaceutical Design* 10(2):145-154 (2004).

98 Kidd, PM. **Autism, an extreme challenge to integrative medicine. Part I: the knowledge base.** *Alternative Medicine Review* August 2002.

99 Manev R, Manev H. **Aminoglycoside antiobiotics and autism: a speculative hypothesis.** *BMC Psychiatry* 1:5-7 (2001).

100 **Autism, Autoimmunity and Immunotherapy**: a Commentary by Vijendra K. Singh, Ph.D. Department of Biology & Biotechnology Center, Utah State University, Logan Scientific Board Member, Autism Autoimmunity Project.

101 Kidd PM. **Autism, an extreme challenge to integrative medicine. Part II: medical management.** *Alternative Medicine Review* December 2002.

102 Wyplosz, B *et al.* **Correlation Between Chlamydia pneumoniae Detection From Coronary Angioplasty Balloons and Atherosclerosis Severity**, *J Am Coll Cardiol, 2006; 47:1229-1231, doi:10.1016/j.jacc.2005.12.037* (Published online 21 February 2006).

103 Lange LG, Schreiner GF. **Immune Mechanisms of Cardiac Disease.** *New England Journal of Medicine*. 330:1129-1135 (1994).

104 Gilliland SE, Nelson CR, Maxwell C. **Assimilation of Cholesterol by Lactobacillus Acidophilus.** *Applied and Environmental Microbiology* 49:377-381 (1985).

105 Frystyk J, Ledet T, Moller N, Flyvbjerg A, Orskov H. **Cardiovascular disease and insulin-like growth factor I.** *Circulation* 106(8):893-895 (2002).

106 Bayes-Genis A, Conover CA, Schwartz RS. **The insulin-like growth factor axis: A review of atherosclerosis and restenosis.** *Circulation Research* 86(2):125-130 (2000).

IGF-1 and -2 function as mediators of cardiovascular disease. The dynamic balance of IGFs, their binding proteins (IGFBP) and the proteases (IGFBP proteases) which remove the binding proteins from the IGFs, activating them, consitutes the IGF axis which determines the extent of IGF-dependent cellular effects. Dysregulation of the IGF axis can lead to coronary athersclerosis through effects on smooth muscle growth, migration, and extracellular matrix synthesis in the atherosclerotic plaque. IGF-1 promotes macrophage chemotaxis, excess LDL cholesterol uptake and release of proinflammatory cytokines.

107 Robert L, Godeau G, Gavignet-Jeannin C, Groult N, Six C, Robert AM. **The Effect of Procyanidolic Oligomers on Vascular Permeability. A Study Using Quantitative Morphology.** *Pathologie Biologie 38:608-616 (1990).*

108 Groziak SM, Miller GD. **Natural bioactive substances in milk and colostrum: effects on the arterial blood pressure system.** *British Journal of Nutrition* 84(Suppl 1):S119-S125 (2000).

109 FitzGerald RJ, Murray BA, Walsh DJ. **Hypotensive peptides from milk proteins.** *Journal of Nutrition* 134(4):980S-988S (2004).

110 Jorde R, Bonaa KH. **Calcium from dairy products, vitamin D intake, and blood pressure: the Tromsø Study.** *American Journal of Clinical Nutrition* 71(6):1530-1535 (2000).

111 Cesarone MR, Belcaro G, Di Renzo A, Dugall M, Cacchio M, Ruffini I, Pellegrini L, Del Boccio G, Fano F, Ledda A, Bottari A, Ricci A, Stuard S, Vinciguerra G. **Prevention of Influenza Episodes With Colostrum Compared With Vaccination in Healthy and High-Risk Cardiovascular Subjects: The Epidemiologic Study in San Valentino.** Clinical and Applied Thrombosis/Hemostasis 13(2):130-136 (2007).

112 Gross N, Carey J, Hamilton J. **Quiet Strides in the War on Cancer.** *Business Week*. p. 150, February 6, 1995.

113 Lidbeck A, Allinger UG, Orrhage KM, Ottova L, Brismar B, Gustafsson JA, Rafter J, Nord CE. **Impact of Lactobacillus Acidophilus Supplements on the Fecal Microflora and Soluble Fecal Bile Acids in Colon Cancer Patients.** *Microbial Ecology in Health and Disease* 4:81-8 (1991).

114 Lidbeck A, Nord CE, Gustafsson JA, Rafter J. **Lactobacilli, Anticarcinogenic Activities and Human Intestinal Microflora.** *European Journal of Cancer Prevention* 1:341-353 (1992).

115 Yamaguchi M, Imai T, Maeda T, Sakata M, Miyake A, Linzer DI. **Cyclic adenosine 3',5'-monophosphate stimulation of placental proliferin and proliferin-related protein secretion.** *Endocrinology* 136(5):2040-2046 (1995).

116 Linzer DI, Nathans D. **A new member of the prolactin-growth hormone gene family expressed in mouse placenta.** *EMBO Journal* 4(6):1419-1423 (1985).

117 Bengtson NW, Linzer DI. **Inhibition of tumor growth by the antiangiogenic placental hormone, proliferin-related protein.** *Molecular Endocrinology* 14(12):1934-43 (2000).

118 Regulier E, Paul S, Marigliano M, Kintz J, Poitevin Y, Ledoux C, Roecklin D, Cauet G, Calenda V, Homann HE. **Adenovirus-mediated delivery of antiangiogenic genes as an antitumor approach.** *Cancer and Gene Therapy* 8(1):45-54 (2001).

119 Yamaguchi M, Ogren L, Barnard R, Imai T, Sawada T, Miyake A, Talamantes F. **Selective inhibition of mouse placental lactogen II secretion by tumour necrosis factor-alpha.** *Journal of Endocrinology* 143(1):95-105 (1994).

120 Blach-Olszewska Z, Janusz M. **Stimulatory effect of ovine colostrinine (a Proline-rich Polypeptide) on interferons and tumor necrosis factor production by murine resident peritoneal cells.** *Archivum immunologiae et therapiae experimentalis (Warszava)* 45(1):43-47 (1997).

121 Inglot AD, Janusz M, Lisowski J. **Colostrinine, a Proline-rich Polypeptide from ovine colostrum, is a modest cytokine inducer in human leukocytes.** *Archivum immunologiae et therapiae experimentalis (Warszava)* 44(4):215-224 (1996).

122 Sekine K, Watanabe E, Nakamura J, Takasuka N, Kim DJ, Asamoto M, Krutovskikh V, Baba-Toriyama H, Ota T, Moore MA, Masuda M, Sugimoto H, Nishino H, Kakizoe T, Tsuda H. **Inhibition of azoxymethane-initiated colon tumor by bovine lactoferrin administration in F344 rats.** *Japanese Journal of Cancer Research* 88(6):523-526 (1997). Rats were treated with azoxymethane, a chemical which induces colon cancer in rats. They were then given bovine lactoferrin orally for 36 weeks. 57.5% of the rats in the control group which received no lactoferrin developed carcinomas, while only 25% of the rats which received 0.2% lactoferrin solutions developed carcinomas. Rats which received a stronger dose of lactoferrin, 2%, had only a 15% rate of tumor development.

123 Tanaka T, Kawabata K, Kohno H, Honjo S, Murakami M, Ota T, Tsuda H. **Chemopreventive effect of bovine lactoferrin on 4-nitroquinoline 1-oxide-induced tongue carcinogenesis in male F344 rats.** *Japanese Journal of Cancer Research* 91(1):25-33 (2000). A more detailed study of the effect of lactoferrin administration on chemically induced carcinomas of the tongue in rats. It was found again that a 2% lactoferrin solution produced better protection against the development of carcinoma than the weaker 0.2% solution, though both provided more protection than the control group. With a 2% solution, only 20% of the rats developed cancer, and they showed 64% less multiple tumors than the control group. It was further determined that the method of action of the lactoferrin was through modification of cell proliferation and detoxifying enzymes, such as glutathione S-transferase and quinone reductase.

124 Kuhara T, Iigo M, Itoh T, Ushida Y, Sekine K, Terada N, Okamura H, Tsuda H. **Orally administered lactoferrin exerts an anti-metastatic effect and enhances production of IL-18 in the intestinal epithelium.** *Nutrition and Cancer* 38(2):192-199 (2000). Oral administration of bovine lactoferrin or its hydrolyzed form caused an increase in CD4+ and CD8+ lymphocytes and asialoGM1+ (a specific type of natural killer cell) in the spleen and blood, and their cytotoxic activities against several types of cancer cell lines

were increased. CD4+ and CD8+ lymphocytes were also increased in intestinal mucosa accompanied by a marked increase in IL-18 production. Using this model, the effects on metastasis of colon carcinoma to the lung was studied and significant inhibition of metastasis was found. The results suggest that the anti-metastatic effect of lactoferrin may be due to enhanced cellular immunity.

125 Tsuda H, Sekine K, Fujita K, Ligo M. **Cancer prevention by bovine lactoferrin and underlying mechanisms – a review of experimental and clinical studies.** *Biochemistry and Cell Biology* 80(1):131-136 (2002). Review article of studies which indicate that bovine lactoferrin is an effective anticancer agent in rat studies, capable of significantly inhibiting colon, esophagus, lung, bladder and tongue carcinogenesis. Following the administration of lactoferrin to animals which had been exposed to a variety of carcinogenic chemicals, phase I enzymes (which seek out carcinogenic materials and "switch them on") were inhibited in colon cancer test subjects while phase II enzyme (which act to detoxify the carcinogens switched on by the phase I enzymes) activity was increased in the tongue cancer study. There was a marked increase in Natural Killer Cell and cytotoxic T-lymphocyte activity in both the mucosal layer of the small intestine and peripheral blood cells, increasing the production of IL-18 and caspase-1 and the subsequent production of interferon-gamma cells. It was also found that lactoferrin has significant anti-Hepatitis C virus activity, and Hepatitis C is a leading cause of liver cancer in Japan.

126 Damiens E, Mazurier J, El Yazidi I, Masson M, Duthille I, Spik G, Boilly-Marer Y. **Effects of human lactoferrin on NK cell cytotoxicity against hematopoietic and epithelial tumor cells.** *Biochimica et Biophysica Acta* 1402(3):277-287 (1998). Human lactoferrin applied at levels found in inflammation was found to boost the cytotoxic activity of natural killer (NK) cells against hematopoietic and breast epithelial tumor cell lines. It also significantly increases the susceptibility to lysis of breast and colon epithelial tumor cell lines but not the hematopoietic tumor cells. Lactoferrin is shown to inhibit epithelial cell proliferation by blocking cell cycle progression.

127 Iigo M, Kuhara T, Ushida Y, Sekine K, Moore MA, Tsuda H. **Orally administered bovine lactoferrin induces caspase-1 and interleukin-18 in the mouse intestinal mucosa: a possible explanation for inhibition of carcinogenesis and metastasis.** *Cytokine* 25(1):36-44 (2004). Oral lactoferrin administration increased the production of IL-18 by intestinal epithelial cells followed by increases in caspase-1 and INF-γ, which potentiate the activity of cytotoxic lymphocytes and natural killer cells in attacking cancer cells.

128 Damiens E, El Yazidi I, Mazurier J, Duthille I, Spik G, Boilly-Marer Y. **Lactoferrin inhibits G1 cyclin-dependent kinases during growth arrest of human breast carcinoma cells.** *Journal of Cell Biochemistry* 74(3):486-498 (1999). It is known that lactoferrin inhibits cell proliferation and suppresses tumor growth. The mechanism of how it does this is unknown, however. In this study, lactoferrin applied to a breast carcinoma cell line arrests

the growth of these cells at the G1 [growth and preparation of the chromosomes for replication] to S [DNA synthesis] transition of the cell cycle. The arrest is associated with a dramatic increase in the levels of Cdk2 [cyclin-dependent kinase 2] and cyclin E and an inhibition of Cdk2 kinase activity. Cdk4 activity is also decreased and Cdk inhibitor p21(CIP1) expression is increased. Lactoferrin also maintains the cell cycle regulator retinoblastoma protein pRb in a hypophosphorylated form. Therefore lactoferrin induces growth arrest by modulating the expression and activity of key G1 regulatory proteins.

129 Kroning R, Jones JA, Hom DK, Chuang CC, Sanga R, Los G, Howell SB, Christen RD. **Enhancement of drug sensitivity of human malignancies by epidermal growth factor.** *British Journal of Cancer* 72(3):615-619 (1995). Study shows that a number of human cancers become more sensitive to chemotherapeutic agents in the presence of epidermal growth factor. Cancers showing increased sensitivity include ovarian carcinoma, cancers of the head, neck, cervix, colon, prostate and pancreas, and non-small-cell lung cancer. Drugs to which the cancers became more sensitized include most common chemotherapeutic agents, such as cisplatin, carboplatin, tetraplatin, taxol, melphalan and 5-fluorouracil.

130 Borissenko M. **Colostrum, growth factors and cancer.** Institute for Colostrum Research, 2004.

131 Nowa and McMichael. **How HIV defeats the immune system.** *Scientific American* Aug:58-65 (1995).

132 Harmsen MC, Swart PJ, Bethune M, Pauwels R, De Clercq E, TheTH, Meijer DK. **Antiviral Effects of Plasma and Milk Proteins: Lactoferrin Shows Potent Activity against Both Human Immunodeficiency Virus and Human Cytomegalovirus Replication In Vitro.** *Journal of Infectious Diseases.* 172:380-8 (1995).

133 Anderson I. **Powdered Milk Cure for Fatal Diarrhea.** *New Scientist,* January 6 1994.

134 Rump JA, Aarndt R, Arnold A, Bendick C, Dichtelmuller H, Franke M, Helm EB, Jager H, Kampmann B, Kolb P. **Treatment of Diarrhoea in Human Immunodeficiency Virus-Infected Patients with Immunoglobulins from Bovine Colostrum.** *Clinical Investigator* 70(7):588-594 (1992).

135 Nord J, Ma P, DiJohn D, Tripori S, Tacket CO. **Treatment with Bovine Hyperimmune Colostrum of Cryptosporidial Diarrhea in AIDS Patients.** *AIDS.* 4(6):581-584 (1990).

136 Mero A, Kahkonen J, Nykanen T, Parviainen T, Jokinen I, Takala T, Nikula T, Rasi S, Leppaluoto J. **IGF-I, IgA, and IgG responses to bovine colostrum supplementation during training.** *Journal of Applied Physiology* 93(2):7323-739 (2002).

137 Nieman DC, Berk LS, Simpson-Westerberg M, Arabatzis K, Youngberg S, Tan SA, Lee JW, Eby WC. **Effects of long-endurance running on immune system parameters and lymphocyte function in experienced marathoners.** *International Journal of Sports Medicine* 10(5):317-323 (1989).

138 Berk LS, Nieman DC, Youngberg WS, Arabatzis K, Simpson-Westerberg M, Lee JW,

Tan SA, Eby WC. **The effect of long endurance running on natural killer cells in marathoners.** *Medicine and Science in Sports and Exercise* 22:207-212 (1990).

139 Sparling SB, Nieman DC, O'Connor PJ. **Selected scientific aspects of marathon racing. An update on fluid replacement, immune function, psychological factors and the gender difference.** *Sports Medicine* 15(2):116-132 (1993).

140 Burke ER. **Colostrum as an Athletic Enhancer and Help for AIDS.** *Nutrition Science News*, May, 1996.

141 Buckley JD, Brinkworth GD, Southcott E, Butler RN. **Bovine colostrum and whey protein supplementation during running training increase intestinal permeability.** *Asia Pacific Journal of Clinical Nutrition* 13(Suppl):S81 (2004).

142 Buckley JD, Abbott MJ, Brinkworth GD, Whyte PB. **Bovine colostrum supplementation during endurance running training improves recovery, but not performance.** *Journal of Science and Medicine in Sport* 5(2):65-79 (2002). Supplementation with colostrum did not increase serum IGF-1 levels or initial performance, but it did significantly improve performance in a second round of performance.

143 Coombes JS, Conacher M, Austen SK, Marshall PA. **Dose effects of oral bovine colostrum on physical work capacity in cyclists.** *Medicine and Science in Sports and Exercise* 34(7):1184-1188 (2002). Colostrum supplementation produced a slight but significant increase in performance in competitive cyclists.

144 Hofman Z, Smeets R, Verlaan G, Lugt R, Verstappen PA. **The effect of bovine colostrum supplementation on exercise performance in elite field hockey players.** *International Journal of Sports Nutrition and Exercise Metabolism* 12(4):461-469 (2002). Colostrum supplementation improved sprint performance of field hockey players compared to whey supplementation.

145 Antonio J, Sanders MS, Van Gammeren D. **The effects of bovine colostrum supplementation on body composition and exercise performance in active men and women.** *Nutrition* 17(3):243-247 (2001). Colostrum supplementation produced a significant increase in lean body mass compared to whey supplementation

146 Mero A, Miikkulainen H, Riski J, Pakkanen R, Aalto J, Takala T. **Effects of bovine colostrum supplementation on serum IGF-I, IgG, hormone, and saliva IgA during training.** *Journal of Applied Physiology* 83(4):1144-1151 (1997). Colostrum supplementation increases levels of IGF-1 in athletes during strength and speed training.

147 Mero A, Kahkonen J, Nykanen T, Parviainen T, Jokinen I, Takala T, Nikula T, Rasi S, Leppaluoto J. **IGF-I, IgA, and IgG responses to bovine colostrum supplementation during training.** *Journal of Applied Physiology* 93(2):732-739 (2002). Although colostrum supplementation increases IGF-1 levels in the blood, this increase is not due to absorption of the IGF-1 from colostrum.

148 Cross CE, Halliwell B, Borish ET, Pryor WA, Ames BN, Saul RL, McCord JM, Harman D. **Oxygen radicals and human disease.** *Annals of Internal Medicine* 107(4):526-545

(1987). Oxygen free radicals, the by-products of normal metabolism, have been implicated in disease processes ranging from carcinogenesis to aging, emphasizing the importance of antioxidants in combating these conditions.

149 Ames BN, Shigenaga MK, Hagen TM. **Oxidants, antioxidants, and the degenerative diseases of aging.** *Proceedings of the National Academy of Sciences USA* 90(17):7915-7922 (1993). Oxidant by-products of metabolism cause significant damage to DNA, proteins and lipids. This damage results in aging and the degenerative diseases associated with aging, such as cancer, cardiovascular disease, immune system decline, brain dysfunction and cataracts. Antioxidant defenses against these diseases decline with age, necessitating the supplementation of antioxidants in the diet.

150 Kurz DJ, Decary S, Hong Y, Trivier E, Akhmedov A, Erusalimsky JD. **Chronic oxidative stress compromises telomere integrity and accelerates the onset of senescence in human endothelial cells.** *Journal of Cell Science* 117:2417-2426 (2004). Oxidative stress due to the buildup of oxidization by-products has been linked to the onset of cell senescence in blood vessel lining cells by disrupting telomere integrity. Telomeres are the "tails" of the chromosomes, the length of which determine the number of cell divisions a cell can undergo before reaching its limit. Glutathione, a powerful natural antioxidant, is crucial in maintaining telomere integrity.

151 Borissenko M. **Glutathione: A powerful anti-oxidant found in colostrum.** NZMP August 2002. Both glutathione and its chemical predecessors are present in large quantities in colostrum. As glutathione is not absorbed directly, glutathione production in the body can only be accomplished by supplementation with its antecedents, cystine, glycine and glutamic acid, all of which are abundant in colostrum.

152 Buescher ES, McIlheran SM. **Antioxidant properties of human colostrum.** *Pediatric Research* 24(1):14-19 (1988). Colostrum reduces ferricytochrome C in polymorphonuclear leucocytes (PMNs) and also disrupts other metabolic and enzymatic activities of PMNs which are crucial in PMN respiratory burst mediation of acute inflammation, showing that colostrum is a powerful antioxidant.

153 Buescher ES, McIlheran SM. **Colostral antioxidants: separation and characterization of two activities in human colostrum.** *Journal of Pediatric Gastroenterology and Nutrition* 14(1):47-56 (1992). Colostrum interferes with the production of PMN respiratory burst products in two ways, ascorbate and uric acid.

154 Boldogh I, Liebenthal D, Hughes TK, Juelich TL, Georgiades JA, Kruzel ML, Stanton GJ. **Modulation of 4HNE-mediated signaling by proline-rich peptides from ovine colostrum.** *Journal of Molecular Neuroscience* 20(2):125-134 (2003). Colostrinin down regulates lipid peroxidation, inhibits glutathione depletion and reduces intracellular levels of reactive oxygen species (ROS). This is one more way that colostrum demonstrates antioxidant activity.

155 Wakabayashi H, Matsumoto H, Hashimoto K, Teraguchi S, Takase M, Hayasawa H.

Inhibition of iron/ascorbate-induced lipid peroxidation by an N-terminal peptide of bovine lactoferrin and its acylated derivatives. *Bioscience, Biotechnology, Biochemistry* 63(5):955-957 (1999). Lactoferrin also plays an important antioxidant role in colostrum by preventing lipid peroxidation.

156 Ulcova-Gallova Z, Fialova P, Krauz V. **[Immunologic factors in human colostrum and milk.]** *Casopis Lekaru Ceskych* 133(9):275-276 (1994). Colostrum was found to contain IgG, IgM, IgD, IgA, sIgA, C3, C4, orosomucoid, prealbumin, alpha 1-antitrypsin, alpha 1-fetoprotein, alpha 2-macroglobulin, haemopexin, haptoglobulin, beta 2-microglobulin, alpha 2-AP glycoprotein, and IgE.

157 Gutteridge JM, Smith A. **Antioxidant protection by haemopexin of haem-stimulated lipid peroxidation.** *Biochemical Journal* 256:861-865 (1988). Haem is a low molecular weight form of iron that is capable of taking part in oxygen radical reactions that can lead to the degradation of proteins, lipids, carbohydrates and DNA. Haemopexin can inhibit such oxidative reactions by as much as 90%.

158 Korhonen H, Syvaoja EL, Ahola-Luttila H, Sivela S, Kopola S, Husu J, Kosunen TU. **Bactericidal effect of bovine normal and immune serum, colostrum and milk against *Helicobacter pylori*.** *Journal of Applied Bacteriology* 78(6):655-662 (1995). Helicobacter pylori is a major cause of gastritis and ulcers in humans. Serum and colostrum from non-immunized Friesian cows were found to be highly bactericidal against *H. pylori*. Post-colostral milk did not show any bactericidal effect against *H. pylori*.

159 Bitzan MM, Gold BD, Philpott DJ, Huesca M, Sherman PM, Karch H, Lissner R, Lingwood CA, Karmali MA. **Inhibition of *Helicobacter pylori* and *Helicobacter mustelae* binding to lipid receptors by bovine colostrum.** *Journal of Infectious Diseases* 177(4):955-961 (1998). *H. pylori* and *H. mustelae* (a gastric pathogen of ferrets) are both bound by lipid receptors (phosphatidylethanolamine, gangliotetraosylceramide and gangliotriaosyl-ceramide) in the gut, allowing them to carry out their pathogenic activities. Bovine colostrum, however, was shown to prevent binding of the pathogens to these lipid receptors even though there was no detectable anti-*H. pylori* antibody activity in the colostrum.

160 Wada T, Aiba Y, Shimizu K, Takagi A, Miwa T, Koga Y. **The therapeutic effect of bovine lactoferrin in the host infected with Helicobacter pylori.** *Scandinavian Journal of Gastroenterology* 34(3):238-243 (1999). Mice infected with *H. pylori* were given a daily dose of bovine lactoferrin for 2-4 weeks. Their intestines were then examined for bacterial content. Numbers of *H. pylori* were reduced to 10% of pre-lactoferrin levels and greatly decreased the numbers of *H. pylori* bound to the intestinal wall. Serum antibody titer to *H. pylori* were reduced to practically zero, indicating that the immune response of the host was no longer recognizing *H. pylori* infection. Therefore it was deduced that lactoferrin has a direct antibacterial effect on *H. pylori* infection and prevents binding of the pathogen to the intestinal lining.

161 Casswall TH, Nilsson HO, Bjorck L, Sjostedt S, Xu L, Nord CK, Boren T, Wadstrom T, Hammarstrom L. **Bovine anti-Helicobacter pylori antibodies for oral immunotherapy.** *Scandinavian Journal of Gastroenterology* 37(12):1380-1385 (2002). Bovine colostrum with high titers against *H. pylori* was given to *H. pylori* infected mice. Comparison of treated mice with control mice showed a 50-66% cure rate for *H. pylori* infection in treated mice. Binding studies also showed that the colostrum prevented binding of the *H. pylori.*

162 Masson PL, Heremans JF, Dive JH. **An iron-binding protein common to many external secretions.** *Clinica Chimica Acta* 14:735 (1966). Lactoferrin inhibits the growth of siderophilic (iron-loving) bacteria and *Candida albicans.*

163 Ogra PL, Losonsky GA, Fishaut M. **Colostrum derived immunity and maternal neonatal interaction.** *Annals of the New York Academy of Sciences* 409:82-92 (1983). Peyer's patches are found throughout the intestinal tract, and groups of similar immunoactive cells are found in the bronchial mucosa. Both the intestinal and bronchial immunoactive cell groups respond to allergens, antigens and pathogens by neutralizing or destroying them. In newborns, these special cell groups are not immediately operative but protection is provided by a variety of immune factors from the mother's colostrum. Antibodies found in colostrum protect against *Eschericia coli, Salmonella, Shigella, Vibrio cholera, Bacteriodes fragilis, Streptococcus pneumoniae, Bordtella pertussis, Clostridium diphtheria, Clostridium tetani, Streptococcus mutans* and *Candida albicans.*

164 Lilius EM, Marnila P. **The role of colostral antibodies in prevention of microbial infections.** *Current Opinion in Infectious Diseases* 14(3):295-300 (2001) . Colostrum offers passive protection against a variety of microbial pathogens in the form of specific immunoglobulin A, G and M antibodies. It is especially effective in the prevention of various gastroenteric infections.

165 Moller W, Lissner R, Nitsche D. **Use of bovine colostral milk as a preparation for the protection of the liver.** US Patent #5,710,132 (1998). Whole bovine colostrum or an immunoglobulin preparation from colostrum are used to protect the liver from bacterial, viral or protozoan diseases, such as *E. coli*, rotavirus or cryptosporidia infection, as well as detoxify the liver by removing toxic protein metabolites such as ammonia. It can also be used to treat the effects of various liver diseases, such as liver inflammation, viral hepatitis, fibrosis of the liver, cirrhosis of the liver, fatty liver, and so forth. These effects include disturbances of the liver's detoxification, excretory, conjugational and synthesizing functions, portal hypertension due to liver disease, and even coma due to liver failure. Supplementation can also be used to relieve stress on the liver due to liver insufficiency as a result of liver parenchyma damage or viral hepatitis, allowing the liver to heal and recover function.

166 Tavakkol, Elder JT, Griffiths CE, Cooper KD, Talwar H, Fisher GJ, Keane KM, Foltin SK, Voorhees JJ. **Expression of growth hormone receptor, insulin-like growth factor I (IGF-I) and IGF-I receptor mRNA and proteins in human skin.** *Journal of*

Investigative Dermatology 99(3):343-349 (1992). Receptors for growth hormone and IGF-I were isolated from human skin, indicating that skin cells may have the ability to react directly to growth hormone stimulation.

167 Hyde C, Hollier B, Anderson A, Harkin D, Upton Z. **Insulin-like Growth Factors (IGF) and IGF-Binding Proteins Bound to Vitronectin Enhance Keratinocyte Protein Synthesis and Migration.** *Journal of Investigative Dermatology* 122(5):1198-1206 (2004). IGF-II binds directly to vitronectin, a component of the extracellular skin matrix, to enhance protein synthesis and migration by skin cells in wound healing and skin regeneration.

168 Bhora Y, et al. **Effect of growth factors on cell proliferation and epithelialization in human skin.** *Journal of Surgical Research* 59(2):236-244 (1995). Fibroblast growth factor (FGF), IGF-I and epithelial growth factor (EGF) are important factors in healing skin wounds. EGF in particular is capable of initiating epithelial growth.

169 El Ghalbzouri A, Hensbergen P, Gibbs S, Kempenaar J, van der Schors R, Ponec M. **Fibroblasts facilitate re-epithelialization in wounded human skin equivalents.** *Laboratory Investigation* 84(1):102-112 (2004). Re-epithelialization of wounds begins with the migration of keratinocytes (skin cells) from the edges of the wound. This migration is dependent on the interaction of the keratinocytes with dermal fibroblasts and extracellular matrix. This migration is accelerated by EGF and keratinocyte growth factor.

170 Moller S, Jensen M, Svensson P, Skakkebaek NE. **Insulin-like growth factor I (IGF-I) in burn patients.** *Burns* 17(4):279-281 (1991). Impaired wound healing in large burns is related to suppressed levels of IGF-I in the burn area.

171 Kasemkijwattana C, Menetrey J, Bosch P, Somogyi G, Moreland MS, Fu FH, Buranapanitkit B, Watkins SS, Huard J. **Use of growth factors to improve muscle healing after strain injury.** *Clinical Orthopedics* 370:272-285 (2000). Muscle injuries, such as strains, are common in athletes. The use of growth factors, such as IGF-I, in treating such injuries is explored.

172 Sato K, Li Y, Foster W, Fukushima K, Badlani N, Adachi N, Usas A, Fu FH, Huard J. **Improvement of muscle healing through enhancement of muscle regeneration and prevention of fibrosis.** *Muscle & Nerve* 28(3):355-372 (2003). IGF-I can improve muscle regeneration in injured muscle.

173 Liang L, Ding YQ. **[Effect of cytokines on repair of tendon injury]** *Zhongguo Xiufu Chongjian Waike Zazhi* (Chinese) 14(5):283-285 (2000). Cytokines, such as the growth factors, can accelerate tendon repair.

174 Molloy T, Wang Y, Murrell G. **The roles of growth factors in tendon and ligament healing.** *Sports Medicine* 33(5):381-394 (2003). The roles of five different growth factors, IGF-I, TGF-β, vascular endothelial growth factor (VEGF), platelet-derived growth factor (PDGF) and basic fibroblast growth factor (bFGF), in healing tendon and ligament injuries is explored. Each plays a different but vital role in the process.

Chapter 5 Notes

175 Roodman GD. **Mechanisms of Bone Metastasis. Review Article.** *New England Journal of Medicine* 350:1655 (2004).

176 Sporn MB, Roberts AB, Shull JH, Smith JM, Ward JM, Sodek J. **Polypeptide transforming growth factors isolated from bovine sources and used for wound healing in vivo.** *Science* 219(4590):1329-1331 (1983). TGF from cows was used to accelerate the healing of experimental wounds in rats by increasing the accumulation of protein, collagen and DNA in the affected area.

177 Holloway NM, Tyler JW, Lakritz J, Carlson SL, Holle J. **Serum immunoglobulin G concentrations in calves fed fresh and frozen colostrum.** *Journal of the American Veterinary Medicine Association* 219(3):357-359 (2001). No significant difference was found between the IgG concentrations of fresh bovine colostrum and frozen and thawed bovine colostrum.

178 Powick, WC. **Inactivation of Vitamin A by rancid fat.** *Journal of Agricultural Research* 31(11):1017-1026 (1925).

179 Godden SM, Smith S, Feirtag JM, Green LR, Wells SJ, Fetrow JP. **Effect of on-farm commercial batch pasteurization of colostrum on colostrum and serum immunoglobulin concentrations in dairy calves.** *Journal of Dairy Science* 86(4):1503-1523 (2003). Pasteurization of high quality colostrum reduces IgG concentrations by 23.6-58.5%.

180 Meylan M, Rings DM, Shulaw WP, Kowalski JJ, Bech-Nielsen S, Hoffsis GF. **Survival of *Mycobacterium paratuberculosis* and preservation of immunoglobulin G in bovine colostrum under experimental conditions simulating pasteurization.** *American Journal of Veterinary Research* 57(11):1580-1585 (1996). Pasteurization produced a mean loss of 12.3% of the IgG in colostrum.

181 Li-Chan E, Kummer A, Losso JN, Kitts DD, Nakai S. **Stability of bovine immunoglobulins to thermal treatment and processing.** *Food Research International* 28(1):9-16 (1995). Pasteurized milk, reconstituted skim milk powder and whey from cheddar cheese all showed high levels of IgG while canned evaporated milk and UHT sterilized milk had little or no IgG.

182 Yolken RH, Kummer A, Losso JN, Kitts DD, Nakai S. **Antibody to human rotavirus in cow's milk.** *New England Journal of Medicine* 312(10):605-610 (1985). Raw and pasteurized milk contain antibodies against rotavirus, an important cause of gastroenteritis and diarrhea in infants. However, infant formulas and other sterile milk preparations had little or no anti-rotaviral activity.

183 Dominguez E, Perez MD, Calvo M. **Effect of heat treatment on the antigen-binding activity of anti-peroxidase immunoglobulins in bovine colostrum.** *Journal of Dairy Science* 80(12):3182-3187 (1997). A negative correlation was made between temperature

and time in the denaturation of IgG, i.e. the higher the temperature, the shorter the time needed for denaturation to occur.

184 Collier RJ, Miller MA, Hildebrandt JR, Torkelson AR, White TC, Madsen KS, Vicini JL, Eppard PJ, Lanza GM. **Factors affecting insulin-like growth factor-I concentration in bovine milk.** *Journal of Dairy Science* 74(9):2905-2911 (1991). IGF-1 levels are highest in colostrum and lower in mature milk. Concentration was not altered by pasteurization (79°C for 45 seconds) but was undetectable at higher temperatures (121°C for 5 minutes) used for infant formula preparation and in commercial infant formula.

185 Paulsson MA, Svensson U, Kishore AR, Naidu AS. **Thermal behavior of bovine lactoferrin in water and its relation to bacterial interaction and antibacterial activity.** *Journal of Dairy Science* 76(12):3711-3720 (1993). Lactoferrin which was either unheated or pasteurized showed similar activity, while lactoferrin exposed to UHT treatment decreased its ability to bind to bacterial species and destroyed its ability to inhibit bacterial growth.

Chapter 6 Notes

186 Mietens C, Keinhorst H, Hilpert H, Gerber H, Amster H, Pahud JJ. **Treatment of infantile E. coli gastroenteritis with specific bovine anti-E.coli milk immunoglobulins.** *European Journal of Pediatrics* 132:239-52 (1979).

187 Tacket CO, Losonsky G, Link H, Hoang Y, Guesry P, Hipert H, Levine MM. (1988). **Protection by milk immunoglobulin concentrate against oral challenge with enterogenic Escherichia coli.** *New England Journal of Medicine* 318:1240-1241 (1988).

188 Tzipori CO, Binion SB, Bostwick E, Losonsky G, Roy MJ, Edelman R. **Remission of diarrhoea due to cryptosporidosis in an immunodeficient child treated with hyperimmune bovine colostrum.** *British Medical Journal* 293:1276-1277 (1986).

189 Ebina T, Sato A, Umezu K, Ishida N, Ohyama S, Oizumi A, Kitaoka S, Suzuki H, Kunno T. **Prevention of rotavirus infection by oral administration of cow colostrum containing antihuman rotavirus antibody.** *Medical Microbiology and Immunology* 174: 177-85 (1985).

190 Brussow H, Hipert H, Walther J, Sidoti J, Meitens C, Bachman P. **Bovine milk immunoglobulins for passive immunity to infantile rotavirus gastroenteritus.** *Journal of Clinical Microbiology* 25:982-986 (1987).

191 Hilpert H, Brussow H, Meitens C, Sidoti J, Lerner L, Werchau H. **Use of bovine milk concentrate containing antibody to rotavirus to treat rotavirus gastroenteritis in infants.** *Journal of Infectious Diseases* 156:158-66 (1987).

192 Tacket CO, Binion SB, Bostwick E, Losonsky G, Roy MJ, Edelman R. (1992). **Efficacy of bovine milk immunoglobulin concentrate in preventing illness after Shigella**

flexneri challenge. *American Journal of Tropical Medicine and Hygiene* 47:276-283 (1992).

193 Tyrell D. **Breast feeding and virus infection: the immunity of infant feeding.** New York, Plenum Press, 1980, pp. 55-61.

194 Khazenson, 1980, op. cit.

195 Hilpert H, Gerber H, Amster H, Pahud JJ, Ballabriga A, Arcalis L,Farriaux JP, de Peyer E, Nussle D. **Bovine milk immunoglobulins (Ig) and their possible utilisation in industrially prepared infant's milk formulae.** In: Food and Immunology, Swedish Nutritional Foundation Symposium XIII, L. Hambraeus, L. A. Hanson, and H. McFarlane, eds., pp 182-196. Almquist and Wiksell, Stockholm, 1977.

196 Rona Z. **Bovine Colostrum emerges as immunity modulator.** *American Journal of Natural Medicine* 5(2):19-23 (1998).

197 Kim K, Keller MA, Heiner DC. **Immunoglobulin G subclasses in human colostrum, milk and saliva.** *Acta Paediatrica* 81(2):113-118 (1992). Human colostrum contains 47% IgG1, 44% IgG2, IgG3 <4%, and IgG4 6%.

198 Aalberse RC, Van der Gaag R, Van Leeuwen J. **Serological aspects of IgG4 antibodies I. Prolonged immunisation results in an IgG4-restricted response.** *Journal of Immunology* 130(2):722-726 (1983). Individuals immunized over a period of several years with phospholipase from honey bee venom, grass pollen allergen or house dust mite allergen show a shift in IgG4:IgG1 antibody ration that finally results in an IgG4 dominated antibody response.

199 Seto A, Okabe T, Ito Y. **Immunoglobulin M associated with secretory component and immunoglobulin A deficiency in bovine colostrum.** *American Journal of Veterinary Research* 38(11):1895-1896 (1977). IgM was found in bovine colostrum associated with the secretory component of sIgA.

200 Boes M, Prodeus AP, Schmidt T, Carroll MC, Chen J. **A critical role of natural immunoglobulin M in immediate defense against systemic bacterial infection.** *Journal of Experimental Medicine* 188(12):2381-2386 (1998). Mice were tested for their response to an experimentally induced systemic bacterial infection. 20% of wild mice died within 32 hours, while 70% of IgM deficient mice died within the same time period. When IgM deficient mice were given IgM, their resistance was restored to that of wild mice.

201 Diamond MS, Sitati EM, Friend LD, Higgs S, Shrestha B, Engle M. **A critical role for induced IgM in the protection against West Nile virus infection.** *Journal of Experimental Medicine* 198(12):1853-1862 (2003). Mice deficient in the production of secreted IgM, even though they were still capable of producing surface IgM and other immunoglobulins, were much more susceptible to lethal infection with West Nile virus than wild mice.

202 Thatcher EF, Gershwin LJ. **Colostral transfer of bovine immunoglobulin E and dynamics of serum IgE in calves.** *Veterinary Immunology and Immunopathology* 20(4):325-334 (1989). Blood serum levels of IgE in calves was high for the first week postpartum,

after which levels declined until 12 weeks of age, when they began to increase again. This suggests that passive transfer of IgE from the mother via colostrum is important in providing the calf immune protection during the first weeks of life.

203 Sarfati M, Vanderbeeken Y, Rubio-Trujillo M, Duncan D, Delespesse G. **Presence of IgE suppressor factors in human colostrum.** *European Journal of Immunology* 16(8):1005-1008 (1986). Human colostrum contains IgE-binding factors which inactivate IgE, suggesting an anti-allergy possible role for colostrum.

204 Keller MA, Heiner DC, Myers AS, Reisinger DM. **IgD in human colostrum.** *Pediatric Research* 19(1):122-126 (1985). Concentrations of IgD in human colostrum were measured in a range from 2.2-410 μg/dl (mean concentration 35 μg/dl).

205 Korhonen H, Marnila P, Gill HS. **Milk immunoglobulins and complement factors.** *British Journal of Nutrition* 84(Suppl 1):S75-S80 (2000). In addition to immunoglobulins, bovine colostrum also contains the complement system, which plays a crucial role in the passive immunization of the calf. Complement activity in bovine colostrum and milk has both hemolytic and bactericidal functions.

206 Nakajima S, Baba AS, Tamura N. **Complement system in human colostrum: presence of nine complement components and factors of alternative pathway in human colostrum.** *International Archives of Allergy and Applied Immunology* 54(5):428-433 (1977). All nine components of the complement system (C1-C9) have been found in human colostrum.

207 Lonnerdal B, Iyer S. **Lactoferrin: molecular structure and biological function.** *Annual Review of Nutrition* 15:93-110 (1995).

208 Harmsen MC, Swart PJ, de Bethune MP, Pauwels R, De Clercq E, The TH, Meijer DK. **Antiviral effects of plasma and milk proteins: lactoferrin shows potent activity against both human immunodeficiency virus and human cytomegalovirus replication in vitro.** *Journal of Infectious Diseases* 172(2):380-388 (1995). Native lactoferrin from colostrum and milk completely blocked CMV infection and inhibited the HIV-1 cytopathic effect. Lactoferrin likely exerts its effect at the level of virus adsorption and/or penetration as the effect is no longer seen once the virus is inside target cells.

209 Andersson Y, Lindquist S, Lagerqvist C, Hernell O. **Lactoferrin is responsible for the fungistatic effect of human milk.** *Early Human Development* 59(2):95-102 (2001). Lactoferrin inhibits the growth of *Candida albicans* through its ability to sequester iron.

210 Levay PF, Viljoen M. **Lactoferrin: a general review.** *Haematologica* 80(3):252-267 (1995).

211 Valenti P, Marchetti M, Superti F, Amendolia MG, Puddu P, Gessani S, Borghi P, Belardelli F, Antonini G, Seganti L. **Antiviral activity of lactoferrin.** *Advances in Experimental and Medical Biology* 443:199-203 (1998).

212 Superti F, Ammendolia MG, Valenti P, Seganti L. **Anti-rotaviral activity of milk proteins: lactoferrin prevents rotavirus infection in the enterocyte-like cell**

line HT-29. *Medical Microbiology and Immunology (Berlin)* 186(2-3):83-91 (1997). Antiviral activity against rotavirus of alpha lactalbumin, beta lactoglobulin, apo-lactoferrin (iron-free) and iron saturated lactoferrin were compared to that of mucin, which has known anti-rotaviral activity. Beta lactoglobulin and both forms of lactoferrin showed anti-rotaviral activity with the strongest response elicited by apo-lactoferrin, which hinders viral attachment to cells by binding directly to the viruses. It also markedly inhibits viral antigen synthesis in the viral adhesion stage.

213 Hashizume S, Kuroda K, Murakami H. **Identification of lactoferrin as an essential growth factor for human lymphocytic cell lines in serum-free medium.** *Biochimica et Biophysica Acta* 763(4):377-382 (1983). Lactoferrin is an essential growth factor for lymphocytes. It has higher growth stimulatory activity than transferrin. Bovine lactoferrin was found to be as effective as human.

214 Gahr M, Speer CP, Damerau B, Sawatzki G. **Influence of lactoferrin on the function of human polymorphonuclear leukocytes and monocytes.** *Journal of Leukocyte Biology* 49(5):427-433 (1991). Polymorphonuclear leukocytes (PMN) exposed to lactoferrin from colostrum exhibit increased random motility and are able to produce more superoxide. Monocytes and monocyte-derived macrophages did not exhibit the same effects when exposed to lactoferrin, so this is a specific effect of lactoferrin on PMN.

215 Damiens E, Mazurier J, El Yazidi I, Masson M, Duthille I, Spik G, Boilly-Marer Y. **Effects of human lactoferrin on NK cell cytotoxicity against haematopoietic and epithelial tumour cells.** *Biochimica et Biophysica Acta* 1402(3):277-287 (1998). Lactoferrin has a pronounced effect on NK cell cytotoxicity against cells from hematopoietic and epithelial cell tumor lines.

216 Kuhara T, Yamauchi K, Tamura Y, Okamura H. **Oral administration of lactoferrin increases NK cell activity in mice via increased production of IL-18 and type I IFN in the small intestine.** *Journal of Interferon and Cytokine Research* 26(7):489-499 (2006). Orally administered bovine lactoferrin increases NK cell populations in blood and spleen and enhances interferon-gamma production. It also increases the production of IL-18 and increases the production of interferon-alpha and interferon-beta in the Peyer's Patches in the intestines and mesenteric lymph nodes.

217 Artym, J. **[Antitumor and chemopreventive activity of lactoferrin]** *Post py Higieny i Medycyny Do wiadczalnej* 60:352-369 (2006). Lactoferrin participates in iron homeostasis, immunoregulatory, anti-inflammatory, anti-tumor, and analgesic activity, regulation of bone metabolism, embryonic development, reproductive functions, and others. It demonstrates direct anti-tumor activity, such as lytic, pro-apoptotic (programmed cell death), anti-proliferative, anti-angiogenic, anti-oxidant and chelation of iron. It also has chemo-preventive properties, regulates the activity of phase I and phase II enzymes participating in the activation and detoxification of carcinogens, and regulates the composition of the intestinal microflora. It stimulates the release of a number of cytokines, including IL-1, IL-6,

IL-8, IL-18, INF-γ and TNF-α. It increases the number and activity of T and B lymphocytes and NK cells and increases the phagocytic activity of monocytes and macrophages.

218 Ward PP, Uribe-Luna S, Conneely OM. **Lactoferrin and host defense.** *Biochemistry and Cell Biology* 80(1):95-102 (2002). Lactoferrin is a prominent component of the first line of defense against infection and inflammation. It accomplishes its activity through a variety of methods, most notably iron sequestration and its effect on down-regulating TNF- , which controls the inflammatory cascade.

219 Elrod, KC, Moore WR, Abraham WM, Tanaka RD. **Lactoferrin, a potent tryptase inhibitor, abolishes late-phase airway responses in allergic sheep.** *American Journal of Respiratory Critical Care Medicine* 156(2 Pt 1):375-381 (1997). Lactoferrin released from neutrophil granules inhibits tryptase, which is involved in late-phase bronchoconstriction and airway hyperactivity in asthma.

220 Kuhara T, Iigo M, Itoh T, Ushida Y, Sekine K, Terada N, Okamura H, Tsuda H. **Orally administered lactoferrin exerts an antimetastatic effect and enhances production of IL-18 in the intestinal epithelium.** *Nutrition and Cancer* 38(2):192-199 (2000). A study on the protective effects of lactoferrin supplementation against lung metastasis in experimentally induced colon cancer. In addition to the increase in cytotoxic cells seen in other studies, there was also an increase in IL-18 production in the intestinal epithelium, suggesting it plays a role in mediating the inhibition of the cancers.

221 Baveye S, Elass E, Mazurier J, Spik G, Legrand D. **Lactoferrin: a multifunctional glycoprotein involved in the modulation of the inflammatory process.** *Clinical Chemistry and Laboratory Medicine* 37(3):281-286 (1999).

222 Artym, 2006. op cit.

223 Chipman DM, Sharon N. **Mechanism of lysozyme action.** *Science* 165(892):454-465. Lysozyme degrades the outer wall of gram-positive bacteria by hydrolyzing -1,4 linkages of outer wall constituents.

224 Ellison RT III, Giehl TJ. **Killing of gram-negative bacteria by lactoferrin and lysozyme.** *Journal of Clinical Investigation* 88(4):1080-1091 (1991). Lactoferrin and lysozyme act in concert to kill gram-negative bacteria. Lactoferrin alters the protective outer membrane of the bacteria, allowing lysozyme to penetrate to the inner membrane, disrupting it and causing the bacteria to lyse (burst).

225 Steele WF, Morrison M. **Anti-streptococcal activity of lactoperoxidase.** *Journal of Bacteriology* 97(2):635-639 (1969).

226 Björck L, Rosen C, Marshall V, Reiter B. **Antibacterial activity of the lactoperoxidase system in milk against pseudomonads and other gram-negative bacteria.** *Applied Microbiology* 30(2):199-204 (1975).

227 Pakkanen R, Aalto J. **Review Paper: Growth Factors and Antimicrobial Factors of Bovine Colostrum.** *International Dairy Journal* 1997(7):285-297 (1997). Cows pass immunity from mother to calf via the immune factors in colostrum. It also contains many

growth factors. IGF-1 and IGF-2 are especially important in stimulating cell growth in the gut of the newborn. Both the growth factors and immune factors may become important components of clinical nutrition in the future.

228 Torre C, Jeusette I, Serra M, Brazis P, Puigdemont A. **Bovine colostrum increases proliferation of canine skin fibroblasts.** *Journal of Nutrition* 7(Suppl):2058S-2060S (2006). Bovine colostrum is a rich source of immunoglobulins, insulin-like growth factors, transforming growth factor-β, platelet-derived growth factor, epidermal growth factor, basic fibroblast growth factor, vascular endothelial growth factor, tumor necrosis factor and telomerase. Bovine colostrum stimulates the proliferation of skin fibroblasts in dogs, an important model for topical applications in wound repair and periodontal tissue repair.

229 Donovan SM, Odle J. **Growth factors in milk as mediators of infant development.** *Annual Review of Nutrition* 14:147-167 (1994). Many of the growth factors found in colostrum and milk, such as IGF-1, IGF-II, insulin, relaxin, epidermal growth factor, TGF-a, TGF-β, nerve growth factor and others, are essential to the normal growth and development of the newborn.

230 Borody TJ, Surace R, Warren E. **Tunnel vision in the bowel.** *Centre for Digestive Diseases, Australia* (2001). The growth factors in colostrum help heal intestinal erosions and ulcerations. It also contains anti-inflammatory factors and is nutrient rich.

231 Canalis E, McCarthy TL, Centrella M. **Growth factors and cytokines in bone cell metabolism.** *Annual Review of Medicine* 42:17-24 (1991). Growth factors regulate the growth and differentiated function of cells. Skeletal cells synthesize fibroblast growth factor, platelet-derived growth factor, insulin-like growth factor, transforming growth factor beta, and additional cytokines. Some of the growth factors produced by bone cells primarily stimulate bone cell replication, whereas others also affect the differentiated function of the osteoblast.

232 Canalis E, McCarthy TL, Centrella M. **The role of growth factors in skeletal remodeling.** *Endocrinology and Metabolism Clinics of North America* 18(4):903-918 (1989). Growth factors play a significant role in bone remodeling, normal bone maintenance, fracture repair and wound healing.

233 Molloy T, Wang Y, Murrell G. **The roles of growth factors in tendon and ligament healing.** *Sports Medicine* 33(5):381-394 (2003). Growth factors are one of the most important components of healing. IGF-1 is involved in the early stages following injury in the proliferation and migration of fibroblasts (connective tissue cells) and the increase of collagen production. TGF-β is active during inflammation of the injured area and plays a role in cellular migration and proliferation. VEGF is most active following the inflammatory phase when it stimulates angiogenesis, the growth of blood vessels into the damaged area. PDGF comes into play immediately after injury and acts to stimulate the production of the other growth factors as well as tissue remodeling. FGF is a powerful stimulator of

angiogenesis and cell proliferation and migration. Adding these factors to the wound site, such as through colostrum supplementation, has been shown to speed the healing process.
234 Flidel-Rimon O, Roth P. **Effects of milk-borne colony stimulating factor-1 on circulating growth factor levels in the newborn infant.** *Journal of Pediatrics* 131(5):748-750 (1997). Levels of CSF-1 were 25 times greater in colostrum than in serum at birth.
235 Yagi H, Suzuki S, Noji T, Nagashima K, Kuroume T. **Epidermal growth factor in cow's milk and milk formulas.** *Acta Paediatrica Scandinavica* 75(2):233-235 (1986). EGF was found in both bovine and human milk in very nearly the same amounts.
236 Xiao X, Xiong A, Chen X, Mao X, Zhou X. **Epidermal growth factor concentrations in human milk, cow's milk and cow's milk-based infant formulas.** *Chinese Medical Journal (English)* 115(3):451-454 (2002). EGF content of cow's milk, human term and preterm colostrum and different milk-based formulas. Highest levels of EGF were found in colostrum from mothers with premature infants, suggesting an adaptation to help the premature infants develop their guts faster. EGF levels in cow's milk were similar to that of term human milk. EGF levels in non-hydrolyzed milk-based formulas were much lower than whole milk and undetectable in hydrolyzed formulas.
237 Boonstra J, Rijken P, Humbel B, Cremers F, Verkleij A, van Bergen en Henegouwen P. **The epidermal growth factor.** *Cell Biology International* 19(5):413-430 (1995). Epidermal growth factor (EGF) is a single polypeptide of 53 amino acid residues involved in the regulation of cell proliferation. It exerts its effects in the target cells by binding to the plasma membrane located EGF receptor.
238 Bhora FY, Dunkin BJ, Batzri S, Aly HM, Bass BL, Sidawy AN, Harmon JW. **Effect of growth factors on cell proliferation and epithelialization in human skin.** *Journal of Surgical Research* 59(2):235-244 (1995). EGF, FGF and IGF-1 are all mitogenic in healing wounds of the skin.
239 Dunbar AJ, Priebe IK, Belford DA, Goddard C. **Identification of betacellulin as a major peptide growth factor in milk: purification, characterization and molecular cloning of bovine betacellulin.** *Biochemistry Journal* 344(Pt 3):713-721 (1999). Betacellulin, a member of the Epidermal Growth Factor family, was isolated from bovine milk whey. It is a glycosylated protein. Its presence in milk suggests it may play a role in the growth and development of the neonatal gastrointestinal tract.
240 Bastian SE, Dunbar AJ, Priebe IK, Owens PC, Goddard C. **Measurement of betacellulin levels in bovine serum, colostrum and milk.** *Journal of Endocrinology* 168(1):203-212 (2001). Betacellulin, a member of the Epidermal Growth Factor (EGF) family, was isolated from bovine colostrum, milk and serum. Highest levels were found in fetal bovine serum, suggesting an endocrine role in the bovine fetus.
241 Hironaka T, Ohishi H, Masaki T. **Identification and partial purification of a basic fibroblast growth factor-like growth factor derived from bovine colostrum.**

Journal of Dairy Science 80(3):488-495 (1997). A protein that behaves like FGF was isolated from the cream fraction of bovine colostrum.

242 Canalis, 1989, op cit.

243 Szabo S, Sandor Z. **Basic fibroblast growth factor and PDGF in GI diseases.** *Baillieres Clinical Gastroenterology* 10(1):97-112 (1996). Both bFGF and PDGF play a role in the healing of gastric and duodenal ulcers.

244 Calhoun DA, Maheshwari A, Christensen RD. **Recombinant granulocyte colony-stimulating factor administered enterally to neonates is not absorbed.** *Pediatrics* 112(2):421-423 (2003). G-CSF is present in amniotic fluid, colostrum and milk. It primarily acts locally on cells in the gut.

245 Collier RJ, Miller MA, Hidledbrandt JR, Torkelson AR, White TC, Madsen KS, Vicini JL, Eppad PK, Lanza GF. **Factors affecting insulin-like growth-I concentration in bovine colostrums.** *Journal of Dairy Science* 74(9):2905–2911 (1991). While lower than the concentrations of human milk, bovine colostrum and milk contained IGF-1 in quantities that decreased with time after birth of the calf.

246 Torre, 2006, op cit.

247 Blumenfeld I, Srouji S, Lanir Y, Laufer D, Livne E. **Enhancement of bone defect healing in old rats by TGF-beta and IGF-1.** *Experimental Gerontology* 37(4):553-565 (2002). Bone healing in the elderly is often slow and is dependent on the availability of various hormones and growth factors. Bone defects induced in aged rats healed much more quickly in rats given either TGF-β or IGF-1, with a combination of both producing the fastest healing.

248 Adams GR, Haddad F. **The relationships among IGF-1, DNA content, and protein accumulation during skeletal muscle hypertrophy.** *Journal of Applied Physiology* 81(6):2509-2516 (1996). The muscle of rats respond to functional overload by increased IGF-1 expression. The elevated IGF-1 appear to contribute to the hypertrophy response.

249 Bayes-Genis A, Conover CA, Schwartz RS. **The insulin-like growth factor axis: A review of atherosclerosis and restenosis.** *Circulation Research* 86(2):125-130 (2000). IGF-1, IGF-2 and their binding proteins are secreted by cells of the cardiovascular system. The dynamic balance of these factors, known as the IGF axis, influences vascular smooth muscle growth, migration and extracellular matrix synthesis. Dysregulation of the axis can result in the formation of atherosclerotic plaque and restenosis.

250 Rabinovsky ED. **The multifunctional role of IGF-1 in peripheral nerve regeneration.** *Neurological Research* 26(2):204-210 (2004). The ability of IGF-1 to promote nerve elongation and branching, angiogenesis (growth of blood vessels), the activation of muscle stem cells and so forth affects multiple layers of the regenerative response of peripheral nerves.

251 Xu RJ. **Development of the newborn GI tract and its relation to colostrum/milk intake: a review.** *Reproduction, Fertility and Development* 8(1):35-48 (1996). In the immediate postnatal period, the GI tract undergoes profound growth, morphological

changes and functional maturation. These changes are related to the onset of colostrum ingestion. Both EGF and IGF-I play a role in postal GI development.

252 O'Dell SD, Day IN. **Insulin-like growth factor II (IGF-II).** *International Journal of Biochemistry and Cell Biology* 30(7):767-771 (1998). IGF-2 plays a key role in mammalian growth, regulating fetal cell division and differentiation and possibly metabolic regulation.

253 Aranda P, Sanchez L, Perez MD, Ena JM, Calvo M. **Insulin in bovine colostrum and milk: evolution throughout lactation and binding to caseins.** *Journal of Dairy Science* 74(12):4320-4325 (1991). Highest levels of insulin were found in first milking colostrum (327 µg/l), which fell by 50% over the first 24 hours.

254 Fernandez-Moreno MD, Serrano-Rios M, Prieto JC. **Identification of insulin receptors in epithelial cells from duodenum, jejunum, ileum, caecum, colon and rectum in the rat.** *Diabetes Metabolism* 13(2):135-139 (1987).

255 Blum JW, Baumrucker CR. **Colostral and milk insulin-like growth factors and related substances: mammary gland and neonatal (intestinal and systemic) targets.** *Domesticated Animal Endocrinology* 23(1-2):101-110 (2002). Both IGFs and IGFBPs influence mammary gland biology towards the end of lactation. IGFBP-3, the major IGFBP in cows, binds to both IGF and lactoferrin. With lactoferrin, it can enter the nucleus of epithelial cells and affect apoptotic (programmed cell death) signaling through retinoic-x-receptors as part of mammary gland involution.

256 Bayes-Genis, 2000, op. cit.

257 Shing Y, Klagsbrun M. **Purification and characterization of a bovine colostrum-derived growth factor.** *Molecular Endocrinology* 1(5):335-338 (1987). PDGF was identified in bovine colostrum.

258 Canalis E, Varghese S, McCarthy TL, Centrella M. **Role of platelet derived growth factor in bone cell function.** *Growth Regulation* 2(4):151-155 (1992). PDGF is a mitogen of osteoblasts and probably plays a role in bone remodeling. It also plays a role in inflammation and wound healing.

259 Hollinger JO, Hart CE, Hirsch SN, Lynch S, Friedlaender GE. **Recombinant human platelet-derived growth factor: biology and clinical applications.** *Journal of Bone and Joint Surgery* 90(Suppl 1):48-54 (2008). PDGF functions as a potent chemoattractant and mitogen for osteogenic (bone-forming) cells and promotes angiogenesis (formation of blood vessels), making it valuable in the treatment of bone and soft tissue disorders, such as osteoporosis, diabetes and the effects of smoking.

260 Carlberg M, Larsson O. **Stimulatory effect of PDGF on HMG-CoA reductase activity and N-linked glycosylation contributes to increased expression of IGF-I receptors in human fibroblasts.** *Experimental Cell Research* 223(1):142-148 (1996). PDGF mediates the growth activation of fibroblasts.

261 Szabo, 1996, op cit.

262 Kim HR, Upadhyay S, Li G, Palmer KC, Deuel TF. **Platelet-derived growth factor**

induces apoptosis in growth-arrested murine fibroblasts. *Proceedings of the National Academy of Sciences (USA)* 92(21):9500-9504 (1995). PDGF is a potent mitogen (inducer of cell division) in fibroblasts. When fibroblasts are deprived of serum, however, they stop their development. If then stimulated by PDGF, the cells undergo apoptotic cell death. This suggests that PDGF can influence both cell division and cell death, depending on the state of the cell.

263 Molloy, 2003, op. cit.

264 Okada M, Ohmura E, Kamiya Y, Murakami H, Onoda N, Iwashita M, Wakai K, Tsushima T, Shizume K. **Transforming growth factor (TGF)-alpha in human milk.** *Life Sciences* 48(12):1151-1156 (1991).

265 Wagner CL, Forsythe DW, Pittard WB. **Variation in the biochemical forms of transforming growth factor-alpha present in human milk and secreted by human milk macrophages.** *Biology of the Neonate* 68(5):325-333 (1995). TGF-α, a component of human colostrum and milk, plays a significant role in postnatal gut development.

266 Wagner CL, Forsythe DW, Wagner MT. **The effect of recombinant TGF-alpha, human milk, and human milk macrophage media on gut epithelial proliferation is decreased in the presence of a neutralizing TGF-alpha antibody.** *Biology of the Neonate* 74(5):363-371 (1998).

267 Wagner CL, Forsythe DW. **Effect of human milk and recombinant EGF, TGF-alpha, and IGF-1 on small intestinal cell proliferation.** *Advances in Experimental Medicine and Biology* 478:373-374 (2000).

268 Fallon J, Reid S, Kinyamu R, Opole I, Opole R, Baratta J, Korc M, Endo TL, Duong A, Nguyen G, Karkehabadhi M, Twardzik D, Patel S, Loughlin S. **In vivo induction of massive proliferation, directed migration, and differentiation of neural cells in the adult mammalian brain.** *Proceedings of the National Academy of Sciences (USA)* 97(26):14686-14691 (2000). TGF-α infused directly into damaged rat forebrains resulted in massive proliferation, directed migration and neurodifferentiation (PMD).

269 Saito S, Yoshida M, Ichijo M, Ishizaka S, Tsujii T. **Transforming growth factor-beta (TGF-beta) in human milk.** *Clinical and Experimental Immunology* 94(1):220-224 (1993). Both TGF-β1 and TGF-β2 were found in human milk.

270 Ginjala V, Pakkanen R. **Determination of transforming growth factor-beta 1 (TGF-beta 1) and insulin-like growth factor (IGF-1) in bovine colostrum samples.** *Journal of Immunoassay* 19(2-3):195-207 (1998).

271 Pakkanen, R. **Determination of transforming growth factor-beta 2 (TGF-beta 2) in bovine colostrum samples.** *Journal of Immunoassay* 19(1):23-37 (1998). TGF-β2 is the major form of TGF-β in colostrum.

272 Tokuyama Y, Tokuyama H. **Purification and identification of TGF-beta 2-related growth factor from bovine colostrum.** *Journal of Dairy Research* 60(1):99-109 (1993).

High levels of TGF-β2 activity are found in early bovine colostrum.

273 Purup S, Vestergaard M, Pedersen O, Sejrsen K. **Biological activity of bovine milk on proliferation of human intestinal cells.** *Journal of Dairy Research* 74(1):58-65 (2007). Bovine milk and colostrum contain a number of biologically active components that affect the growth and development of human intestinal tissues, including TGF-β1, TGF-β2, IGF-1, IGF-2 and others.

274 Coffman RL, Lebman DA, Shrader B. **Transforming growth factor beta specifically enhances IgA production by lipopolysaccharide-stimulated murine B lymphocytes.** *Journal of Experimental Medicine* 170(3):1039-1044 (1989).

275 Chen SS, Li Q. **Transforming growth factor-beta 1 (TGF-beta 1) is a bifunctional immune regulator for mucosal IgA responses.** *Cellular Immunology* 128(2):353-361 (1990). TGF- β1 is a potent costimulator with LPS-induced IgA responses while also exerting a profound immunosuppressive effect on IL-5 induced IgA synthesis. TGF-β1 is produced by intestinal epithelial cells that may help ensure the integrity of the mucosal surface.

276 Centrella M, McCarthy TL, Canalis E. **Skeletal tissue and transforming growth factor beta.** *FASEB Journal* 2(15):3066-2073 (1988). TGF-β regulates replication and differentiation of mesenchymal precursor cells, chondrocytes, osteoblasts and osteoclasts. Its activity is controlled at many different levels by both local and systemic agents. It is vital to skeletal growth during development, maintenance of bone mass in adults, and healing of fractures.

277 Centrella M, McCarthy TL, Canalis E. **Effects of transforming growth factors on bone cells.** *Connective Tissue Research* 20(1-4):267-275 (1989). TGF-β controls abundance and biochemical function of osteoclasts and osteoblasts.

278 Torre, 2006, op cit.

279 Molloy, 2003, op cit.

280 Bessler H, Straussberg R, Hart J, Notti I, Sirota L. **Human colostrum stimulates cytokine production.** *Biology of the Neonate* 69(6):376-382 (1996). Human colostrum stimulates the production of IL-1, IL-3 and IL-6 in blood monocytes.

281 Bocci V, von Bremen K, Corradeschi F, Luzzi E, Paulesu L. **What is the role of cytokines in human colostrum?** *Journal of Biological Regulators and Homeostatic Agents* 5(4):121-124 (1991). Colostrum contains IL-1, IL-6, TNF-α and interferon-γ which may exert an important immunostimulatory role particularly on oropharyngeal-associated lymphoid tissue. Oral supplementation with cytokines may be of benefit to aged or immunodeficient people.

282 Goto M, Maruyama M, Kitadate K, Kirisawa R, Obata Y, Koiwa M, Iwai H. **Detection of interleukin-1 beta in sera and colostrum of dairy cattle and in sera of neonates.** *Journal of Veterinary Medical Science* 59(6):437-441 (1997). IL-1β was present in high volumes in bovine milk for 20 days prepartum and 3 days postpartum.

283 Hagiwara K, Kataoka S, Yamanaka H, Kirisawa R, Iwai H. **Detection of cytokines in bovine colostrum.** *Veterinary Immunology and Immunopathology* 76(3-4):183-190 (2000). IL-1β, IL-6, TNF-α, INF-γ and IL-1 receptor antagonist (IL-1ra) were found in higher concentrations in bovine colostrum than in mature milk. These appear to play a role in neonatal immunity.

284 Zizka J, Kverka M, Novotna O, Stankova I, Lodinova-Zadnikova R, Kocourkova I, Sterzl I, Prokesova L. **Perinatal period cytokines related to increased risk of future allergy development.** *Folia Microbiologica (Praha)* 52(5):549-555 (2007). Cytokine levels were tested in the colostrum, cord blood and amniotic fluid of healthy and allergic mothers. Differences in levels of IL-5, IL-10, TGF-β, TNF-α, EGF and eotaxin were found. Allergic mothers and children also tended to have higher levels of IL-4.

285 Zizka, 2007, ibid

286 Rudloff HE, Schmalstieg FC Jr, Palkowetz KH, Paszkiewicz EJ, Goldman AS. **Interleukin-6 in human milk.** *Journal of Reproductive Immunology* 23(1):13-20 (1993). IL-6 was isolated from human milk (colostrum) collected within the first day postpartum.

287 Hashira S, Okitsu-Negishi S, Yoshino K. **Interleukin 8 in the human colostrum.** *Biology of the Neonate* 82(1):34-38 (2002). IL-8 was produced by colostral cells *in vitro*.

288 Garofalo R, Chheda S, Mei F, Palkowetz KH, Rudloff HE, Schmalstieg FC, Rassin DK, Goldman AS. **Interleukin-10 in human milk.** *Pediatric Research* 37(4pt1):444-449 (1995). IL-10 was found in both aqueous and lipid phases of human milk (colostrum)

289 Bryan DL, Hawkes JS, Gibson RA. **Interleukin-12 in human milk.** *Pediatric Research* 45(6):858-859 (1999). Concentrations of IL-12 in human colostrum, transitional milk and mature Interleukin-12 in human milk were studied, with highest concentrations being found in colostrum, declining over time to mature milk.

290 Takahata Y, Takada H, Nomura A, Ohshima K, Nakayama H, Tsuda T, Nakano H, Hara T. **Interleukin-18 in human milk.** *Pediatric Research* 50(2):268-272 (2001). IL-18 levels were found to be highest in colostrum compared to transitional and mature milk. IL-18 levels were correlated to high concentrations of soluble Fas ligand. Levels of IL-18 were significantly higher in mothers with preterm delivery and pregnancy problems, indicating that IL-18 plays a significant role in host defense of high-risk infants.

291 Bocci, 1991, op. cit.

292 Bocci, 1991, op. cit.

293 Buescher ES, McWilliams-Koeppen P. **Soluble tumor necrosis factor-alpha (TNF-alpha) receptors in human colostrum and milk bind to TNF-alpha and neutralize TNF-alpha bioactivity.** *Pediatric Research* 44(1):37-42 (1998). TNF-α receptors in colostrum and milk bind to TNF-α and have the ability to block its activity. As TNF-α is the controlling factor in the inflammatory cascade, the ability of TNF-α receptors to turn it off signifies that this is one of the main anti-inflammatory mechanisms in colostrum and milk.

294 Kumura H, Miura A, Sato E, Tanaka T, Shimazaki K. **Susceptibility of bovine osteopontin to chymosin.** *Journal of Dairy Research* 71(4):500-504 (2004). Osteopontin is found in bovine colostrum.

295 Nagatomo, T, Ohga S, Takada H, Nomura A, Hikino S, Imura M, Ohshima K, Hara T. **Microarray analysis of human milk cells: persistent high expression of osteopontin during the lactation period.** *Clinical and Experimental Immunology* 138(1):47-53 (2004). Osteopontin is expressed in human milk at high levels beginning with the first milk or colostrum. It reaches a peak in early (transitional) milk. It may play a role in the immunological development of infants by activating T-lymphocytes.

296 Ashkar S, Weber GF, Panoutsakopoulou V, Sanchirico ME, Jansson M, Zawaideh S, Rittling SR, Denhardt DT, Glimcher MJ, Cantor H. **Eta-1 (osteopontin): an early component of type-1 (cell-mediated) immunity.** *Science* 287(5454):860-864 (2000). Cell-mediated (type-1) immunity is necessary for immune protection against most intracellular pathogens and, when excessive, can result in organ-specific autoimmune destruction. Mice deficient in the expression of the Eta-1 (osteopontin) gene have severely impaired type-1 immunity to both viral and bacterial infections. Osteopontin apparently acts through regulation of macrophage IL-10 and IL-12 expression through its interaction with the CD44 and integrin receptors respectively.

297 Vidal, K, van den Broek P, Lorget F, Donnet-Hughes A. **Osteoprotegerin in human milk: a potential role in the regulation of bone metabolism and immune development.** *Pediatric Research* 55(6):1001-1008 (2004). Osteoprotegerin, a cytokine member of the Tumor Necrosis Factor superfamily, is found in human milk and colostrum as well as bovine colostrum and milk. It inhibits osteoclast activity and helps regulate the immune system. It may help explain the mechanism of antiresorptive effect of milk on bone, helping prevent osteoporosis. Its presence in colostrum may help prevent immune and bone disorders in the newborn.

298 Maheshwari A, Christensen RD, Calhoun DA. **ELR+ CXC chemokines in human milk.** *Cytokine* 24(3):91-102 (2003). CXC chemokines with the glutamic acid-leucine-arginine motif (ELR) are found in human milk and are crucial mediators in neutrophil-dependent inflammation. All except NAP2/CXCL7 are found in higher concentrations in milk than in serum and are secreted by mammary epithelial cells. They may help protect intestinal epithelial cells.

299 Bottcher MF, Jenmalm MC, Bjorksten B. **Cytokine, chemokine and secretory IgA levels in human milk in relation to atopic disease and IgA production in infants.** *Pediatric Allergy and Immunity* 14(1):35-41 (2003). Levels of IL-4, -5, -6, -8, -10, -13, -16, IFN-γ, TGF-β1, TGF-β2, RANTES, eotaxin and SIgA were measured in colostrum and mature milk in relation to the development of positive skin prick tests for allergies and allergic symptoms in infants up to 2 years.

300 Srivastava MD, Srivastava A, Brouhard B, Saneto R, Groh-Wargo S, Kubit J. **Cytokines in**

human milk. *Research Communications in Molecular Pathology and Pharmacology* 93(3):263-287 (1996). Chemokines present in milk and colostrum included GRO-alpha, MCP-1, RANTES and IL-8.

301 Takahata Y, Takada H, Nomura A, Nakayama H, Ohshima K, Hara T. **Detection of interferon-gamma-inducible chemokines in human milk.** *Acta Paediatrica* 92(6):659-665 (2003). Levels of IP-10 and MIG were significantly higher in colostrum and transitional milk than in mature milk. IP-10 and MIG were produced both by mammary epithelial and milk cells. IP-10 and MIG may contribute to the migration and activation of intestinal T-lymphocytes in the early neonatal period.

302 Srivastava, 1996, op. cit.

303 Takahata, 2003, op. cit.

304 Bottcher, 2003, op. cit.

305 Staroscik, 1983, op. cit.

306 Janusz, 1993, op. cit.

307 Elahi S, Buchanan RM, Attah-Poku S, Townsend HG, Babiuk LA, Gerdts V. **The host defense peptide beta-defensin 1 confers protection against *Bordetella pertussis* in newborn piglets.** *Infection and Immunity* 74(4):2338-2352 (2006).

308 Armogida SA, Yannaras NM, Melton AL, Srivastava MD. **Identification and quantification of innate immune system mediators in human breast milk.** *Allergy and Asthma Proceedings* 25(5):297-304 (2004). Mediators of the innate immune system were found in human colostrum and milk, including defensins, cathelicidins, and toll-like receptors.

309 Filipp D, Alizadeh-Khiavi K, Richardson C, Palma A, Paredes N, Takeuchi O, Akira S, Julius M. **Soluble CD14 enriched in colostrum and milk induces B cell growth and differentiation.** *Proceedings of the National Academy of Sciences (USA)* 98(2):603-608 (2001).

310 Pasare C, Medzhitov R. **Toll-like receptors: linking innate and adaptive immunity.** *Microbes and Infection* 6(15):1382-1387 (2004). Toll-like receptors are the principal means of detection and response to microbial infections, including bacteria, viruses, fungi and protozoa. Initial recognition by the Toll-like receptors sets off a complex series of signaling events that sets off the immune response to the infection.

311 LeBouder E, Rey-Nores JE, Rushmere NK, Grigorov M, Lawn SD, Affolter M, Griffin GE, Ferrara P, Schiffrin EJ, Morgan BP, Labeta MO. **Soluble forms of Toll-like receptor (TLR)-2 capable of modulating TLR2 signaling are present in human plasma and breast milk.** *Journal of Immunology* 171(12):6680-6689 (2003). Failure of the innate immune response to bacterial infection can lead to septic shock and death. Toll-like receptors play a crucial role in the innate immune response and is found in human colostrum and milk.

312 Murakami M, Dorschner RA, Stern LJ, Lin KH, Gallo RL. **Expression and secretion of**

cathelicidin antimicrobial peptides in murine mammary glands and human milk. *Pediatric Research* 57(1):10-15 (2004). Antimicrobial peptides belonging to the cathelicidin family have recently been identified as being important components of the mammalian immune response. These peptides were found in both mouse and human milk and colostrum. They have antimicrobial activity against both gram-negative and gram-positive bacteria.

313 Newburg, DS. **Human milk glycoconjugates that inhibit pathogens.** *Current Medical Chemistry* 6(2):117-127 (1999). The protection offered by human milk may not be limited to just secretory IgA. Milk and colostrum contain numerous complex carbohydrates, including glycoproteins, glycolipids, glycosaminoglycans, mucins and oligosaccharides. Those with homology to cell surface glycoconjugate pathogen may inhibit pathogen binding by competing for binding sites. One of the fucosyloligo-saccharides inhibits *E. coli* toxin. Another inhibits infection by *Campylobacter jejuni.* Milk oligo-saccharides inhibit the binding of *Streptococcus pneumoniae* and enteropathogenic *E. coli.* Lactadherin inhibits rotavirus. A mannosylated glycopeptide inhibits binding by enterohemorrhagic *E. coli.* A glycosaminoglycan prevents binding of gp120 (a form of HIV) to CD4, the first step in HIV infection. Milk mucin inhibits binding of S-fimbriated *E. coli.* Ganglioside GM1 reduces diarrhea due to cholera toxin and *E. coli* labile toxin. Glycosphingolipid Gb3 binds to shiga toxin.

314 Kawasaki Y, Isoda H, Tanimoto M, Dosako S, Idota T, Ahiko K. **Inhibition by lactoferrin and kappa-casein glycomacropeptide of binding of Cholera toxin to its receptor.** *Bioscience, Biotechnology and Biochemistry* 56(2):195-198 (1992). Both lactoferrin and GMP from cow's milk inhibited the binding of Cholera toxin to a cultured cell line and ganglioside GM1.

315 Kawasaki Y, Isoda H, Shinmoto H, Tanimoto M, Dosako S, Idota T, Nakajima I. **Inhibition by kappa-casein glycomacropeptide and lactoferrin of influenza virus hemagglutination.** *Bioscience, Biotechnology and Biochemistry* 57(7):1214-1215 (1993).

316 Brody EP. **Biological activities of bovine glycomacropeptide.** *British Journal of Nutrition* 84(Suppl 1):S39-S46 (2000). Glycomacropeptide (GMP) has been found to be able to bind cholera and E. coli endotoxins, inhibit bacterial and viral adhesion, suppress gastric secretions, promote the growth of bifidobacteria and modulation of the immune system.

317 Makowski L, Brittingham KC, Reynolds JM, Suttles J, Hotamisligil GS. **The fatty acid binding protein, aP2, coordinates macrophage cholesterol trafficking and inflammatory activity: Macrophage expression of aP2 impacts peroxisome proliferator-activated receptor gamma and I-kappa kinase activities.** *Journal of Biological Chemistry* 280(13):12888-12895 (2005). The fatty acid-binding protein aP2 regulates two molecular pathways in macrophages to coordinate cholesterol uptake and inflammatory activity.

318 Sawyer L, Kontopidis G. **The core lipocalin, bovine beta-lactoglobulin.** *Biochemica et Biophysica Acta* 1482(1-2):136-148 (2000).

319 Superti F, Ammendolia MG, Valenti P, Seganti L. **Anti-rotaviral activity of milk proteins: lactoferrin prevents rotavirus infection in the enterocyte-like cell line HT-29.** *Medical Microbiology and Immunology (Berlin)* 186(2-3):83-91 (1997). Antiviral activity against rotavirus of alpha lactalbumin, beta lactoglobulin, apo-lactoferrin (iron-free) and iron saturated lactoferrin were compared to that of mucin, which has known anti-rotaviral activity. Beta lactoglobulin and both forms of lactoferrin showed anti-rotaviral activity with the strongest response elicited by apo-lactoferrin, which hinders viral attachment to cells by binding directly to the viruses. It also markedly inhibits viral antigen synthesis in the viral adhesion stage.

320 Ulcova-Gallova Z, Fialova P, Krauz V. **[Immunologic factors in human colostrum and milk].** *Casopis Lekaru Ceskych* 133(9):275-276 (1994). Colostrum was found to contain IgG, IgM, IgD, IgA, sIgA, C3, C4, orosomucoid, prealbumin, alpha 1-antitrypsin, alpha 1-fetoprotein, alpha 2-macroglobulin, haemopexin, haptoglobulin, beta 2-microglobulin, alpha 2-AP glycoprotein, and IgE.

321 Sorensson J, Ohlson M, Bjornson A, Haraldsson B. **Orosomucoid has a cAMP-dependent effect on human endothelial cells and inhibits the action of histamine.** *American Journal of Physiology – Heart and Circulatory Physiology* 278(5):H1725-1731 (2000). Orosomucoids negate the effect of histamine on human capillary endothelial cells and uses cAMP as a secondary messenger.

322 Kang SW, Lim SW, Choi SH, Shin KH, Chun BG, Park IS, Min BH. **Antisense oligonucleotide of clusterin mRNA induces apoptotic cell death and prevents adhesion of rat ASC-17D Sertoli cells.** *Molecules and Cells* 10(2):193-198 (2000). When the production of clusterin is blocked by antisense oligonucleotides of clusterin mRNA, cultured Sertoli cells are unable to attach to the Petri dish and therefore die. This indicates that clusterin plays an important role in cell-cell and cell-substratum interactions.

323 Carver JA, Rekas A, Thorn DC, Wilson MR. **Small heat-shock proteins and clusterin: intra- and extracellular molecular chaperones with a common mechanism of action and function?** *IBUMB Health* 55(12):661-668 (2003). So-called small heat shock (stress) proteins (sHsps) and clusterin both function as molecular chaperones, although they are not chemically related and sHsps are found intracellularly while clusterin is mostly found extracellularly. They act to prevent the aggregation and precipitation of target proteins under stress conditions, such as elevated temperature and redox reactions. Both are found in increased concentrations in disease states that involve protein misfolding and the deposition of highly structured protein aggregates (amyloid fibrils), such as Alzheimer's, Creutzfeld-Jakob and Parkinson's diseases.

324 Ulcova-Gallova, 1994, op cit.

325 Gutteridge JM, Smith A. **Antioxidant protection by haemopexin of haem-stimulated lipid peroxidation.** *Biochemical Journal* 256:861-865 (1988). Haem is a low molecular weight form of iron that is capable of taking part in oxygen radical reactions that

can lead to the degradation of proteins, lipids, carbohydrates and DNA. Haemopexin can inhibit such oxidative reactions by as much as 90%.

326 Tolosano E, Altruda F. **Hemopexin: structure, function, and regulation.** *DNA and Cell Biology* 21(4):297-306 (2002). Hemopexin's main role appears to be to act as an antioxidant after blood heme overload. It does not appear to participate in iron metabolism to any significant degree.

327 Smith A, Eskew JD, Borza CM, Pendrak M, Hunt RC. **Role of heme-hemopexin in human T-lymphocyte proliferation.** *Experimental Cell Research* 232(2):246-254 (1997). Heme-hemopexin supports and stimulates proliferation of human acute T-lymphoblastic (MOLT-3) cells, precursor cells to mature T-lymphocytes. MOLT-3 cells express approximately 58,000 hemopexin receptors per cell, about 20% of which are on the cell surface. Heme-hemopexin appears to act not only as an iron source, but the binding of the molecule to the receptor triggers a signaling pathway involved in the regulation of cell growth, stimulating the cells to proliferate.

328 Suzuki K, Namiki H. **[Serum hemopexin: suppressive effect on neutrophil functions and prospect of clinical application to autoimmune conditions]** *Nippon Rinsho* 62(3):577-586 (2004). Serum hemopexin suppresses neutrophil adhesion and phagocytosis by a mechanism unrelated to its haem-binding ability.

329 Suzuki K, Kobayashi N, Doi T, Hijikata T, Machida I, Namiki H. **Inhibition of Mg++-dependent adhesion of polymorphonuclear leukocytes by serum hemopexin: differences in divalent-cation dependency of cell adhesion in the presence and absence of serum.** *Cell Structure and Function* 28(4):243-253 (2003). Hemopexin has a strong inhibitory effect on the binding of polymorphonuclear leukocytes to fibrinogen or serum-coated surfaces. In the presence of Ca++, however, adhesion was not affected.

330 Arredouani MS, Kasran A, Vanoirbeek JA, Berger FG, Baumann H, Ceuppens JL. **Haptoglobin dampens endotoxin-induced inflammatory effects both *in vitro* and *in vivo*.** *Immunology* 114(2):263-271 (2005). Haptoglobin regulates monocyte activation following LPS stimulation. The increase in haptoglobin in the acute phase reaction may represent a feedback effect which dampens the severity of cytokine release and protects against endotoxin-induced damage.

331 Schmidt J, Kuhlenschmidt MS. Microbial adhesion of *Cryptosporidium parvum*: Identification of a colostrum-derived inhibitory lipid. *Molecular Biochemistry and Parasitology* 162(1):32-39 (2008).

332 Schlimme E, Martin D, Meisel H. **Nucleosides and nucleotides: natural bioactive substances in milk and colostrum.** *British Journal of Nutrition* 84(Suppl 1):S59-S68 (2000).

333 Carver JD, Cox WI, Barness LA. **Dietary nucleotide effects upon murine natural killer cell activity and macrophage activation.** *Journal of Parenteral and Enteral Nutrition* 14(1):18-22 (1990). Weanling mice fed a diet that included nucleotides exhibited

increased NK cell activity and lower macrophage activation than control animals fed a diet with no extra nucleotides.

334 Carver JD. **Dietary nucleotides: effects on the immune and gastrointestinal systems.** *Acta Paediatrica Supplement* 88(430):83-88 (1999). Infants fed diets with nucleotide supplementation have a lower incidence of diarrhea, higher antibody levels following *Haemophilus influenzae* vaccination, and higher NK cell activity.

335 Juul SE, Christensen RD. **Absorption of enteral recombinant human erythropoietin by neonates.** *Annals of Pharmacotherapy* 37(6):782-786 (2003). EPO is a component of colostrum, but its function is unknown. To test whether or not EPO in colostrum is absorbed in sufficient quantities to stimulate erythropoiesis, recombinant human erythropoietin was given orally to infants. Circulating amounts of EPO, however, did not increase.

336 Gyawu P, Pope GS. **Oestrogens in milk.** *Journal of Steroid Biochemistry* 19(1C):877-882. Both estrogen and progesterone are found in colostrum and milk.

337 Baram T, Koch Y, Hazum E, Fridkin M. Gonadotropin-releasing hormone in milk. *Science* 198(4314):300-302 (1977). GnRH has been found in the colostrum and milk of man, cow, and rat. TRH is also present, though in much lower quantities.

338 Zhang T, Iguchi K, Mochizuki T, Hoshino M, Yanaihara C, Yanaihara N. **Gonadotropin-releasing hormone-associated peptide immunoreactivity in bovine colostrum.** *Proceedings of the Society for Experimental Biology and Medicine* 194(3):270-273 (1990). The presence of a peptide associated with GnRH in colostrum suggests that the GnRH precursor is synthesized and processed in the mammary gland.

339 Oda S, Satoh H, Sugawara T, Matsunaga N, Kuhara T, Katoh K, Shoji Y, Nihei A, Ohta M, Sasaki Y. **Insulin-like growth factor-I, GH, insulin and glucagon concentrations in bovine colostrum and in plasma of dairy cows and neonatal calves around parturition.** *Comparative Biochemistry and Physiology A* 94(4):805-808.

340 Aranda, 1991, op cit.

341 Pinotti L, Rosi F. **Leptin in bovine colostrum and milk.** *Hormone and Metabolic Research* 38(2):89-93 (2006). Leptin concentration is 56% lower in colostrum than in mature milk.

342 Amarant T, Fridkin M, Koch Y. **Luteinizing hormone-releasing hormone and thyrotropin-releasing hormone in human and bovine milk.** *European Journal of Biochemistry* 127(3):647-650 (1982). Both human and bovine milk and colostrum had high levels of LHRH and TRH.

343 Eriksson L, Valtonen M, Laitinen JT, Paananen M, Kaikkonen M. **Diurnal rhythm of melatonin in bovine milk: pharmacokinetics of exogenous melatonin in lactating cows and goats.** *Acta Veterinaria Scandinavica* 39(3):301-310 (1998). Levels of melatonin in the colostrum and milk of cows and goats follow the diurnal rhythm of melatonin in the blood with a short delay.

344 Koldovsky O, Thornburg W. **Hormones in milk.** *Journal of Pediatric Gastroenterology and Nutrition* 6(2):172-196 (1987). Hormones in colostrum and milk include EGF, Erythropoietin, GnRH, growth hormone, prolactin, thyroid hormones and others.

345 Gyawu, 1983, op cit.

346 Koldovsky, 1987, op cit.

347 Lippert TH, God B, Voelter W. **Immunoreactive relaxin-like substance in milk.** *IRCS Journal of Medical Science* 9:925 (1981). First report of relaxin in bovine and human milk/colostrum. Levels in bovine milk/colostrum were 2916 ng/l, while in human milk levels were between 195 and 438 ng/l between days 3 and 6 postpartum and blood serum levels of relaxin decreased from 83-32 ng/l between days 3 and 6, disappearing entirely after day 7, indicating that the mammary gland is the primary source of the relaxin. Relaxin is most likely involved in nipple development in the mother rather than having any significant effect on the newborn.

348 Rao RK, Lam K, Philipps AF, Williams C, Lake M, Koldovsky O. **Presence of multiple forms of peptidase inhibitors in rat milk.** *Journal of Pediatric Gastroenterology and Nutrition* 17(4):414-420 (1993). Peptides such as somatostatin, epidermal growth factor, TGF-α and insulin-like growth factors are found in the colostrum of many species.

349 Baram, 1977, op cit.

350 Guth PS. **Kinins produced from bovine colostrum by kallikrein and saliva.** *British Journal of Pharmacology* 14:549-552 (1959).

351 Tauzin J, Miclo L, Gaillard JL. **Angiotensin-I-converting enzyme inhibitory peptides from tryptic hydrolysate of bovine alphaS2-casein.** *FEBS Letters* 531(2):369-374 (2002).

352 Pihlanto-Leppala A, Koskinen P, Piilola K, Tupasela T, Korhonen H. **Angiotensin I-converting enzyme inhibitory properties of whey protein digests: concentration and characterization of active peptides.** *Journal of Dairy Research* 67(1):53-64 (2000).

353 Ijäs H, Collin M, Finckenberg P, Pihlanto-Leppala A, Korhonen H, Korpela R, Vapaatalo H, Nurminen M-L. **Antihypertensive opioid-like milk peptide α-lactorphin: lack of effect on behavioral tests in mice.** *International Dairy Journal* 14(3):201-205 (2004). α-lactorphin, a peptide derived from milk whey, lowers blood pressure in hypertensive rats without the sedative effects of other opioid-like peptides.

354 Dawes J, Clezardin P, Pratt DA. **Thrombospondin in milk, other breast secretions, and breast tissue.** *Seminars in Thrombosis and Hemostasis* 13(3):378-384 (1987). Thrombospondin, a protein important in cell-cell and cell-matrix communication and wound repair, and a potent inhibitor of angiogenesis and tumor growth, is found in high concentrations in colostrum and mature milk. Highest concentrations are found in colostrum.

355 Saumet A, de Jesus N, Legrand C, Dubernard V. **Association of thrombospondin-1**

with the actin cytoskeleton of human thrombin-activated platelets through an alphaIIbbeta3- or CD36-independent mechanism. *Biochemistry Journal* 363(Pt 3):473-482 (2002). Thrombospondin-1 participates in platelet aggregation by binding to the surface of the platelets.

356 Isenberg JS, Romeo MJ, Yu C, Yu CK, Nghiem K, Monsale J, Rick ME, Wink DA, Frazier WA, Roberts DD. **Thrombospondin-1 stimulates platelet aggregation by blocking the antithrombotic activity of nitric oxide/cGMP signaling.** *Blood* 111(2):613-623 (2008). Thrombospondin-1 promotes platelet aggregation by overcoming the antithrombic activity of nitric oxide.

357 Bal dit Sollier C, Drouet L, Pignaud G, Chevallier C, Caen J, Fiat AM, Izquierdo C, Jolles P. **Effect of kappa-casein split peptides on platelet aggregation and on thrombus formation in the guinea-pig.** *Thrombosis Research* 81(4):427-437 (1996). GMP inhibits platelet aggregation and fibrinogen binding, preventing the formation of arterial thrombosis, a leading cause of stroke and heart attack.

358 Chabance B, Jolles P, Izquierdo C, Mazoyer E, Francoual C, Drouet L, Fiat AM. **Characterization of an antithrombotic peptide from kappa-casein in newborn plasma after milk ingestion.** *British Journal of Nutrition* 73(4):583-590 (1995). Both human and bovine kappa-caseinoglycopeptides were found in the blood serum of infants after ingestion of either bovine or human milk and colostrum, suggesting these bioactive peptides are produced by the digestion of milk.

359 Chabance B, Qian ZY, Migliore-Samour D, Jolles P, Fiat AM. **Binding of the bovine caseinoglycopeptide to the platelet membrane glycoprotein GPIb alpha.** *Biochemistry and Molecular Biology International* 42(1):77-84 (1997). Bovine kappa-caseinoglycopeptide inhibits platelet aggregation by binding to a specific membrane protein on the platelets which is involved in platelet aggregation.

360 Christensen T, Wiegers T, Hermansen J, Sottrup-Jensen L. **Plasma-derived protease inhibitors in bovine milk.** *International Dairy Journal* 5:439-449 (1995). Seven plasma-derived inhibitors, α2-macroglobulin, α2-antiplasmin, antithrombin III, C1-inhibitor, inter-α-trypsin inhibitor, bovine plasma elastase inhibitor (EI) and bovine plasma trypsin inhibitor (TI), have been identified in bovine colostrum and milk.

361 Stassen JM, Arnout J, Deckmyn H. **The hemostatic system.** *Current Medicinal Chemistry* 11(17):2245-2260 (2004). The hemostatic system comprises platelet aggregation, coagulation and fibrinolysis. Fibrinolysis is controlled by plasminogen activators inhibitor (PAI-1), α2-antiplasmin, α2-microglobulin and thrombin-activated fibrinolysis inhibitor (TAFI).

362 Christensen, 1995, op cit.

363 Stassen, 2004, op cit.

364 Christensen, 1995, op cit.

365 Olds RJ, Lane DA, Mille B, Chowdhury V, Thein SL. **Antithrombin: the principal**

inhibitor of thrombin. *Seminars in Thrombosis and Hemostasis* 20(4):353-372 (1994).

366 Habata Y, Fujii R, Hosoya M, Fukusumi S, Kawamata Y, Hinuma S, Kitada C, Nishizawa N, Murosaki S, Kurokawa T, Onda H, Tatemoto K, Fujino M. **Apelin, the natural ligand of the orphan receptor APJ, is abundantly secreted in the colostrum.** *Biochemica et Biophysica Acta* 1452(1):25-35 (1999). Apelin, a peptide secreted in large amounts in bovine colostrum and milk, is a ligand for the seven-transmembrane domain receptor 7TMR APJ (angiotensin receptor-like 1). As apelin was found to partially suppress cytokine production by mouse spleen cells in response to T cell receptor/CD3 cross-linking, it may play a role in immunomodulation.

367 Szokodi I, Tavi P, Foldes G, Voutilainen-Myllyla S, Ilves M, Tokola H, Pikkarainen S, Piuhola J, Rysa J, Toth M, Ruskoaho H. **Apelin, the novel endogenous ligand of the orphan receptor APJ, regulates cardiac contractility.** *Circulation Research* 91(5):434-440 (2002). Both apelin and the orphan receptor APJ are produced in large quantities in the heart. Apelin is one of the most potent stimulators of cardiac contraction known.

368 Kleinz MJ, Davenport AP. **Emerging roles of apelin in biology and medicine.** *Pharmacology and Therapeutics* 107(2):198-211 (2005). Apelin is involved in the regulation of cardiac function and fluid homeostasis and as a substrate for ACE II. It also has the ability to block HIV infection by blocking the HIV coreceptor APJ.

369 Quigley, JD III, Martin KR, Dowlen HH. **Concentrations of trypsin inhibitor and immunoglobulins in colostrum of Jersey cows.** *Journal of Dairy Science* 78(7):1573-1577 (1995). Mean concentration of trypsin inhibitor in bovine colostrum was 56 mg of trypsin inhibited/ml colostrum. Its function is thought to involve protection of colostrum components from digestion in the gastrointestinal tract.

370 Telemo E, Westrom BR, Ekstrom G, Karlsson BW. **Intestinal macromolecular transmission in the young rat: influence of protease inhibitors during development.** *Biology of the Neonate* 52(3):141-148 (1987). The absorption of large macromolecules in neonatal rats was enhanced when combined with either soy or porcine colostrum protease inhibitor.

371 von Fellenberg R, Horber H. **[Multiple protease inhibitors in colostrum and in bovine udder tissue and their possible functional significance].** *Schweizer Archiv für Tierheilkunde* 122(3):159-168 (1980).

372 Lindberg T. **Protease inhibitors in human milk.** *Pediatric Research* 13(9):969-972 (1979). Protease inhibitors, including trypsin, chymotrypsin and elastase, were found in colostrum, with highest levels on the first day postpartum.

373 Uruena C, Telleria JJ, Blanco-Quiros A, Arranz E, Gomez-Carrasco JA. **Alpha-1 antichymotrypsin levels are actively increased in normal colostrum.** *Journal of Pediatric Gastroenterology and Nutrition* 26(4):376-379 (1998). A survey of antiproteases in human colostrum was undertaken. Antithrombin II, inter-α trypsin inhibitor and α-2 macroglobulin were undetectable, and antitrypsin levels were at only 6% of serum levels.

α-1 antichymotrypsin levels were higher than expected, however (0.39±0.34 g/l), 41% of serum levels. The protein also differed from serum antichymotrypsin in electrophoretic mobility and Western blot analysis. This indicates that it is probably produced by mammary epithelial cells.

374 Lindberg, 1979, op cit.

375 Pineiro A, Brock JH, Esparza I. **Isolation and properties of bovine colostral trypsin inhibitor.** *Annales de Reserches Veterinaires* 9(2):281-286 (1978). An inhibitor of bovine trypsin was isolated. It was active against both bovine and rat trypsin and weakly active against bovine chymotrypsin.

376 Lindberg, 1979, op cit.

377 Veselsky L, Cechova D, Jonakova V. **Secretion and immunochemical properties of the trypsin inhibitor from bovine colostrum.** *Hoppe Seylers Zeitschrift für Physiologische Chemie* 359(8):873-878 (1978). A trypsin inhibitor was isolated from bovine colostrum. It is only secreted by the mammary gland during the time colostrum is secreted and is not present in mature milk.

378 Cheung PY, Sawicki G, Gross S, Van Aerde J, Radomski M. **Differential expression of matrix metalloproteinases and the tissue inhibitor in human milk.** *Proceedings of the Western Pharmacology Society* 44:97-98 (2001). Both MMP-2 (matrix metalloproteinase-2) and TIMP-4 (tissue inhibitor of metalloproteinase-4) are expressed in human milk from days 1-30. MMP-2 was at its highest levels on Day 1, while TIMP-4 peaked at Day 7.

379 Pons SM, et al. **Triacylglycerol composition in colostrum, transitional and mature human milk.** *European Journal of Clinical Nutrition* 54(12):878-882 (2000). Triglyceride profiles for colostrum, transitional and mature human milk were distinctive. However, the predominant triglycerides in colostrum (49%) were also predominant in transitional (34%) and mature (42%) milk.

380 Ronneberg R, Skara B. **Essential fatty acids in human colostrum.** *Acta Paediatrica* 81(10):779-783 (1992). Major fatty acids present included palmitic acid (24.3%) and oleic acid (39.7%). The main polyunsaturated fatty acid was linoleic acid (11.5%). Others included linolenic acid (0.7%) and docosahexaenoic acid (0.6%). The ratio of polyunsaturated to saturated fatty acids was 0.42.

381 Shope RE, Gowen JW. **Cholesterol and cholesterol ester content of bovine colostrum.** *Journal of Experimental Medicine* 48(1):21-24 (1928). Colostrum is rich in cholesterol, which then decreases in content as the mammary gland switches to transitional and mature milk.

382 Haug A, Hostmark AT, Harstad OM. **Bovine milk in human nutrition – a review.** *Lipids in Health and Disease* 6:25 (2007).

383 Lazarou J, Pomerantz BH, Corey PN. . **Incidence of adverse drug reactions in hospitalized patients: a meta-analysis of prospective studies..** *Journal of the*

American Medical Association (JAMA) 279(15):1200-1205 (1998).
384 Ainarson TR. . **Drug-related hospital admissions.**. *Annals of Pharmacotherapy*; 127(7):832-840 (2003).
385 Chen TS, Chang FY. **Clinical characteristics of Helicobacter pylori-negative duodenal ulcer disease.** *Hepatogastroenterology* 55(86-87):1615-1618 (2008).
386 van Leerdam ME. **Epidemiology of acute upper gastrointestinal bleeding.** *Best Practice & Research. Clinical Gastroenterology* 22(2):209-224 (2008).
387 Bowen B, Yuan Y, James C, Rashid F, Hunt RH. **Time course and pattern of blood loss with ibuprofen treatment in healthy subjects.** *Clinical Gastroenterology and Hepatology* 3(11):1075-1082 (2005).
388 Bowen B, Yuan Y, James C, Rashid F, Hunt RH. **Time course and pattern of blood loss with ibuprofen treatment in healthy subjects.** *Clinical Gastroenterology and Hepatology* 3(11):1075-1082 (2005).
389 Hollenz M, Stolte M, Leodolter A, Labenz J. **NSAID-associated dyspepsia and ulcers: a prospective cohort study in primary care.** *Digestive Diseases* 24(1-2):189-194 (2006).

Chapter 8 Notes

390 Janusz M, Staroscik K, Zimecki M, Wieczorek Z, Lisowski J. **A Proline-rich Polypeptide (PRPs) with immunoregulatory properties isolated from ovine colostrum. Murine thymocytes have on their surface a receptor specific for PRPs.** *Archivum immunologiae et therapiae experimentalis (Warszava)* 34(4):427-436 (1986). PRPs has immunoregulatory properties. It induces the maturation of thymocytes into mature helper or suppressor T cells. There is a specific receptor for PRPs on the surface of thymocytes.

391 Wieczorek Z, Zimecki M, Spiegel K, Lisowski J, Janusz M. **Differentiation of T cells into helper cells from immature precursors: identification of a target cell for a Proline-rich Polypeptide (PRPs).** *Archivum immunologiae et therapiae experimentalis (Warszava)* 37(3-4):313-322 (1989). The precursors of helper T cells belong to a minor thymocyte subset bearing the Thy-1 +/-, H-2+, L3T4-, lyt 2-, CD3- phenotype. PRPs induced the production of antigens consistent with mature helper T cells.

392 Zimecki M, Staroscik K, Janusz M, Lisowski J, Wieczorek Z. **The inhibitory activity of a Proline-rich Polypeptide (PRPs) on the immune response to polyvinylpyrrolidone (PVP).** *Archivum immunologiae et therapiae experimentalis (Warszava)* 31(6):895-903 (1983). PRPs administered to a test animal before immunization with PVP inhibits the immune response to this antigen. PRPs did this by increasing the activity of suppressor T cells and by increasing the generation of new suppressor T cells.

393 Kubis A, Marcinkowska E, Janusz M, Lisowski J. **Studies on the mechanism of action**

of a Proline-rich Polypeptide complex (PRPs): effect on the stage of cell differentiation. *Peptides* 26(11):2188-2192 (2005). PRPs affects the differentiation and maturation of cells of the monocyte/ macrophage lineage and may regulate in this way the inflammatory processes in which these cells participate.

394 Julius MH, Janusz M, Lisowski J. **A colostral protein that induces the growth and differentiation of resting B lymphocytes.** *Journal of Immunology* 140(5):1366-371 (1988). PRPs induced resting B cells and supported their progression through the cell cycle to form mature B cells. It had the same action on splenocytes.

395 Bishop GA, Haxhinasto SA, Stunz LL, Hostager BS. **Antigen-specific B-lymphocyte activation.** *Critical Reviews in Immunology* 23(3):159-197 (2003). B cells have the exclusive ability to produce and secrete immunoglobulins of various types. They also function in antigen presentation and the production of a number of cytokines and chemokines.

396 Zablocka A, Janusz M, Rybka K, Wirkus-Romanowska I, Kupryszewski G, Lisowski J. **Cytokine-inducing activity of a proline-rich polypeptide complex (PRPs) from ovine colostrum and its active nonapeptide fragment analogs.** *European Cytokine Network* 12(3):462-467 (2001). PRPs induces the production of INF-γ, TNF-α, IL-6 and IL-10 in human whole blood cultures.

397 Kruzel ML, Janusz M, Lisowski J, Fischleigh RV, Georgiades JA. **Towards an understanding of biological role of colostrinin peptides.** *Journal of Molecular Neuroscience* 17(3):379-389 (2001). PRPs (colostrinin) is a potent inducer of leukocyte proliferation and of certain cytokines.

398 Janusz M, Lisowski J. **Proline-rich Polypeptide (PRPs)--an immunomodulatory peptide from ovine colostrum.** *Archivum immunologiae et therapiae experimentalis (Warszava)* 41(5-6):275-279 (1993). PRPs increases the permeability of blood vessels in the skin and causes the differentiation of thymocytes into mature T cells.

399 See DM, Gurnee K, LeClair M. **An In Vitro Screening Study of 196 Natural Products for Toxicity and Efficacy.** *Journal of the American Nutraceutical Association* 2(1):25-39 (1999). A comparative study of 196 natural products showed that many demonstrated toxicity and cytochrome p450 activity (indicative of liver toxicity) while having little or no beneficial action. Some natural products, including *Echinacea*, and glyconutrient-containing products, showed the highest degree of NK cell stimulation. Bovine colostrum showed significant enhancement of NK cell cytotoxicity.

400 See DM. **Transfer Factor™ testing – transfer factor study with 20 cancer patients.** http://www.immune-system-iq.com/research.htm. 20 cancer patients (levels 3 and 4) with average life expectancy of 3.7 months received 9 capsules of Transfer Factor Plus™ along with other general nutrients. After 8 months, 16 of the 20 were still alive and were either in remission, improving or stabilized. Baseline for NK cell activity was 6.4. After 4 weeks, it increased to 25.7 and after 6 months to 27.6, an increase of 400%.

401 See D, Mason S, Roshan R. **Increased tumor necrosis factor alpha (TNF-α) and**

natural killer cell (NK) function using an integrative approach in late stage cancers. *Immunological Investigations* 31(2):137-153 (2002). A combination of natural products was shown to increase the cytotoxicity of NK cell TNF-α while decreasing DNA damage in patients with late-stage cancer. 20 patients with stage IV end-stage cancer were evaluated using Transfer Factor Plus (3 tabs 3 times/day), IMU-Plus (40 gm/day), IV (50-100 gm/day) and oral (12 gm/day) ascorbic acid, Agaricus Blazeii Murill teas 10 gm/day), Immune Modulator Mix, nitrogenated soy extract, and Andrographis Paniculata (500 mg twice daily). The 16 survivors of the study showed significantly higher NK function and TNF-α levels over baseline. Side effects were limited to occasional diarrhea and nausea, while quality of life improved for all survivors over the six month period of the study. http://www.informaworld.com/10.1081/IMM-120004804

Chapter 10 Notes

402 Wrana JL, Attisano L, Carcamo J, Zentella A, Doody J, Laiho M, Wang XF, Massague J. **TGF beta signals through a heteromeric protein kinase receptor complex.** *Cell* 71(6):1003-1014 (1992).

Chapter 12 Notes

403 Lawrence HS, Borkowsky W. **Transfer factor: current status and future prospects.** *Biotherapy* 9:1-5 (1996).

404 Kim S, Lira SM, Dalal MA, Verity MA, Voskuhl RR. **Estriol ameliorates autoimmune demyelinating disease.** *Neurology* 52(6):1230-1237 (1999).

405 Formby B. **Immunologic response in pregnancy. Its role in endocrine disorders of pregnancy and influence on the course of maternal autoimmune conditions.** *Endocrinology and Metabolic Clinics of North America* 24(1):187-205 (1995).

406 Bjorksten B. **Environment and infant immunity.** *Proceedings of the Nutrition Society* 58(3):729-732 (1999).

407 Nicolini A, Ferrari P, Spinelli R, Carpi A, Sagripanti A, Amborgi F. **Cell-mediated immunity in breast cancer patients.** *Biomedicine and Pharmacotherapy* 50(8):337-343 (1996).

408 Bansal AS, Bruce J, Devine PL, Scells B, Zimmermann PV. **Serum cytokines and tumor markers in patients with non-small cell carcinoma of the lung.** *Disease Markers* 13(3):195-199 (1997).

409 Aziz M, Akhtar S, Malik A. **Evaluation of cell-mediated immunity and circulating immune complexes as prognostic indicators in cancer patients.** *Cancer Detection*

and Prevention 22(2):87-99 (1998).

410 Czarnechi D, Zaleberg J, Kulinshaya E, Kaz T. **Impaired cell-mediated immunity of apparently normal patients who had multiple skin cancers.** *Cancer* 76(2):228-231 (1995).

411 Mallmann P, Krebs D. **[The effect of immunotherapy with thymopentin on the parameters of cellular immunity and the clinical course of gynecologic tumor patients.]** *Onkologie* 12(Suppl 3):15-21 (1989).

412 Mallmann P, Krebs D. **Investigations on cell-mediated immunity in patients with breast and ovarian carcinomas receiving a combination of chemotherapy and immunotherapy with thymopentin.** *Methods and Findings in Experimental Clinical Pharmacology* 12(5):333-340 (1990).

413 Kitahara T, Takeaka T, Yoshino M. **Infection and immunosuppression in cancer patients.** *Gan To Kagaku Ryoho* 16(4 Pt 2-1):1108-1114 (1989).

414 O'Byrne KJ, Dalgleish AG, Browning MJ, Steward WP, Harris AL. **The relationship between angiogenesis and the immune response in carcinogenesis and the progression of malignant disease.** *European Journal of Cancer* 36(2000):151-169, September 21 (1999).

415 Lawrence HS. **Transfer factor in cellular immunity.** The Harvey Lecture Series 68. New York: Academic Press, 1987.

416 Pizza G, De Vinci C, Cuzzocrea D, Menniti D, Aiello E, Maver P, Corrado G, Romagnoli P, Dragoni E, LoConte G, Riolo U, Palareti A, Zucchelli P, Fornarola V, Viza D. **A preliminary report on the use of transfer factor for treating stage D3 hormone-unresponsive metastatic prostate cancer.** *Biotherapy* 9(3-1):123-132 (1996).

417 Pilotti V, Mastrotilli M, Pizza G, De Vinci C, Busutti L, Palareti A, Gozzetti G, Cavallari A. **Transfer factor as an adjuvant to non-small cell lung cancer (NSCLC) therapy.** *Biotherapy* 9:117-121 (1996).

418 Jirova D, Sperlingova I, Halaskova M, Bendova H, Dabrowska L. **Immunotoxic effects of carbon tetrachloride: the effect on morphology and function of the immune system in mice.** *Central European Journal of Public Health* 4(1):16-20 (1996).

419 Heo Y, Lee WT, Lawrence DA. **In vivo the environmental pollutants lead and mercury induce oligoclonal T cell responses skewed toward type-2 reactivities.** *Cellular Immunology* 179(2):185-195 (1997).

420 Khan A. **Transfer Factor in viral diseases.** *The Lancet* 1(8059):328-329 (1978).

421 Milich DR, Chen MK, Hughes JL, Jones JE. **The secreted hepatitis precove antigen can modulate the immune response to the nucleocapsid: a mechanism for persistence.** *Journal of Immunology* 160:2013-2021 (1998).

422 Tsai SL, Liaw TF, Chen MH, Huang LY, Kuo GC. **Detection of type-2 like T helper cells in hepatitis C detection: implications for hepatitis C virus chronicity.** *Hepatology* 25:449-458 (1997).

423 Ferrer-Argote VE, Romero-Cabello R, Hernandez-Medoza L, Arista-Viveros A, Rojo-Medina J, Balseca-Olivera F, Fierro M, Gonzalez-Constandse R. **Successful treatment of severe complicated measles with non-specific transfer factor.** *In Vivo* 8:555-558 (1994).

424 McCormick DP, Lim-Melia E, Sneed K, Baldwin CD, Chonmaitice T. **Detection of respiratory viruses in middle ear fluids of children with otitis media infections.** *Pediatric Infectious Disease Journal* 19(3):256-258 (2000).

425 Ramilio O. **Role of respiratory viruses in acute otitis media: implications for management of AOM.** *Pediatric Infectious Disease* 18(12):1125-1129 (1999).

426 Khan A, Sellars W, Grater W, Graham M, Pflanzer J, Antonetti A, Bailey J, Hill NO. **The usefulness of transfer factor in asthma associated with frequent infections.** *Annals of Allergy* 40(4):229-232 (1978).

427 Ibid.

428 Khan A. **The syndrome of asthma, recurrent viral infections and T-cell immuno-deficiency: investigations and management.** *Annals of Allergy* 43(2):69-72 (1979).

429 Clerici M, Merola M, Ferrario E, Trabattoni D, Villa ML, Stefanon B, Venzon DJ, Shearer GM, De Palo G, Clerici E. **Cytokine production patterns in cervical intraepithelial neoplasis: association with human papillomavirus infection.** *Journal of the National Cancer Institute* 89(3):245-250 (1997).

430 Grohn P. **Transfer factor in chronic and recurrent respiratory tract infections in children.** *Acta Paediatrica Scandinavica* 66:211-217 (1977).

431 De Vinci C, Pizza G, Cuzzocrea D, Menniti D, Aiello E, Maver P, Corrado G, Romagnoli P, Dragoni E, LoConte G, Riolo U, Masi M, Severini G, Fornarola V, Viza D. **Use of transfer factor for the treatment of recurrent non-bacterial female cystitis (NBRC): a preliminary report.** *Biotherapy* 9(1-3):133-138, 1996.

432 Masi M, De Vinci C, Baricordi OR. **Transfer factor in chronic mucocutaneous candidiasis.** *Biotherapy* 9(1-3):97-103 (1996).

433 Matyniak JE, Reiner SL. **T helper phenotype and genetic susceptibility in experimental Lyme disease.** *Journal of Experimental Medicine* 181(3):1251-1254 (1995).

434 Lawrence HS, Borkowsky W. **Transfer Factor: current status and future prospects.** *Biotherapy* 9:1-5 (1996).

435 Hana I, Vrubel J, Pekarek J, Cech K. **The influence of age on transfer factor treatment of cellular immunodeficiency, chronic fatigue syndrome and/or chronic viral infections.** *Biotherapy* 9(1-3):91-95 (1996).

436 Ablashi DV, Levine PH, De Vinci C, Whitman JE Jr, Pizza G, Viza D. **Use of anti HHV-6 transfer factor for the treatment of two patients with chronic fatigue syndrome (CFS): two case reports.** *Biotherapy* 9(1-3):81-86 (1996).

437 Pizza G, Viza D, De Vinci C, Palareti A, Cuzzocrea D, Fornarola V, Baricordi R. **Orally administered HSV-specific transfer factor(TF) prevents genital or labial herpes relapses.** *Biotherapy* 9(1-3):67-72 (1996).

438 Meduri R, Campos E, Scorolli L, De Vinci C, Pizza G, Viza D. **Efficacy of transfer in treating patients with recurrent ocular herpes infections.** *Biotherapy* 9(1-3):61-66 (1996).

439 Basten A, Pollard JD, Stewart GJ, Frith JA, McLeod JG, Walsh JC, Garrick R, van der Brink CM. **Transfer Factor in treatment of multiple sclerosis.** *Lancet* 2(8201):931-934 (1980).

440 Long KZ, Santos JI. **Vitamins and the regulation of the immune response.** *Pediatric Infectious Disease Journal* 18:283-290 (1999).

441 Ibid.

442 Wu B. **Effect of acupuncture on the regulation of cell-mediated immunity in the patients with malignant tumors.** *Chen Tzu Yen Chiu* 20(3):67-71 (1995).

443 Lawrence HS. **Immune Regulation in Transfer Factors.** New York: Academic Press, p. 613, 1979.

444 Khan A, Sellars WA, Gabela P, Thometz D. **Transfer factor, thymosin and E rosettes.** *New England Journal of Medicine* 292:868 (1975).

445 See D, Gurnce K, Leclair M. **An *in vitro* screening study of 196 natural products for toxicity and efficacy.** *Journal of the American Medical Association* 2(1) (1999).

446 Khan A. **Transfer factor in viral diseases.** *Lancet* 1(8059):328-329 (1978).

447 Bjerring P, Thestrup-Pedersen K, Zachariae H. **Treatment of Kaposi's varicelliform eruption with adenine arabinoside (Vira-A) and transfer factor.** *Acta Dermato-Venereologica* 62(1):85-87 (1982). Kaposi's varicelliform eruptions are a skin condition caused by herpes virus. Use of an antiviral drug, Vira-A, and transfer factor (PRPs) had a beneficial effect on halting the spread and alleviating the severity of the infection.

448 Pizza G, Meduri R, De Vinci C, Scorolli L, Viza D. **Transfer factor prevent relapses in herpes keratitis patients: a pilot study.** *Biotherapy* 8(1):63-68 (1994). 33 patients suffering from herpes eye infections were treated with HSV-specific PRPs (PRPs). The rate of relapses was reduced from 20.1 before treatment to 0.51 after (6 of 33 patients suffered a relapse).

449 Pizza G, Viza D, De Vinci C, Palareti A, Cuzzocrea D, Fornarola V, Baricordi R. **Orally administered HSV-specific transfer (TF) prevents genital or labial herpes relapses.** *Biotherapy* 9(1-3):67-72 (1996). 22 patients suffering from genital herpes and 22 from labial herpes were treated with bovine HSV-specific transfer factor (PRPs). Untreated patients suffered a relapse rate of 61.2 while those receiving treatment had a relapse rate of 21.4.

450 Meduri R, Campos E, Scorolli L, De Vinci C, Pizza G, Viza D. **Efficacy of transfer factor in treating patients with recurrent ocular herpes infections.** *Biotherapy* 9(1-3):61-66 (1996). Cellular immunity plays an important role in recurrent herpes eye infections. Patients treated with HSV-specific transfer facot (PRPs) showed a significant increase in cell-mediated immune response as measured by the lymphocyte stimulation test and

leukocyte migration test. Relapse rates went from 13.2 to 4.17. There were no reported side effects.

451 De Vinci C, Pizza G, Cuzzocrea D, Menniti D, Aiello E, Maver P, Corrado G, Romagnoli P, Dragoni E, LoConte G, Riolo U, Masi M, Severini G, Fornarola V, Viza D. **Use of transfer factor for the treatment of recurrent non-bacterial female cystitis (NBRC): a preliminary report.** *Biotherapy* 9(1-3):133-138 (1996). Non-bacterial recurrent cystitis (NBRC) is associated with impaired cell-mediated immunity to both *Candida* and herpes virus. Use of HSV-specific and *Candida*-specific transfer factor (PRPs) showed that specific PRPs could control NBRC and alleviate the symptoms.

452 Estrada-Parra, S, Chavez-Sanchez R, Ondarza-Aguilera R, Correa-Meza B, Serrano-Miranda E, Monges-Nicolau A, Calva-Pellicer C. **Immunotherapy with transfer factor of recurrent herpes simplex type I.** *Archives of Medical Research* 26(Spec. No.):S87-S92 (1995). Transfer factor (PRPs) proved to be the most effective agent when used as immunotherapy against recurrent herpes simplex type I virus.

453 Estrada-Parra S, Nagaya A, Serrano E, Rodriguez O, Santamaria V, Ondarza R, Chavez R, Correa B, Monges A, Cabezas R, Calva C, Estrada-Garcia I. **Comparative study of transfer factor and acyclovir in the treatment of herpes zoster.** *International Journal of Immunopharmacology* 20(10):521-535 (1998). Herpes zoster, or shingles, is a skin disease caused by varicella herpes virus (VHV) and can lie latent for long periods of time. A comparison study was performed between transfer factor (PRPs) and acyclovir, an antiviral drug which has shown the most promise against VHV in 28 patients. Patients who received PRPs had a much more favorable clinical course. Those receiving PRPs showed an increase in interferon-gamma levels and CD4+ lymphocytes. This was not seen in patients receiving acyclovir. This result is very significant and confirms the immunomodulatory properties of PRPs.

454 Raise E, Guerra L, Viza D, Pizza G, De Vinci C, Schiattone ML, Rocaccio L, Cicognani M, Gritti F. **Preliminary results in HIV-1-infected patients treated with transfer factor (TF) and zidovudine (ZDV).** *Biotherapy* 9(1-3):49-54 (1996). Patients with persistent generalized lymphadenopathy or ARC (AIDS-related complex) were treated with HIV-1-specific transfer factor (PRPs) in combination with Zidovudine, an antiviral medication. Patients who received both PRPs and Zidovudine had higher levels of white blood cells, CD8 lymphocytes and IL-2 compared to those on Zidovudine alone. The combination seemed to be safe and well tolerated.

455 Ferrer-Argote VE, Romero-Cabello R, Hernandez-Mendoza L, Arista-Viveros A, Rojo-Medina J, Balseca-Olivera F, Fierro M, Gonzalez-Constandse R. **Successful treatment of severe complicated measles with non-specific transfer factor.** *In Vivo* 8(4):555-557 (1994). Severe complicated measles has a high mortality rate and no specific treatment. 10 patients, one with encephalitis, were treated with PRPs. 9 of 10 survived and were cured. The patient with encephalitis showed no neurologic effects two weeks after receiving the last dose.

456 De Vinci C, Levine PH, Pizza G, Fudenberg HH, Orens P, Pearson G, Viza D. **Lessons from a pilot study of transfer factor in chronic fatigue syndrome.** *Biotherapy* 9(1-3):87-90 (1996). Of 20 chronic fatigue patients given transfer factor (PRPs), 12 showed improvement.

457 Iseki M, Aoyama T, Koizumi Y, Ojima T, Murase Y, Osano M. **[Effects of transfer factor on chronic hepatitis B in childhood]** *Kansenshogaku Zasshi* 63(12):1329-1332 (1989). Nine children with chronic hepatitis B received transfer factor (PRPs) for 3-17 months. Of these, 4 became hepatitis-B negative. After 22-48 months, 6 of the 9 were negative. No side effects were observed.

458 Vasily DB, Miller OF, Fudenberg HH, Goust JM, Wilson GB. **Epidermodysplasia verruciformis: response to therapy with dialyzable leukocyte extract [PRPs] derived from household contacts.** *Journal of Clinical and Laboratory Immunology* 14(1):49-57 (1984). EV is characterized by severely depressed suppressor T cell levels. Treatment with PRPs showed a gradual yet definite resolution of symptoms.

459 Wilson GB, Metcalf JF, Fudenberg HH. **Treatment of *Mycobacterium fortuitum* pulmonary infection with transfer factor (TF): new methodology for evaluating TF potency and predicting clinical response.** *Clinical Immunology and Immunopathology* 23(2):478-491 (1982).

460 Fabre RA, Perez TM, Aguilar LD, Rangel MJ, Estrada-Garcia I, Hernandez-Pando R, Estrada-Parra S. **Transfer factors as immunotherapy and supplement of chemotherapy in experimental pulmonary tuberculosis.** *Clinical and Experimental Immunology* 136(2):215-223 (2004). Treatment with either mouse or human transfer factors (PRPs) restores Th1 cytokines and TNF- levels to levels usually seen only at the initial infection, allowing the body to fight off the tuberculosis bacteria.

461 Louie E, Borkowsky W, Klesius PH, Haynes TB, Gordon S, Bonk S, Lawrence HS. **Treatment of cryptosporidiosis with oral bovine transfer factor.** *Clinical Immunology and Immunopathology* 44(3):329-334 (1987).

462 McMeeking A, Borkowsky W, Klesius PH, Bonk S, Holzman RS, Lawrence HS. **A controlled trial of bovine dialyzable leukocyte extract for cryptosporidiosis in patients with AIDS.** *Journal of Infectious Diseases* 161(1):108-112 (1990). A trial using bovine dialyzable leukocyte extract (PRPs) in AIDS patients suffering from cryptosporidial diarrhea was promising with 6 of 7 patients showing improvement or complete elimination of symptoms and oocytes.

463 Tanphaichitra D. **Cellular immunity in typhoid fever, Legionnaires' disease, amebiasis: role of transfer factor and Levamisole in typhoid fever.** *Developments in Biological Standardization* 53:35-40 (1983). Both typhoid fever and Legionnaires' disease impair cellular immunity. Typhoid fever patients treated with transfer factor (PRPs) improved faster in general condition, fever and cellular immunity.

464 Tanphaichitra D. **Tropical disease in the immunocompromised host: melioidosis**

and pythiosis. *Reviews of Infectious Diseases* 11(Suppl 7):S1629-S1643 (1989). Transfer factor (PRPs) was used to restore cellular immunity in AIDS patients suffering from recurrent melioidosis.

465 Feigin RD, Shackelford PG, Eisen S, Spitler LE, Pickering LK, Anderson DC. **Treatment of mucocutaneous candidiasis with transfer factor.** *Pediatrics* 53(1):63-70 (1974).

466 Masi M, De Vinci C, Baricordi OR. **Transfer factor in chronic mucocutaneous candidiasis.** *Biotherapy* 9(1-3):97-103 (1996).

467 Spitler LE, Dau PC. **Immunotherapy in infectious disease, autoimmunity and cancer.** *Acta Neurologica Scandinavica Supplement* 63:227-237 (1977).

468 Zachariae H, Ellegaard J, Grunnet E, Thestrup-Pedersen K. **Transfer factor in mycosis fungoides: three years experience.** *Dermatologica* 160(1):1-6 (1980). Patients treated with transfer factor (PRPs) showed partial or complete remission of symptoms in 7 cases out of 13 studied. T lymphocyte levels returned to normal levels in these patients, and serum IgE levels decreased.

469 Pizza G, De Vinci C, Viza D. **Immunotherapeutic approaches for renal cancer.** *Folia Biologica (Praha)* 48(5):167-181 (2002).

470 Pizza G, De Vinci C, Cuzzocrea D, Menniti D, Aiello E, Maver P, Corrado G, Romagnoli P, Dragoni E, LoConte G, Riolo U, Palareti A, Zucchelli P, Fornarola V, Viza D. **A preliminary report on the use of transfer factor for treating stage D3 hormone-unresponsive metastatic prostate cancer.** *Biotherapy* 9(1-3):123-132 (1996).

471 Pilotti V, Mastrorilli M, Pizza G, De Vinci C, Busutti L, Palareti A, Gozzetti G, Cavallari A. **Transfer factor as an adjuvant to non-small cell lung cancer (NSCLC) therapy.** *Biotherapy* 9(1-3):117-121 (1996).

472 Fujisawa T, Yamaguchi Y. **Postoperative immunostimulation after complete resection improves survival of patients with stage I non-small cell lung carcinoma.** *Cancer* 78(9):1892-1898 (1996).

473 Phillips J, Boiucheix C, Pizza G, Sartorio C, Viza D. **Effect of in vitro produced transfer factor on Hodgkin patients.** *British Journal of Haematology* 38(3):430-431 (1978).

474 Gonzalez RL, Wong P, Spitler LE. **Adjuvant immunotherapy with transfer factor in patients with melanoma metastatic to lung.** *Cancer* 45(1):57-63 (1980).

475 Levin AS, Byers VS, Fudenberg HH, Wybran J, Hackett AJ, Johnston JO, Spitler LE. **Osteogenic sarcoma. Immunologic parameters before and during immunotherapy with tumor-specific transfer factor.** *Journal of Clinical Investigation* 55(3):487-499 (1975).

476 Boldogh I, Aguilera-Aguirre L, Bacsi A, Choudhury BK, Saavedra-Molina A, Kruzel M. **Colostrinin [PRP] Decreases Hypersensitivity and Allergic Responses to Common Allergens.** *International Archives of Allergy and Immunology* 146(4):298-306 (2008).

477 Keech A. **Peptide Immunotherapy: The Use of Bovine Colostrum Proline-rich**

Polypeptides in Cytokine Modulation for the Alternative Relief of Allergic Symptoms. *Journal of Allergy and Clinical Immunology* 119(1): S260-S260 (2008).

478 Navarro Cruz D, Serrano Miranda E, Orea M, Estrada Parra S, Teran Ortiz L, Gomez Vera J, Flores Sandoval G. **[Transference factor in moderate and severe atopic dermatitis]** *Revista Alergia Mexico* 43(5):116-123 (1996).

479 Khan A, Sellars WA, Pflanzer J, Hill JM, Thometz D, Haenke J. **Asthma and T cell immuno-deficiency: improvement with transfer factor and immunopeptide.** *Annals of Allergy* 37(4):264-274 (1976).

480 Khan A, Sellars W, Grater W, Graham MF, Pflanzer J, Antonetti A, Bailey J, Hill NO. **The usefulness of transfer factor in asthma associated with frequent infections.** *Annals of Allergy* 40(4):229-232 (1978). 15 patients with asthma and suffering from repeated respiratory infections received transfer factor (PRPs). A marked decrease in respiratory infections and striking improvement in asthma resulted.

481 Zimecki M. **A Proline-rich Polypeptide from ovine colostrum: colostrinin with immuno-modulatory activity.** *Advances in Experimental Medicine and Biology* 606:241-250 (2008). PRPs, originally isolated from ovine (sheep) colostrum, promote T lymphocyte maturation into mature T helper cells and also recruit suppressor T cells in the suppression of autoimmune conditions. They also regulate cytokine production in the blood. In addition, they delay the progress of Alzheimer's and similar dementias.

482 Lawrence HS. **Transfer factor and autoimmune disease.** *Annals of the New York Academy of Sciences* 124(1):56-60 (1965).

483 Dutta RC. **Peptide immunomodulators versus infection; an analysis.** *Immunology Letters.* 83(3):153-61 (2002). Immune stimulators have been found to be useful in helping to fight off infections, while immunosuppressors have been found useful in autoimmune conditions and transplants.

484 Zimecki M, Hraba T, Janusz M, Lisowski J, Wieczorek Z. **Effect of a Proline-rich Polypeptide (PRPs) on the development of hemolytic anemia and survival of New Zealand black (NZB) mice.** *Archivum Immunologiae et Therapiae Experimentalis (Warszava)* 39(5-6):461-467 (1991).

485 Hraba T, Wieczorek Z, Janusz M, Lisowski J, Zimecki M. **Effect of Proline-rich Polypeptide on experimental autoimmune response to erythrocytes.** *Archivum Immunologiae et Therapiae Experimentalis (Warszava)* 34(4):437-443 (1986).

486 Hughes RA. **Immunological treatment of multiple sclerosis.** *Journal of Neurology* 230(2):73-80 (1983). PRPs slowed the progression of the disease whereas interferon and levamisole did not.

487 Nitsch A, Nitsch FP. **Clinical Use of Bovine Colostrum.** *Journal of Orthomolecular Medicine* 13(2) (1998). Low molecular weight components of colostrum (PRPs) were used in a clinical study for the treatment of rheumatoid arthritis with promising results.

488 Fudenberg HH, Strelkauskas AJ, Goust JM, Osborne D, Fort D, Vasily D. **"Discoid" lupus**

erythematosus: dramatic clinical and immunological response to dialyzable leukocyte extract [PRPs]. *Transactions of the Association of American Physicians* 94:279-291 (1981).

489 Wolf RE, Fudenberg HH, Welch TM, Spitler LE, Ziff M. **Treatment of Behçet's syndrome with transfer factor.** *Journal of the American Medical Association* 238(8):869-871 (1977). Of five patients treated with PRPs, three showed great improvement, on moderate improvement, and one was unresponsive.

490 Franzoni E, Masi M, Conte R, Giovannini A, Malferrari C, Scanabissi E, Specchia F, Ricci G. **Behçet syndrome: report of two early-onset cases treated with transfer factor.** *Italian Journal of Neurological Science* 5(1):93-96 (1984).

491 Lloyd AR, Hickie I, Brockman A, Hickie C, Wilson A, Dwyer J, Wakefield D. **Immunologic and psychologic therapy for patients with chronic fatigue syndrome: a double-blind, placebo-controlled trial.** *American Journal of Medicine* 94(2):197-203 (1993). Treatment of chronic fatigue syndrome using both psychological cognitive therapy and dialyzable leukocyte extract (PRPs) resulted in improvement of the condition generally, but there was no specific response found.

492 Vezendi S, Schroder I. **Transfer factor therapy of thoracic sarcoidosis.** *Allergologia et Immunopathologia* 17(1):35-37 (1989). Treatment of patients with thoracic sarcoidosis has generally proven beneficial, probably due to the ability of transfer factor (PRPs) to stimulate the immune system.

493 Fudenberg HH, Whitten HD, Arnaud P, Khansari N, Tsang KY, Hames CG. **Immune diagnosis of a subset of Alzheimer's disease with preliminary implications for immunotherapy.** *Biomedicine and Pharmacotherapy* 38(6):290-297 (1984).

494 Leszek J, Inglot AD, Janusz M, Lisowski J, Krukowska K, Georgiades JA. **Colostrinin: a Proline-rich Polypeptide (PRP) complex isolated from ovine colostrum for treatment of Alzheimer's disease. A double-blind, placebo-controlled study.** *Archivum Immunologiae et Therapiae Experimentalis (Warszava)* 47(6):377-385 (1999).

495 Leszek J, Inglot AD, Janusz M, Byczkiewicz F, Kiejna A, Georgiades J, Lisowski J. **Colostrinin Proline-rich Polypeptide complex from ovine colostrum--a long-term study of its efficacy in Alzheimer's disease.** *Medical Science Monitor* 8(10):193-196 (2002).

496 Bilikiewicz A, Gaus W. **Colostrinin (a naturally occurring, proline-rich, polypeptide mixture) in the treatment of Alzheimer's disease.** *Journal of Alzheimer's Disease* 6(1):17-26 (2004).

497 Mokran V, Simko M, Nyulassy S. **[Epileptic seizures and immune disorders]** *Bratislavské Lekárske Listy* 98(4):229-233 (1997). Out of 125 epileptic patients, only 3.2% showed no disturbances of immunity, indicating that immunomodulatory therapy might be effective in controlling the disorder.

498 Simko M, Mokran V, Nyulassy S. **[Immunomodulatory therapy of epilepsy with**

transfer factor] *Bratislavské Lekárske Listy* 98(4):234-237 (1997). Eight epileptic patients treated for 3 months with transfer factor (PRPs) had significant reduction of epileptic episodes.

499 Levin AS, Spitler LE, Fudenberg HH. **Transfer factor I: methods of therapy.** *Birth Defects Original Articles Series* 11(1):445-448 (1975). Approximately 50% of patients with a variety of immunodeficiency disorders are induced to a clinically acceptable level of cell-mediated immunity when given transfer factor (PRPs).

500 Chan MC, Cheung CY, Chui WH, Tsao SW, Nicholls JM, Chan YO, Chan RW, Long HT, Poon LL, Guan Y, Peiris JS. **Proinflammatory cytokine responses induced by influenza A (H5N1) viruses in primary human alveolar and bronchial epithelial cells.** *Respiratory Research* 6:135 (2005).

501 Pizza G, Amadori M, Ablashi D, De Vinci C, Viza D. **Cell mediated immunity to meet the avian influenza A (H5N1) challenge.** *Medical Hypotheses* 67(3):601-608 (2006).

Chapter 13 Notes

502 UNAIDS/WHO AIDS Epidemic Update 2007.

503 United Nations Department of Economic and Social Affairs/Population Division report: **The Impact of AIDS** (2004). http://www.un.org/esa/population/publications/AIDSimpact/AIDSWebAnnounce.htm

504 Keech A, Nwabuko U, Chikezie C, Wogu GUE. **Peptide Immunotherapy: A New Direction in HIV/AIDS Treatment.** *In press*

Appendix Notes

505 **An Examination of Immune Response Modulation in Humans by Ai/E'°® Utilizing A Double Blind Study.** Immune Consultants, Tucson, Arizona, January 2001.

506 Caligiuri MA. **Human natural killer cells.** *Blood* 112(3):461-469 (2008).

507 Kirkpatrick CH. **Structural nature and functions of transfer factors.** *Annals of the New York Academy of Sciences* 685:362-368 (1993).

508 Whitcomb ME, Rocklin RE. **Transfer factor therapy in a patient with progressive primary tuberculosis.** *Annals of Internal Medicine* 79(2):161-166 (1973).

509 Brambell FWR. In: **The Transmission of Passive Immunity From Mother to Young.** Vol. 18. Elsevier Publishing Co., New York, 1969.

510 Penhale WJ, LoganEF, Selman IE, Fisher EW, McEwan AD. **Observations on the adsorption of colostral immunoglobulins by neonatalcalf and their significance in colibacillosis.** *Ann. Rech. Vet.* 4: 223-229 (1973).

511 Smith T, Little RB. **The significance of colostrum to the newborn calf.** *Journal of Experimental Medicine* 36: 181-186 (1922).

512 McEwan AD, Fisher EW, Selman IE. **Observations on the immunoglobulin level of neonatal calves and their relationship to disease.** *Journal of Comparative Pathology* 80: 259-263 (1970).

513 McGuire TC, Pfeiffer NE, Weikel JM, Bartsch RG. **Failure of colostral immunoglobulin transfer in calves dying from infectious disease.** *Journal of the American Veterinary Medicince Association* 169: 713-716 (1976).

514 Pahud JJ, Hilbert H, Schwartz K, Amster H, Smiley M. **Bovine milk antibodies in the treatment of enteric infections and their ability to eliminate virulence factors from pathogenic *E. coli*.** In: The Ruminant Immune System, edited by J. E. Butler, pp 591-600. Plenum, New York, 1981.

515 Hilpert H, Gerber H, Amster H, Pahud JJ, Ballabriga A, Arcalis L, Farriaux JP, de Peyer E, Nussle, D. **Bovine milk immunoglobulins (Ig) and their possible utilisation in industrially prepared infant's milk formulae.** In: Food and Immunology, Swedish Nutritional Foundation Symposium XIII, Hambraeus L, Hanson LA, McFarlane H, eds, pp 182-196. Almquist and Wiksell, Stockholm. 1977.

516 Chaplin DD. **Overview of the human immune response.** *Journal of Allergy and Clinical Immunology* 117(Suppl. 2):S430-S435 (2006).

517 Mosmann TR, Cherwinski, H, Bond, MW, Giedlin MA, Coffman RL. **Two types of murine helper T cell clone. I. Definition according to profiles of lymphokine activities and secreted proteins.** *Journal of Immunology* 136:2348-2357 (1986).

518 Mosmann TR, Coffman RL. **TH1 and TH2 cells: different patterns of lymphokine secretion lead to different functional properties.** *Annual Reviews of Immunology* 7:145-173 (1989).

519 Mosmann TR, Sad S. **The expanding universe of T-cell subsets: Th1, Th2 and more.** *Immunology Today* 17:138-146 (1996).

520 Abbas AK, Murphy KM, Sher A. **Functional diversity of helper T lymphocytes.** *Nature* 383:787-793 (1996).

521 McGuirk, P, Mills, KH. **Pathogen-specific regulatory T cells provoke a shift in the Th1/Th2 paradigm in immunity to infectious diseases.** *Trends in Immunology* 23:450-455 (2002).

Appendix C Notes

Bovine Lactoferrin

522 Kanyshkova TG, Buneva VN, Nevinsky GA. **Lactoferrin and its biological functions.** *Biochemistry (Moscow)* 66(1):1-7 (2001).

523 Sanchez L, Calvo M, Brock JH. **Biological role of lactoferrin.** *Archives of Disease in Childhood* 67(5):657-661 (1992).

524 Kensler TW, Tsuda H, Wogan GN. **United States-Japan workshop on new rodent models for the analysis and prevention of carcinogenesis.** *Cancer Epidemiology, Biomarkers and Prevention* 8(11):1033-1037 (1999).

525 Ushida Y, Sekine K, Kuhara T, Takasuka N, Iigo M, Tsuda H. **Inhibitory effects of bovine lactoferrin on intestinal polyposis in the Apc(Min) mouse.** *Cancer Letters* 134(2):141-145 (1998).

526 Ushida Y, Sekine K, Kuhara T, Takasuka N, Iigo M, Maeda M, Tsuda H. **Possible chemopreventive effects of bovine lactoferrin on esophagus and lung carcinogenesis in the rat.** *Japanese Journal of Cancer Research* 90(3):262-267 (1999).

527 Tanaka K, Ikeda M, Nozaki A, Kato N, Tsuda H, Saito S, Sekihara H. **Lactoferrin inhibits hepatitis C virus viremia in patients with chronic hepatitis C: a pilot study.** *Japanese Journal of Cancer Research* 90(4):367-371 (1999).

528 Wang D, Pabst KM, Aida Y, Pabst MJ. **Lipopolysaccharide-inactivating activity of neutrophils is due to lactoferrin.** *Journal of Leukocyte Biology* 57:865-874 (1995)

529 Arnold RR, Cole MF, McGhee JR. **A bactericidal effect for human lactoferrin.** *Science* 197(4300):263-265 (1977).

530 Arnold RR, Brewer M, Gauthier JJ. **Bactericidal activity of human lactoferrin: sensitivity of a variety of microorganisms.** *Infection and Immunity* 28(3):893-898 (1980).

531 Debbabi H, Dubarry M, Rautureau M, Tome D. **Bovine lactoferrin induces both mucosal and systemic immune response in mice.** *Journal of Dairy Research* 65:283-29 (1998).

532 Samaranayake YH, Samaranayake LP, Wu PC, So M. **The antifungal effect of lactoferrin and lysozyme on *Candida krusei* and *Candida albicans*.** *APMIS* 105:875-883 (1997).

533 Mattsby-Baltzer I, Roseanu A, Motas C, Elverfors J, Engberg I, Hanson LA. **Lactoferrin or a fragment thereof inhibits the endotoxin-induced interleukin-6 response in human monocytic cells.** *Pediatric Research* 40(2):257-262 (1996).

534 Teraguchi S, Shin K, Ozawa K, Nakamura S, Fukuwatari Y, Tsuyuki S, Namihira H, Shimamura S. **Bacteriostatic effect of orally administered bovine lactoferrin on proliferation of Clostridium species in the gut of mice fed bovine milk.** *Applied Environmental Microbiology* 61(2):501-506 (1995).

535 Zagulski T, Lipinski P, Zagulska A, Broniek S, Jarzabek Z. **Lactoferrin can protect mice against a lethal dose of E. coli in experimental infection *in vivo*.** *British Journal of Experimental Pathology* 70:697-704 (1989).

536 Lee, WJ, Farmer JL, Hilty M, Kim YB. **The protective effects of lactoferrin feeding against endotoxin lethal shock in germfree piglets.** *Infection and Immunity* 66(4):1421-1426 (1998).

537 Naidu A, Arnold RR. **Lactoferrin interaction with salmonella potentiates antibiotic susceptibility *in vitro*.** *Diagnostic Microbiology and Infectious Disease* 20(2):69-75 (1994).

538 Wakabayashi H, Abe S, Okutomi T, Tansho S, Kawase K, Yamaguchi H. **Cooperative anti-Candida effects of lactoferrin or its peptides in combinations with azole antifungal agents.** *Microbiological Immunology* 40(11):821-825 (1996).

539 Harmsen MC, Swart PJ, de Bethune MP, Pauwels R, De Clercq E, The TH, Meijer DK. **Antiviral effects of plasma and milk proteins: lactoferrin shows potent activity against both human immunodeficiency virus and human cytomegalovirus replication *in vitro*.** *Journal of Infectious Diseases* 172:380-388 (1995).

540 Marchetti M, Pisani S, Antonini G, Valenti P, Seganti L, Orsi N. **Metal complexes of bovine lactoferrin inhibit in vitro replication of herpes simplex virus type 1 and 2.** *Biometals* 11(2):89-94 (1998).

541 Kawasaki Y, Isoda H, Shinmoto H, Tanimoto M, Dosako S, Idota T, Nakajima I. **Inhibition of kappa-casein glycomacropeptide and lactoferrin of influenza virus hemagglutination.** *Bioscience, Biotechnology and Biochemistry* 57(7):1214-1215 (1993).

542 Superti F, Ammendolia MG, Valenti P, Seganti L. **Antirotaviral activity of milk proteins: lactoferrin prevents rotavirus infection in the enterocyte-like cell line HT-29.** *Medical Microbiology and Immunology* 186(2-3):83-91 (1997).

543 Shimizu K, Matsuzawa H, Okada K, Tazume S, Dosako S, Kawasaki Y, Hashimoto K, Koga Y. **Lactoferrin-mediated protection of the host from murine cytomegalovirus infection by a T-cell dependent augmentation of natural killer cell activity.** *Archives of Virology* 141(10):1875-1889 (1996).

544 Yi M, Kaneko S, Yu DY, Murakami S. **Hepatitis C virus envelope proteins bind lactoferrin.** *Journal of Virology* 71(8):5997-6002 (1997).

545 Cohen MS, Mao J, Rasmussen GT, Serody JS, Britigan BE. **Interaction of lactoferrin and lipopolysaccharide (LPS): effects on the antioxidant property of lactoferrin an the ability of LPS to prime human neutrophils for enhanced superoxide formation.** *Journal of Infectious Diseases* 166(6):1375-1378 (1992).

546 Zimecki M, Mazurier J, Machnicki M, Wieczorek Z, Montreuil J, Spik G. **Immunostimulatory activity of lactoferrin and maturation of CD4-, CD8- murine thymocytes.** *Immunology Letters* 30(1):119-123 (1991).

Growth Factors

547 Shing YW, Klagsbrun M. **Human and Bovine Milk Contain Different sets of Growth Factors.** *Endocrinology* 115(1):273-282 (1984).

548 Iacoppetta BJ, Grieu F, Horisberger M, Sunahara G I. **Epidermal Growth Factor in Human and Bovine Milk.** *Acta Paediatrica* 81(4):287-291 (1992).

549 Shamay, A, Cohen N, Niwa M, Gertler A. **Effects of Insulin-Like Growth Factor I on Deoxyribonucleic Acid Synthesis and Galactopoiesis in Bovine Undifferentiated and Lactating Mammary Tissue.** *Endocrinology* 123(2):804-809 (1988).

550 Baumrucker CR, Blum JW. **Secretion of Insulin-Like Growth Factors in Milk and their Effect on the Neonate.** *Livestock Production Science* 35: 49-72 (1993).

551 Xu RJ, Mellor DJ, Birtles MJ, Breier BH, Gluckman PD. **Effects of Oral IGF-I or IGF-II on Digestive Organ Growth in Newborn Piglets.** *Biology of the Neonate* 66(5):280-287 (1994).

552 Baumrucker CR, Hadsell DL, Blum JW. **Effects of Dietary Insulin-Like Growth Factor I on Growth and Insulin-Like Growth Factor Receptors in Neonatal Calf Intestine.** *Journal of Animal Science* 72(2):428-433 (1994).

553 Baumrucker CR, Blum JW. **Effects of Dietary Recombinant Human Insulin-Like Growth Factor-I on Concentration of Hormones and Growth Factors in the Blood of Newborn Calves.** *Journal of Endocrinology* 140(1):15-21 (1994).

554 Humbel RE. **Insulin-Like Growth Factors, Somatomedins, and Multiplication Stimulating Activity: Chemistry.** *Hormonal Proteins and Peptides*, Edited by Choh, HL, Volume XII, pp 57-72, 1984.

555 Mero A, Mikklulainen H, Riski J, Pakkanen R, Aalto J, Takala T. **Effects of Bovine Colostrum Supplementation on Serum IGF-1, IgG, Hormone and Saliva IgA During Training.** *Journal of Applied Physiology* 83(4):1144-1151 (1997).

556 Buckley JD, Abbott M, Martin S, Brinkworth G, Whyte P. **Effect of an Oral Bovine Colostrum Supplement on Running Performance.** Abstract from: 1988 Australian Conference of Science and Medicine in Sport, Adelaide, South Australia, October, 1988.

557 Buckley JD, Brinkworth GD, Bourdon PC, Gulbin J, Stilwell EJ, David A, Myers N. **Oral Supplementation with Bovine Colostrum Improves Rowing Performance in Elite Female Rowers.** Abstract presented at the 5th I.O.C. World Congress on Sports Sciences, Sydney, Australia. October, 1999.

558 Buckley JD, Abbott M, Brinkworth GD, Whyte P. **Oral Supplementation with Bovine Colostrum Increases Vertical Jump Performance.** Abstract presented at the 4th Annual Congress of the European College of Sports Science. Rome, Italy, July, 1999.

559 Barton-Davis ER, Shoturma DI, Musaro A, Rosenthal N, Sweeney HL. **Viral Mediated Expression of Insulin-Like Growth Factor I Blocks the Aging-Related Loss**

of Skeletal Muscle Function. *Proceedings of the National Academy of Sciences USA* 95(26):15603-15607 (1998).

560 Hammerman MR. **Insulin-Like Growth Factors and Aging.** *Endocrinology and Metabolism Clinics of North America* 16(4):995-1011 (1987).

561 Cohen P, Ocrant I, Fielder PJ, Neely EK, Gargosky SE, Deal CI, Ceda GP, Youngman O, Pham H, Lamonson G. **Insulin-like Growth Factors (IGFs): Implications for Aging.** *Psychoneuroendocrinology* 17(4):335-342 (1992).

562 Swerdloff RS, Wang C, Hines M, Gorski R. **Effect of Androgens on the Brain and Other Organs During Development and Aging.** *Psychoneuroendocrinology* 17(4):375-383 (1992).

563 George-Nascimento C, Lowenson J., Borissenko M, Calderon A, Medina-Selby A, Kuo J, Clarke S, Randolph A. **Replacement of a Labile Aspartyl Residue Increases the Stability of Human Epidermal Growth Factor.** *Biochemistry* 29(41):9584-9591 (1990).

564 Hall K, Bang P, Brismar K. **[Insulin-like Growth Factors. Future Treatment in Catabolism?]** *Lakartidningen* 92(26-27):2666-2671 (1995).

IGF-1 and Cancer—Not!

565 Spagnoli A, Rosenfeld RG. **The mechanisms by which growth hormone brings about growth. The relative contributions of growth hormone and insulin-like growth factors.** *Endocrinology and Metabolic Clinics of North America* (3):615-631 (1996)

566 Liu JL, LeRoith D. **Insulin-like growth factor I is essential for post-natal growth in response to growth hormone.** *Endocrinology* 140(11):5178-84 (1999).

567 Butler AA, Yakar S, Gewolb IH, Karas M, Okubo Y, LeRoith D. **Insulin-like growth factor-I receptor signal transduction: at the interface between physiology and cell biology.** *Comparative Biochemistry and Physiology B Biochemistry and Molecular Biology* 121(1):19-26 (1998)

568 Hwa V, Oh Y, Rosenfeld RG. **The insulin-like growth factor binding protein (IGFBP) superfamily.** *Endocrinology Reviews* 20(6):761-787 (1999).

569 Werner H, Hernandez-Sanchez C, Karnieli E, LeRoith D. **The regulation of IGF-I receptor gene expression.** *International Journal of Biochemistry and Cell Biology* 27(10):987-994 (1995).

570 LeRoith D. **Insulin-like growth factor receptors and binding proteins.** *Baillieres Clinical Endocrinology and Metabolism* 10(1):49-73 (1996).

571 Kelly KM, Oh Y, Gargosky SE, Gucev Z, Matsumoto T, Hwa V, Ng L, Simpson DM, Rosenfeld RG. **Insulin-like growth factor-binding proteins (IGFBPs) and their regulatory dynamics.** *International Journal of Biochemistry and Cell Biology* 28(6):619-637 (1996).

572 Hasegawa T, Hasegawa Y, Rosenfeld, RG, Cohen P. **Insulin-like growth factor binding**

protein-4 accumulation is negatively correlated with growth rate in TM-3 cells. *Growth Hormone and IGF Research* 8(4):277-282 (1998)

573 Rosenfeld RG, Hwa V, Wilson L, Lopez-Bermejo A, Buckway C, Choi WK, Devi G, Ingermann A, Graham D, Minniti G, Spagnoli A, Oh Y. **The insulin-like growth factor binding protein superfamily: new perspectives.** *Pediatrics* 1999 Oct; 104(4):1018-1021 (1999).

574 Chan JM, Stampfer MJ, Giovannucci E, Gann PH, Ma J, Wilkenson P, Hennekens CH, Pollak M. **Plasma insulin-like growth factor-I and prostate cancer risk: a prospective study.** *Science* 279(5350):563-566 (1998).

575 Wolk A, Mantzorous CS, Anderrson SO, Bergstrom R, Signorello LB, Adami HO, Trichopoulos D. **Insulin-like growth factor-I and prostate cancer risk: a population-based, case-control study.** *Journal of the National Cancer Institute* 90(12):911-5 (1998).

576 Chan JM, Giovannucci E, Anderrson SO, Yuen J, Adami HO, Wolk A. **Dairy products, calcium, phosphorous, vitamin D, and risk of prostate cancer.** *Cancer Causes Control* 9(6):559-566 (1998).

577 Hwa V, Tomasini-Sprenger C, Bermejo AL, Rosenfeld RG, Plymate SR. **Characterization of insulin-like growth factor-binding protein-related protein-1 in prostate cancer.** *Journal of Clinical Endocrinology and Metabolism* 83(12):4355-62 (1998).

578 Sprenger CC, Damon SE, Hwa V, Rosenfeld RG, Plymate SR. **Insulin-like growth factor binding protein-related protein 1 (IGFBP-rP1) is a potent tumor suppressor protein for prostate cancer.** *Cancer Research* 59(10):2370-5 (1999)

579 Papa V, Hartmann KK, Rosenthal SM, Maddux BA, Siiteri PK, Goldfine ID. **Progestins induce down-regulation of insulin-like growth factor-I (IGF-I) receptors in human breast cancer cells: potential autocrine role of IGF-II.** *Molecular Endocrinology* 5(5):709-717 (1991).

580 Goldfine ID, Papa V, Vigneri R, Siiteri P, Rosenthal S. **Progestin regulation of insulin and insulin-like growth factor I receptors in cultured human breast cancer cells.** *Breast Cancer Research and Treatment* 22(1):69-79 (1992).

581 Frittitta L, Vigneri R, Papa V, Goldfine ID, Grasso G, Trischitta V. **Structural and functional studies of insulin receptors in human breast cancer.** *Breast Cancer Research and Treatment* 25(1):73-78 (1993).

582 Papa V, Gliozzo B, Clark GM, McGuire WL, Moore D, Vigneri R, Goldfine ID, Pezzino V. **Insulin-like growth factor-I receptors are overexpressed and predict a low risk in human breast cancer.** *Cancer Research* 53(16):3736-3740 (1993).

583 Papa V, Milazzo G, Goldfine ID, Waldman FM, Vigneri R. **Sporadic amplification of the insulin receptor gene in human breast cancer.** *Journal of Endocrinology Investigation* 20(9):531-6 (1997).

584 Yang DH, Kim HS, Wilson EM, Rosenfeld RG, Oh Y. **Identification of glycosylated 38-**

kDa connective tissue growth factor (IGFBP related protein 2) and proteolytic fragments in human biological fluids, and up-regulation of IGFBP-rP2 expression by TGF-beta in Hs578T human breast cancer cells. *Journal of Clinical Endocrinology and Metabolism* 83(7):2593-6 (1998).

585 Gliozzio B, Sung CK, Scalia P, Papa V, Frasca F, Sciacca L, Giorgino F, Milazzo G, Goldfine ID, Vigneri R,Pezzino V. **Insulin-stimulated cell growth in insulin receptor substrate-1-deficient ZR-75-1 cells is mediated by a phosphatidylinositol-3-kinase-independent pathway.** *Journal of Cell Biochemistry* 70(2):268-280 (1998).

586 Bohlke K, Cramer DW, Trichopoulos D, Mantzorous CS. **Insulin-like growth factor-I in relation to premenopausal ductal carcinoma in situ of the breast.** *Epidemiology* 1998 Sep; 9(5):570-573 (1998).

587 Yamanaka Y, Fowlkes JL, Wilson EM, Rosenfeld RG, Oh Y. **Characterization of insulin-like growth factor binding protein-3 (IGFBP-3) binding to human breast cancer cells: kinetics of IGFBP-3 binding and identification of receptor binding domains of the IGFBP-3 molecule.** *Endocrinology* 140(3):1319-1328 (1999).

588 Ma J, Pollak MN, Giovannucci E, Chan JM, Tao Y, Hennekens CH, Stampfer MJ. **Prospective study of colorectal cancer risk in men and plasma levels of insulin-like growth factor (IGF)-I and IGF binding protein-3.** *Journal of the National Cancer Institute* 91(7):620-5 (1999).

589 How HK, Yeoh A, Quah TC, Oh Y, Rosenfeld RG, Lee KO. **Insulin-like growth factor binding proteins IGFBPs and IGFBP-related protein-1 levels in cerebrospinal fluid of children with acute lymphoblastic leukemia.** *Journal of Clinical Endocrinology and Metabolism* 84(4):1283-1287 (1999).

590 Vorwerk P, Wex H, Hohmann B, Oh Y, Rosenfeld RG, Mittler U. **CTGF (IGFBP-rP2) is specifically expressed in malignant lymphoblasts of patients with acute lymphoblastic leukemia (ALL).** *British Journal of Cancer* 83(6):756-760 (2000).

591 Sueoka N, Lee HY, Wiehle S, Cristiano RJ, Fang B, Ji L, Roth JA, Cohen P, Kurie JM. Insulin-like growth factor binding protein-6 activates programmed cell death in non-small cell lung cancer cells. *Oncogene* 19(38):4432-4436 (2000).

592 Chan (1998), op cit.

593 Bohlke (1998), op cit.

594 Yamanaka (1998), op cit.

595 Ma (1999), op cit.

596 Sprenger (1999), op cit.

597 Yang (1998), op cit.

598 Sueoka (2000), op cit.

599 Mantozoros CS, Tzonou A, Signorello LB, Stampfer M, Trichopoulos D, Adami HO. **Insulin-like growth factor-1 in relation to prostate cancer and benign prostatic hyperplasia.** *British Journal of Cancer* 76(9):1115-1118 (1997).

600 Goldfine (1992), op cit.

601 Yang (1998), op cit.

602 Cohen P, Nunn SE, Peehl DM. **Transforming growth factor-beta induces growth inhibition and IGF-binding protein-3 production in prostatic stromal cells: abnormalities in cells cultured from benign prostatic hyperplasia tissues.** *Journal of Endocrinology* 164(2):215-23 (2000).

603 Travers SH, Labarta JI, Gargosky SE, Rosenfeld RG, Jeffers BW. **Insulin-like growth factor binding protein-I levels are strongly associated with insulin sensitivity and obesity in early pubertal children.** Journal of Clinical Endocrinology and Metabolism 83(6):1935-1939 (1998).

604 Burvin R, LeRoith D, Harel H, Zloczower M, Marbach M, Karnieli E. **The effect of acute insulin-like growth factor-II administration on glucose metabolism in the rat.** *Growth Hormone and IGF Research* 8(3):205-210 (1998).

605 Spagnoli A, Chiarelli F, Vorwerk P, Boscherini B, Rosenfeld RG. **Evaluation of the components of insulin-like growth factor (IGF) and IGF binding protein (IGFBP) system in adolescents with type 1 diabetes and persistent microalbuminuria: relationship with increased excretion of IGFBP-3 18 kD N-terminal fragment.** *Clinical Endocrinology (Oxford)* 51(5):587-96 (1999).

606 Travers (1998), op cit.

607 Signorello LB, Wuu J, Tzonou A, Trichopoulos D, Mantozoros CS. **Hormones and hair patterning in men: a role for insulin-like growth factor 1.** *Journal of the American Academy of Dermatology* 40(2):200-203 (1999).

608 de Lacerda L, Carvalho JA, Stannard B, Werner H, Boguszewski MC, Sandrini R, Malozowski SN, LeRoith D, Underwood, LE. **In vitro and in vivo responses to short-term recombinant human insulin-like growth factor-1 (IGF-1) in a severely growth-retarded girl with ring chromosome 15 and deletion of a single allele for IGF-1 receptor gene.** *Clinical Endocrinology (Oxford)* 51(5):541-550 (1999).

609 Butler AA, Blakesley VA, Poulaki V, Tsokos M, Wood TL, LeRoith D. **Stimulation of tumor growth by recombinant insulin-like growth factor-I (IGF-I) is dependent on the dose and level of IGF-I receptor expression.** *Cancer Research* 58(14):3021-3027 (1998).

610 Grimberg A, Cohen P. **Role of insulin-like growth factors and their binding proteins in growth control and carcinogenesis.** *Journal of Cell Physiology* 183(1):1-9 (2000).

611 Werner H, Karnieli E, Rauscher FJ, LeRoith D. **Wild-type and mutant p53 differentially regulate transcription of the insulin-like growth factor-I receptor gene. Proceedings of the National Academy of Sciences USA** 93(16):8318-23 (1996).

612 Mannhardt B, Weinzimmer SA, Wagner M, Fiedler M, Cohen P, Jansen P, Zwerschke W.

Human papillomavirus type 16 E7 oncoprotein binds and inactivates growth-inhibitory insulin-like growth factor binding protein-3. *Molecular and Cell Biology* 20(17):6483-95 (2000).

Glutathione: A Powerful Antioxidant Found In Colostrum

613 Glutathione. **Alternative Health Care.** 2(4) May 1999. http://www.healthalternative.org/vol2.htm 24 June 2002.

614 Bounous G. **Whey Protein Concentrate (WPC) and Glutathione Modulation in Cancer Treatment.** *Anticancer* 20(6C):4785-4792 (2000).

615 Kennedy RS, Konokil GP, Bounous G, Baruchel S. **The Use of a Protein Concentrate in the Treatment of Pathogens with Metastatic Carcinoma: A Phase I-II Clinical Study.** *Anticancer Research* 15:2643-2650 (1995).

616 Petrosino SP. **The Benefits of Glutathione (GSH).** The Nutrition Advisor. http://NutritionAdvisor.com 20 June 2002.

617 Parodi PW. **Cow's Milk Components With Anti-Cancer Potential.** *Australian Journal of Dairy Technology* 56:65-73 (2001).

618 Zhang YH, Kramer TR, Taylor PR, Li JY, Blot WJ, Brown CC, Guo W, Dawsey SM, Li B. **Possible immunologic involvement of antioxidants in cancer prevention.** *American Journal of Clinical Nutrition* 62(6 Suppl):1477S-1482S (1995).

619 Buescher ES, McIlheran SM. **Antioxidant Properties of Human Colostrum.** *Pediatrics Research* 24(1)14-19 (1988).

620 Lands LC, Grey VL, Smountas AA. **The Effect of Supplementation With a Cysteine Donor on Muscular Performance.** *Journal of Applied Physiology* 87(4):1381-1385 (1999).

621 Reeds PJ, Burrin DG, Stoll B, Jahoor F, Wykes L, Henry J, Frazer M. **Enteral Glutamate is the Preferential Source of Mucosal Glutathione Synthesis in the Piglet.** *American Journal of Physiology* 273(2 Pt.1):E408-E415 (1997).

622 Micke P, Beeh KM, Sclaak JK, Buhl R. **Oral Supplementation With Whey Proteins Increases Plasma Glutathione Levels of HIV-Infected Patients.** *European Journal of Clinical Investigation* 31(20):171-178 (2001).

623 **Health-Enhancing Properties of Dairy Ingredients—Composition of Whey.** *Dairy Council Digest* June 24, 2002.

Complex Lipids

624 Lambersten G, Christiansen EN. **Milk Fat: Nutrition And Product Development.** *Scandinavian Journal of Nutrition* 41:88-90 (1997). http://www.snf.ideon.se/sjn/temanr/pdf-filer/297milk%20fat.pdf

625 Paltauf F, Hermetter A. **Phospholipids: Natural, Semi-synthetic, Synthetic.** In:

Phospholipids, Hanin and Pepeu (eds.). New York, Plenum Press, 1990, pp 1-12.

626 Laegreid A, Otnaess AB, Fuglesang J. **Human and Bovine Milk: Comparison and Enterotoxin-Inhibitory Activity.** *Pediatric Research* 20(5):416-421 (1986).

627 Malmsten M, Bergenståhl B, Nyberg L, Odham G. **Sphingomyelin from Milk: Characterization of Liquid Crystalline, Liposome and Emulsion Properties.** JAOCS 71(9):1021-1026 (1994).

628 Holmgren J., Sveneerholm AM, Ahren C. **Non-Immunoglobulin Fraction of Human Milk Inhibits Bacterial Adhesion (Hemagglutination) and Enterotoxin Binding of *Escherichia coli* and *Vibrio cholerae*.** *Infection and Immunity* 33(1):136-141 (1981).

629 Hannun YA, Linardic CM. **Sphingolipid breakdown products: anti-proliferative and tumor-suppressor lipids.** *Biochimica et Biophysica Acta* 1154(3-4):223-236 (1993).

630 Dillehay DL, Webb SK, Schmelz EM, Merrill AH Jr. **Dietary sphingomyelin inhibits 1,2-dimethylhydrazine-induced colon cancer in CF1 mice.** *Journal of Nutrition* 124(5):615-620 (1994).

631 Modrak DE, Rodriguez MD, Goldenberg DM, Lew W, Blumenthal R. **Sphingomyelin Enhances Chemotherapy Efficacy and Increases Apoptosis in Human Colonic Tumor Xenografts.** *International Journal of Oncology* 20(2):379-384 (2002).

632 Takamizama K, Iwamori M, Mutai M, Nagai Y. 1986. **Gangliosides of Bovine Buttermilk. Isolation and Characterization of a Novel Monosialoganglioside with a Branching Structure.** *Journal of Biological Chemistry* 261(12): 5625-5630 (1986).

633 Sinforiana E, Agostinis C, Merlo P, Gualtieri S, Mauri M, Mancuso A. **Cognitive Decline in Aging Brain.** *Clinical Trials Journal* 24(1):115-124 (1987).

634 Kidd, PM. **Phosphatidylserine Offers Nutritional Support for Brain Function.** *Vitamin Retailer* January, 1999.

635 Amaducci L. The SMID Group. **Phosphatidylserine in the treatment of Alzheimer's disease: results of a multicenter study.** *Psychopharmacology Bulletin* 24(1):130–134 (1988).

636 Caffarra P, Santamaria V. **The effects of phosphatidylserine in patients with mild cognitive decline: an open trial.** *Clinical Trials Journal* 24(1):109-114 (1987).

637 Cenacchi T, Bertoldin T, Farina C, Fiori MG, Crepaldi G. **Cognitive decline in the elderly: A double-blind, placebo-controlled multicenter study on efficacy of phosphatidylserine administration.** *Aging* 5:123-133 (1993).

638 Funfgeld EW, Nedwick P. **Neurohomologous phosphatidylserine in Parkinson's patients with associated disorders of cerebral metabolism.** *Clinical Trials Journal* 24(1):42-61 (1987).

639 Nunzi MG, Milan F, Guidolin D, Zanotti A, Toffano G. **Therapeutic properties of Phosphatidylserine in the Aging Brain.** In: *Phospholipids*, Hanin and Pepeu (eds.). New York: Plenum Press, 1990.

640 Villardita C, Grioli S, Salmeri G, Nicoletti F, Pennisi G. **Multicenter Clinical Trial of**

Brain Phosphatidylserine in Elderly Patients With Intellectual Deterioration. *Clinical Trials Journal* 24(1):84-93 (1987).

641 Pakula R, Konikoff FM, Rubin M, Ringel Y, Peled Y, Tietz A, Gilat T. **The Effects of Dietary Phospholipids Enriched with Phosphatidylethanolamine on Bile and Red Cell Membrane Lipids in Humans.** *Lipids* 31(3):295-303 (1996).

642 Holub BJ. **The nutritional significance, metabolism, and function of myo-inositol and phosphatidylinositol in health and disease.** *Advances in Nutrition Research* 4:107-141 (1982).

Lactose Intolerance, Dairy Products, and Colostrum

643 Sahi T. **Genetics and epidemiology of adult-type hypolactasia.** *Scandinavian Journal of Gastroenterology Supplement* 202:7-20 (1994).

644 Scrimshaw NS, Murray EB. **The acceptability of milk and milk products in populations with a high prevalence of lactose intolerance.** *American Journal of Clinical Nutrition* 48(4 Suppl):1079-1159 (1988).

645 Vesa TH, Korpela RA, Sahi T. **Tolerance to small amounts of lactose in lactose maldigesters.** *American Journal of Clinical Nutrition* 64(2):197-201 (1996).

646 Suarez FL, Savaiano D, Arbisi P, Levitt MD. **Tolerance to the daily ingestion of two cups of milk by individuals claiming lactose intolerance.** *American Journal of Clinical Nutrition* 65(5):1502-1506 (1997).

647 Gilliland SE, Kim HS. **Effect of viable starter culture bacteria in yogurt on lactose utilization in humans.** *Journal of Dairy Science* 67:1-6 (1984).

648 Jennes R, Sloan RE. **The composition of milks of various species: a review.** *Dairy Science Abstracts* 32:599-612.

649 Kolars JC, Levitt MD, Aouji M, Savaino DA. **Yogurt—an autodigesting source of lactose.** *New England Journal of Medicine* 310(1):1-3 (1984).

650 Hertzler SR, Huynh BC, Savaiano DA. **How much lactose is low lactose?** *Journal of the American Dietary Association* 96(3):243-246 (1996).

Colostrum Plus Probiotics, Prebiotics, and Complex Lipids The Ideal Combination

651 Smith T, Little RB. **The significance of colostrum to the newborn calf.** *Journal of Experimental Medicine* 36:181-186 (1922).

652 McGuire TC, Pfeiffer NE, Weikel JM, Bartsch RG. **Failure of colostral immunoglobulin transfer in calves dying from infectious disease.** *Journal of the American Veterinary Medical Association* 169:713-716 (1976).

653 Brambell FWR. **The Transmission of Passive Immunity From Mother to Young.**

Proceedings of the Nutrition Society 28:35-41 (1969).

654 McEwan AD, Fisher EW, Selman IE. **Observations on the immunoglobulin level of neonatal calves and their relationship to disease.** *Journal of Comparative Pathology* 80: 259-263 (1970).

655 Hilpert H, Gerber H, Amster H, Pahud JJ, Ballabriga A, Arcalis L, Farriaux JP, de Peyer E, Nussle, D. **Bovine milk immunoglobulins (Ig): Their possible utilization in industrially prepared infant's milk formulae.** In: Food and Immunology, Swedish Nutritional Foundation Symposium XIII, Hambraeus, Hanson and McFarlane (eds.), pp 182-196. Stockholm: Almquist and Wiksell, 1977.

656 Penhale WJ, Logan EF, Selman IE, Fisher EW, McEwan, AD. **Observations on the adsorption of colostral immunoglobulins by neonatal calf and their significance in colibacillosis.** *Annales de Recherches Vétérinaires* 4:223-229 (1973).

657 Pahud JJ, Hilbert H, Schwartz K, Amster H, Smiley M. **Bovine milk antibodies in the treatment of enteric infections and their ability to eliminate virulence factors from pathogenic E. coli.** In: *The Ruminant Immune System*, edited by J. E. Butler, pp 591-600. New York: Plenum Press, 1981.

658 Tacket CO, Losonsky G, Link H, Hoang Y, Guesry P, Hilpert H, Levine MM. **Protection by milk immunoglobulin concentrate against oral challenge with enterogenic *Escherichia coli*.** *New England Journal of Medicine* 318(19):1240-1241 (1988).

659 Tacket CO, Binion SB, Bostwick E, Losonsky G, Roy MJ, Edelman R. **Efficacy of bovine milk immunoglobulin concentrate in preventing illness after *Shigella flexneri* challenge.** *American Journal of Tropical Medicine and Hygiene* 47(3):276-283 (1992).

660 Mietens C, Keinhorst H, Hilpert H, Gerber H, Amster H, Pahud JJ. **Treatment of infantile E. coli gastroenteritis with specific bovine anti-E. coli milk immunoglobulins.** *European Journal of Pediatrics* 132: 239-52 (1979).

661 Brussow H, Hilpert H, Walther J, Sidoti J, Meitens C, Bachman P. **Bovine milk immunoglobulins for passive immunity to infantile rotavirus gastroenteritis.** *Journal of Microbiology* 25: 982-986 (1987).

662 Ebina T, Sato A, Umezu K, Ishida N, Ohyama S, Oizumi A, Kitaoka S, Suzuki H, Kunno T. **Prevention of rotavirus infection by oral administration of cow colostrum containing antihuman rotavirus antibody.** *Medical Microbiology and Immunology* 174(4):177-185 (1985).

663 Hilpert H, Brussow H, Meitens C, Sidoti J, Lerner L, Werchau H. **Use of bovine milk concentrate containing antibody to rotavirus to treat rotavirus gastroenteritis in infants.** *Journal of Infectious Diseases* 156(1):158-166 (1987).

664 Tzipori CO, Binion SB, Bostwick E, Losonsky G, Roy MJ, Edelman R. **Remission of diarrhoea due to cryptosporidiosis in an immunodeficient child treated with hyperimmune bovine colostrum.** *British Medical Journal Clinical Research Edition* 293(6557):1276-1277 (1986).

665 McConnell MA, Buchanan G, Borissenko MV, Brooks HJL. **A Comparison of IgG and IgG1 Activity in an Early Milk Concentrate from Non-Immunized Cows and a Milk from Hyperimmunized Animals.** *Food Research International* 34:255-261 (2001).

666 Pascall IC, Surani MA, Barton SC, Vaughan TJ, Brown KD. **Directed expression of simian virus 40 T-antigen in transgenic mice using the epidermal growth factor gene promoter.** *Journal of Molecular Endocrinology* 12(3):313-325 (1994).

667 Baird A. **Fibroblast growth factors: activities and significance of non-neurotrophin neurotrophic growth factors.** *Current Opinions in Neurobiology* 4(1):78-86 (1994).

668 **Hormonal Proteins and Peptides.** *Growth Factors*, Vol. XII, Choh, H.L. (ed) 1984.

669 Tannock GW. **Normal Microflora.** *An introduction to the Microbes Inhabiting the Human Body*, Chapman & Hill, 1995.

670 Payne MJ. **Probiotic Organisms.** *Recent Advances in Microbiology* 3:215-254 (1995).

671 Sanders ME. **Probiotics.** *Food Technology* 53(11):67-77 (1999).

672 Shahani KM, Chandan RC. **Nutritional and healthful aspects of cultured and culture-containing dairy foods.** *Journal of Dairy Science* 62(10):1685-1694 (1979).

673 Friend BA, Shahani KM. **Nutritional and therapeutic aspects of lactobacilli.** *Journal of Applied Nutrition* 36:125-53 (1984).

674 Gomes AM, Malcata FX. **Bifidobacterium spp. and Lactobacillus acidophilus: biological, biochemical, technological and therapeutical properties relevant for use as probiotics.** *Trends in Food Science & Technology* 10:139-157 (1999).

675 Siitonen S, Vapaatalo H, Salminen S, Gordin A, Saxelin M, Wikberg R, Kirkkola AL. **Effect of Lactobacillus GG yoghurt in prevention of antibiotic associated diarrhea.** *Annals of Medicine* 22(1):57-59 (1990).

676 Oksanen PJ, Salminen S, Saxelin M, Hamalainen P, Ihantola-Vormisto A, Muurasniemi-Isoviita L, Nikkari S, Oksanen T, Porsti I, Salminen E. **Prevention of travellers' diarrhea by Lactobacillus GG.** *Annals of Medicine* 22(1):53-56 (1990).

677 Isolauri E, Juntunen M, Rautanen T, Sillanaukee P, Koivula T. **A human Lactobacillus strain (*Lactobacillus casei* sp. Strain GG) promotes recovery from acute diarrhea in children.** *Pediatrics* 88(1):90-97 (1991).

678 Seki M, Igarashi T, Fukuda Y, Simamura S, Kaswashima T, Ogasa K. **The effect of Bifidobacterium cultured milk on "regularity" among an aged group.** *Nutritional Foodstuff* 31:379-387 (1978).

679 Nanji AA, Khettry U, Sadrzadeh SM. **Lactobacillus feeding reduces endotoxemia and severity of experimental alcoholic liver (disease).** *Proceedings of the Society for Experimental Biology and Medicine* 205:243-247 (1994).

680 Gade J, Thorn P. **Paraghurt for patients with irritable bowel syndrome. A controlled clinical investigation from general practice.** *Scandinavian Journal of Primary Health Care* 7(1):23-26 (1989).

681 Kruis W, Schutz E, Fric P, Fixa B, Judmaier G, Stolte M. **Double-blind comparison of an oral *Escherichia coli* preparation and mesalazine in maintaining remission of ulcerative colitis.** *Alimentary Pharmacology and Therapeutics* 11(5):853-858 (1997).

682 Majamaa H, Isolauri E. Probiotics: a novel approach in the management of food allergy. *Journal of Allergy and Clinical Immunology* 99:179-185 (1997).

683 Aso Y, Akazan H. **Prophylactic effect of a *Lactobacillus casei* preparation on the recurrence of superficial bladder cancer.** *Urologica Internationalis* 49(3):125-129 (1992).

684 Alm L. **Effect of fermentation on B-vitamin content of milk in Sweden.** *Journal of Dairy Science* 65:353-9 (1982).

685 Tomomatsu H. (1994) **Health Effects of Oligosaccharides.** Food Technology 48:61-65 (1994).

686 Tungland BC. **A Natural Prebiotic.** *The World of Food Ingredients*, September 1998.

687 Urashima T, Saito T., Ohmisya K, Shimazaki K. **Structural Determination of Three Neutral Oligosaccharides in Bovine Colostrum, including the Novel Trisaccharide; GalNAc alpha 1-3Gal beta 1-4Glc.** *Biochimica et Biophysica Acta* 1073(1):225-229 (1990).

688 O'Carroll P. **Formulating yogurt.** *The World of Food Ingredients*, April 1997.

689 Deis DR. **New Directions for Cultured Dairy Products.** Food Product Design Elements. 25 March 2001. http://www.foodproductdesign.com/archive/200/0300de.html

690 van den Broek A. **Functional Foods: The Japanese Approach.** *International Food Ingredients* 1(2):4-9 (1993)

691 Klont R, Mannion P. **Inulin and Oligofructose.** *The World of Food Ingredients*, September 1998.

692 Sensus Product Bulletins, P.O. Box 1308, 4700 BH Roosendaal, The Netherlands (1997).

693 Brandt L. **New Inulin Offers High Performance.** *Prepared Foods*, May 1998.

694 Remesy C, Levrat M, Gamet L, Demigne CD. **Cecal fermentations in rats fed oligosaccharides (inulin) are modulated by dietary calcium level.** *American Journal of Physiology* 264(5 Pt 1):G855-G862 (1993).

695 Paltauf F, Hermetter A. **Phospholipids: Natural, Semi-synthetic, Synthetic.** In: *Phospholipids*, Hanin and Pepeu (eds.). New York, Plenum Press, 1990, pp 1-12.

696 Lambersten G, Christiansen EN. **Milk Fat: Nutrition And Product Development.** *Scandinavian Journal of Nutrition* 41:88-90 (1997). http://www.snf.ideon.se/sjn/temanr/pdf-filer/297milk%20fat.pdf

697 Laegreid A, Otnaess AB, Fuglesang J. **Human and Bovine Milk: Comparison and Enterotoxin-Inhibitory Activity.** *Pediatric Research* 20(5):416-421 (1986).

698 Takamizama K, Iwamori M, Mutai M, Nagai Y. 1986. **Gangliosides of Bovine Buttermilk. Isolation and Characterization of a Novel Monosialoganglioside with a Branching Structure.** *Journal of Biological Chemistry* 261(12): 5625-5630 (1986).

699 Malmsten M, Bergenståhl B, Nyberg L, Odham G. **Sphingomyelin from Milk: Characterization of Liquid Crystalline, Liposome and Emulsion Properties.** JAOCS 71(9):1021-1026 (1994).

700 Holmgren J., Sveneerholm AM, Ahren C. **Non-Immunoglobulin Fraction of Human Milk Inhibits Bacterial Adhesion (Hemagglutination) and Enterotoxin Binding of *Escherichia coli* and *Vibrio cholerae*.** *Infection and Immunity* 33(1):136-141 (1981).

701 Hannun YA, Linardic CM. **Sphingolipid breakdown products: anti-proliferative and tumor-suppressor lipids.** *Biochemica et Biophysica Acta* 1154(2-3):223-236 (1993).

702 Dillehay DL, Webb SK, Schmetz EM, Merrill AH Jr. **Dietary sphingomyelin inhibits 1,2-dimethylhydrazine-induced colon cancer in CF1 mice.** *Journal of Nutrition* 124(5):615-620 (1994).

703 Modrak DE, Rodriguez MD, Goldenberg DM, Lew W, Blumenthal R. **Sphingomyelin Enhances Chemotherapy Efficacy and Increases Apoptosis in Human Colonic Tumor Xenografts.** *International Journal of Oncology* 20(2):379-384 (2002).

704 Kidd PM. **Phosphatidylserine Offers Nutritional Support for Brain Function.** *Vitamin Retailer,* January 1999.

705 Nunzi MG, Milan F, Guidolin D, Zanotti A, Toffano G. **Therapeutic properties of Phosphatidylserine in the Aging Brain.** In: *Phospholipids*, Hanin and Pepeu (eds.). New York: Plenum Press, 1990.

706 Sinforiana E, Agostinis C, Merlo P, Gualtieri S, Mauri M, Mancuso A. **Cognitive Decline in Aging Brain.** *Clinical Trials Journal* 24(1):115-124 (1987).

707 Villardita C, Grioli S, Salmeri G, Nicoletti F, Pennisi G. **Multicenter Clinical Trial of Brain Phosphatidylserine in Elderly Patients With Intellectual Deterioration.** *Clinical Trials Journal* 24(1):84-93 (1987).

708 Amaducci L. **Phosphatidylserine in the treatment of Alzheimer's disease: results of a multicenter study.** *Psychopharmacology Bulletin* 24(1):130–134 (1988).

709 Caffarra P, Santamaria V. **The effects of phosphotidylserine in patients with mild cognitive decline: an open trial.** *Clinical Trials Journal* 1987; 24(1): 109–114.

710 Cenacchi T, Bertoldin T, Farina C, Fiori MG, Crepaldi G. **Cognitive decline in the elderly: A double-blind, placebo-controlled multicenter study on efficacy of phosphatidylserine administration.** *Aging* 5(2):123-133 (1993).

711 Funfgeld EW, Nedwidek P. **Neurohomologous phosphatidylserine in Parkinson's patients with associated disorders of cerebral metabolism.** *Clinical Trials Journal* 24(1):42–61 (1987).

712 Pakula R, Konikoff FM, Rubin M, Ringel Y, Peled Y, Tietz A, Gilat T. **The Effects of Dietary Phospholipids Enriched with Phosphatidylethanolamine on Bile and Red Cell Membrane Lipids in Humans.** *Lipids* 31(3):295-303 (1996).

713 Cohen BM, Babb SM, Yurgelun-Todd D. **Brain choline uptake and cognitive function in middle age.** *Biological Psychiatry* 41:905 (1997).

714 Holub BJ. **The nutritional significance, metabolism, and function of myo-inositol and phosphatidylinositol in health and disease.** *Advances in Nutrition Research* 4:107-141 (1982).

Pasteurization

715 University of Guelph. **Pasteurization module.** http://www.foodsci.uoguelph.ca/dairyedu/pasteurization.html 17/05/02

716 **Grade "A" Pasteurized Milk Ordinance.** 1999 Revision. U.S. Department of Health & Human Services. Public Health Services, Food and Drug Administration, Washington DC, United States of America.

717 International Dairy Foods Association. **Regulation and Food Safety, Current Systems for Thermal Processing.** www.idfa.org/reg/fda/fedhaccp.htm 11/06/02.

718 Korhonen H. **Immune Milk Preparations—Novel Means for Prevention and Treatment of Human Microbial Diseases.** September 2000, Agricultural Research Centre, Food Research, FIN-31600 Jokioinen, Finland.

719 **Dairy Heat Treatment.** Discussion Paper 35. Ministry of Agriculture and Forestry, Wellington, New Zealand.

720 Chen CC, Tu YY, Chang HM. **Thermal Stability of Bovine Milk Immunoglobulin G (IgG) and the Effect of Added Thermal Protectants on the Stability.** *Journal of Food Science* 65(2):188-193 (2000).

721 Li-Chan E, Kummer A, Losso JN, Kitts DD, Nakai S. (1995). **Stability of Bovine Immunoglobulins to Thermal Treatment and Processing.** *Food Research International* 28:9-16 (1995).

722 Mainer G, Dominguez E, Randrup M, Sanchez L, Calvo M. **Effect of Heat Treatment on Anti-Rotavirus Activity of Bovine Colostrum.** *Journal of Dairy Research* 66:131-137 (1999).

723 Dominguez E, Perez MD, Calvo M. **Effect of Heat Treatment on the Antigen-Binding Activity of Anti-Peroxidase Immunoglobulins in Bovine Colostrum.** *Journal of Dairy Science* 80(12):3182-3187 (1997).

724 Wei H, Loimaranta V, Tenovuo J, Rokka S, Syvaoja EL, Korhonen H, Joutsjoki V, Marnila P. **Stability and Activity Specific Antibodies Against Streptococcus mutans and Streptococcus sobrinus in Bovine Milk Fermented with Lactobacillus Strain GG or Treated at Ultra-High Temperature.** *Oral Microbiological Immunology* 17(1):9-15 (2002).

Freeze Drying vs Spray Drying

725 **Food Processing and Preservation.** Microsoft Encarta Online Encyclopedia 2000.

726 **How Food Preservation Works.** Marshal Brian's How Stuff Works http://www.howstuffworks.com.

727 Jennings TA. **Overview of the Lyophilization Process.** INSIGHT 1(9):1-6 (2000). http://www.phase-technology.com.

728 McConnell MA, Buchan GAA, Borissenko MV, Brooks HJL. **A Comparison of IgG and IgG1 Activity in an Early Milk Concentrate from Non-Immunized Cows and a Milk from Hyperimmunized Animals.** *Food Research International* 34:255-261 (2001).

729 Mujumdar AS. **Handbook for Industrial Drying.** 1987, New York: Marcel Dekker.

730 Donnelly PE, Petch SF, McLaren RD, Oakley AP. **Development of a Dried Colostrum.** *Proceedings of the New Zealand Society of Animal Production* 48:143-146 (1988).

731 Scopes RK. **Protein Purification: Principles and Practice.** Springer Advanced Texts in Chemistry, 1988; C.R. Cantor (ed), 2nd edition, pp. 237- 252.

732 Borissenko M, Bryce M. **The Effect of Spray Drying versus Freeze Drying on IGF-1 Levels in Colostrum.** Manuscript in progress.

733 Hilpert H, Gerber H, Amster H, Pahud JJ, Ballabriga A, Arcalis L, Farriaux JP, de Peyer E, Nussle D. **Bovine milk immunoglobulins (Ig) their possible utilization in industrially prepared infant's milk formulae.** In: Food and Immunology, Swedish Nutritional Foundation Symposium XIII, edited by L Hambraeus, LA Hanson, and H McFarlane, pp 182-196. Almquist and Wiksell, Stockholm, 1977.

734 Xu RJ, Mellor DJ, Birtles MJ, Breier BH, Gluckman PD. **Effects of Oral IGF-1 or IGF-II on Digestive Organ Growth in Newborn Piglets.** *Biology of the Neonate* 66(5):280-287 (1994).

735 Baumrucker CR, Hadsell DL, Blum JW. **Effects of Dietary Insulin-Like Growth Factor I on Growth and Insulin-Like Growth Factor Receptors in Neonatal Calf Intestine.** *Journal of Animal Science* 72(2):428-433 (1994).

736 Baumrucker CR, Blum JW. **Secretion of Insulin-Like Growth Factors in Milk and their Effect on the Neonate.** *Livestock Production Science* 35: 49-72 (1993).

737 Mero A, Mikklulainen H, Riski J, Pakkanen R, Aalto J, Takala T. **Effects of Bovine Colostrum Supplementation on Serum IGF-1, IgG, Hormone and Saliva IgA During Training.** *Journal of Applied Physiology* 83(4):1144-1151 (1997).

738 Mietens C, Keinhorst H, Hilpert H, Gerber H, Amster H, Pahud JJ. **Treatment of infantile E. coli gastroenteritis with specific bovine anti-E. coli milk immunoglobulins.** *European Journal of Pediatrics* 132(4):239-252 (1979).

739 Brussow H, Hilpert H, Walther J, Sidoti J, Meitens C, Bachman P. **Bovine milk immunoglobulins for passive immunity to infantile rotavirus gastroenteritis.** *Journal of Clinical Microbiology* 25(6):982-6 (1987).

740 Ebina T, Sato A, Umezu K, Ishida N, Ohyama S, Oizumi A, Aikawa K, Katagiri S, Katsushima N, Imai A. **Prevention of rotavirus infection by oral administration of cow colostrum containing antihuman rotavirus antibody.** *Medical Microbiology and Immunology* 174(4):177-85 (1985).

741 Tacket CO, Binion SB, Bostwick E, Losonsky G, Roy MJ, Edelman R. (1992). **Efficacy of**

bovine milk immunoglobulin concentrate in preventing illness after *Shigella flexneri* challenge. *American Journal of Tropical Medicine and Hygiene* 47(3):276-283 (1992).

742 Hilpert H, Brussow H, Meitens C, Sidoti J, Lerner L, Werchau H. **Use of bovine milk concentrate containing antibody to rotavirus to treat rotavirus gastroenteritis in infants.** *Journal of Infectious Diseases* 156(1):158-166 (1987).

743 Tzipori S, Roberton D, Chapman C. **Remission of diarrhoea due to cryptosporidiosis in an immunodeficient child treated with hyperimmune bovine colostrum.** *British Medical Journal Clinical Research Edition* 293(6557):1276-1277(1986).

744 McConnell MA, Buchan G, Borissenko MV, Brooks HJL. (1998). **A Comparative Study Of Immunoglobulin Levels in Four Colostrum Derived Milks.** Abstract presented at the Joint Annual Meeting of The New Zealand Microbiology Society and The New Zealand Society for Biochemistry and Molecular Biology. Masterton, New Zealand, November, 1998.

745 McConnell MA, Buchanan G, Borissenko MV, Brooks HJL. **A Comparison of IgG and IgG1 Activity in an Early Milk Concentrate from Non-Immunized Cows and a Milk from Hyperimmunized Animals.** *Food Research International* 34:255-261 (2001).

746 **Health-Enhancing Properties of Dairy Ingredients—Composition of Whey.** *Dairy Council Digest* June 24, 2002. http://www.nationaldairycouncil.org/lvl04/nutrib/digest/dairydigest_722b.htm 24/6/02.

747 **Antioxidant Activity of Colostrum.** http://www.doctors-choice.com/activity.html 22 June, 2002

748 Buescher ES, McIlheran SM. **Antioxidant Properties of Human Colostrum.** *Pediatrics Research* 24(1)14-19 (1988).

749 Micke P, Beeh KM, Sclaak JK, Buhl R. **Oral Supplementation With Whey Proteins Increases Plasma Glutathione Levels of HIV-Infected Patients.** *European Journal of Clinical Investigations* 31(20):171-178 (2001).

750 **Glutathione.** *Alternative Health Care.* Volume Two, Article Four, May 1999. http://www.healthalternative.org/vol2.htm 24 June 2002.

751 Borissenko M. **Glutathione—A Powerful Antioxidant Found in Colostrum. Science Review.** *Institute of Colostrum Research* August 2002 www.colostrumresearch.org

752 Petrosino SP. **The Benefits of Glutathione (GSH).** *The Nutrition Advisor.* http://NutritionAdvisor.com 20 June 2002.

753 **The-Analysis-Glutathione.** http://www.digitalnaturopath.com/treat/treat/T147297.html 24 June, 2002.

754 Parodi PW. **Cow's Milk Components With Anti-Cancer Potential.** *Australian Journal of Dairy Technology* 56:65-73 (2001).

755 Bounous G. **Whey Protein Concentrate (WPC) and Glutathione Modulation in Cancer Treatment.** *Anticancer* 20(6C):4785-4792 (2000).

756 Lands LC, Grey VL, Smountas AA. T**he Effect of Supplementation With a Cysteine**

Donor on Muscular Performance. *Journal of Applied Physiology* 87(4):1381-1385 (1999).

757 Leppäluoto J, Rasi S, Martikkala V, Puukka M. **Bovine Colostrum Supplementation Enhances Physical Performance on Maximal Exercise Tests.** 2000 Pre-Olympic Congress Sports Medicine and Physical Education International Congress on Sport Science. Brisbane, Australia. 7-13 September, 2000.

758 Coombes JS, Conacher M, Austen SK, Marshall PA. **Dose effects of Oral Bovine Colostrum Supplementation on Physical Work Capacity in Cyclists.** 2000 Pre-Olympic Congress Sports Medicine and Physical Education International Congress on Sport Science. Brisbane, Australia. 7-13 September, 2000.

759 Buckley JD, Abbott M, Martin S, Brinkworth G, Whyte P. **Effect of an Oral Bovine Colostrum Supplement on Running Performance.** Abstract from: 1988 Australian Conference of Science and Medicine in Sport, Adelaide, South Australia, October, 1988.

760 Murdie A, Cummins R, McKay J. **Effect of Bovine Colostrum on Immunological Status of Competitive Swimmers.** Global Bioactives Summit, July 25-7, 2001, Hamilton, New Zealand.

761 Griffin F, Hopkins W, Rehrer N, Thomson C, Walmsley A. **The Effects of Dietary Supplementation with Bovine Colostrum on the Training, Immunologic Status, and Performance of Competitive Distance Runners.** Annual Sport Science New Zealand Conference, September 2-30, 2001, Wellington, New Zealand.

762 Coombes JS, Conacher M, Austen SK, Marshal PA. **Dose Effects of Oral Bovine Colostrum on Physical Work Capacity in Cyclists.** *Medicine & Science in Sports & Exercise* 34(7):1184-88 (2002).

763 Burke E. **Colostrum as an Athletic Enhancer and Help for AIDS.** *Nutrition Science News.* May, 1996.

764 Kuipers H, van Breda E, Verlaan G, Smeets R. **Effects of Oral Bovine Colostrum Supplementation on Serum Insulin-Like Growth Factor-1 Levels.** *Nutrition* 18(7-8):566-567 (2002).

765 Baumrucker CR, Blum JW. **Effects of Dietary Recombinant Human Insulin-Like Growth Factor-1 on Concentration of Hormones and Growth Factors in the Blood of Newborn Calves.** *Journal of Endocrinology* 140(1):15-21 (1994).

766 Humbel RE. **Insulin-Like Growth Factors, Somatomedins, and Multiplication Stimulating Activity: Chemistry.** *Hormonal Proteins and Peptides*, Edited by Choh, HL, Volume XII, pp 57-72, 1984.

767 Antonio J, Sanders MS, Van Gammeren D. **The Effects of Bovine Colostrum Supplementation on Body Composition and Exercise Performance in Active Men and Women.** *Nutrition* (3):243-7 (2001).

768 Barton-Davis ER, Shoturma DI, Musaro A, Rosenthal N, Sweeney HL. **Viral Mediated Expression of Insulin-Like Growth Factor 1 Blocks the Aging-Related Loss**

of Skeletal Muscle Function. *Proceedings of the National Academy of Sciences USA* 95(26):15603-15607 (1998).

769 Buckley JD, Abbott M, Brinkworth GD, Whyte P. **Oral Supplementation with Bovine Colostrum Increases Vertical Jump Performance.** Abstract presented at the 4th Annual Congress of the European College of Sports Science. Rome, Italy. July, 1999.

770 Buckley JD, Abbott M, Brinkworth GD, Whyte P. **Bovine Colostrum Supplementation During Training Increases Vertical Jump Performance.** 2000 Pre-Olympic Congress Sports Medicine and Physical Education International Congress on Sport Science. Brisbane, Australia. 7-13 September, 2000.

771 Buckley JD, Brinkworth GD, Bourdon PC, Gulbin J, Stilwell EJ, David A, Myers N. **Oral Supplementation with Bovine Colostrum Improves Rowing Performance in Elite Female Rowers.** Abstract presented at the 5th I.O.C. World Congress on Sports Sciences, Sydney, Australia. October, 1999.

772 Sen CK, Atalay M, Hanninen O. **Exercise-Induced Oxidative Stress: Glutathione Supplementation and Deficiency.** *Journal of Applied Physiology* 77(5):2177-87 (1994).

773 Sjodin B, Hellsten-Westing Y, Apple FS. **Biochemical Mechanisms for the Oxygen Free Radical Formation During Exercise.** *Sports Medicine* 10(4):236-254 (1990).

774 Lands LC, Grey VL, Smountas AA. **Effect of Supplementation With A Cysteine Donor On Muscular Performance.** *Journal of Applied Physiology* 87(4):1381-1385 (1999).

775 Wilson T, Liggins GC, Joe L. **Purification and characterization of a uterine phospholipase inhibitor that loses activity after labor onset in women.** *American Journal of Obstetrics and Gynecology* 160(3):602-606 (1989).

776 Wilson T, Liggins GC, Aimer GP, Skinner SJ. **Partial purification and characterization of two compounds from amniotic fluid which inhibit phospholipase activity in human endometrial cells.** *Biochemistry and Biophysics Research Communications* 131(1):22-29 (1985).

777 Wilson T, Christie DL. **Gravidin, an endogenous inhibitor of phospholipase A2 activity, is a secretory component of IgA.** *Biochemistry and Biophysics Research Communications* 176(1):447-452 (1991).

778 Playford RJ, Floyd DN, Macdonald CE, Calnan DP, Adenekan RO, Johnson W, Goodlad RA, Marchbank T. **Bovine Colostrum is a Health Food Supplement which Prevents NSAID Induced Gut Damage.** *Gut* 44(5):653-658 (1999).

779 Playford RJ, Macdonald CE, Calnan DP, Floyd DN, Poda T, Wicks AC, Bashir O, Marchbank T. **Co-administration of the Health Food Supplement, Bovine Colostrum, Reduces the Acute Non-Steroidal Anti-Inflammatory Drug-Induced Increase in Intestinal Permeability.** *Clinical Science (London)* 100(6):627-633 (2001).

780 Playford RJ, Macdonald CE, Johnson WS. **Colostrum and Milk-Derived Peptide Growth Factors for the Treatment of Gastrointestinal Disorders.** *American Journal of Clinical Nutrition* 72(1):5-14 (2000).

781 Mero A. **Bovine Colostrum.** *Sports Dietary Supplements Update.* 13/6/02, http://www.esportmed.comsdsu/content/viewnotes.cfm?sis=31.

782 **Drugs in Sport Update.** *Australian Sports Drug Agency (ASDA) Newsletter* Spring 1998 Edition, Volume 2, Issue 3. http://www.nevdgp.org.au/geninf/health_info_search.htm 9/09/02.

783 Paton CD, Hopkins WG. **Performance Enhancement at the Fifth IOC World Congress on Sport Sciences.** *Sport Science* 3(3) (1999). http://www.sportsci.org/jour/9903/cdpwghIOC.html 9/09/02.

784 Hopkins WG, Hawley JA, Burke LM. **Design and Analysis of Research on Sport Performance Enhancement.** *Medicine & Science in Sports & Exercise* 31(3):472-85 (1999).

785 **Olympic Movement Anti-Doping Code, Appendix A: Prohibited Classes of Substances and Prohibited Methods.** 1 April 2000. http://www.nevdgp.org.au/geninf/asda/drugsin1.html 30/9/02.

786 **Substitutes Appendix A of the OMAC 1999—Olympic Movement Anti-Doping Code, Appendix A: Prohibited Classes of Substances and Prohibited Methods—2003.** 1 January 2003. http://www.usantidoping.org/files/2003IOCprohibited.pdf, published 27 September 2002 3/10/02.

787 **ASDA Drugs in Sport: Information on Substances** http://www.asda.org.au/au/dis.html 13 December 2002.

Leptin

788 Houseknecht KL, Mantzoros CS, Kuliawat R, Hadro E, Flier JS, Kahn BB. **Evidence for leptin binding to proteins in serum of rodents and humans: modulation with obesity.** *Diabetes* 45(11):1638-1643 (1996).

789 Golden PL, Maccagnan TJ, Pardridge WM. **Human blood-brain barrier leptin receptor. Binding and endocytosis in isolated human brain microvessels.** *Journal of Clinical Investigation* 99(1):14-18 (1997).

790 Diamond FB, Eichler DC, Duckett G, Jorgenson EV, Shulman D, Rot AW. **Demonstration of a leptin binding factor in human serum**. *Biochemistry and Biophysics Research Communications* 233:818-822 (1997).

791 Maffei M, Halaas J, Ravussin E, Pratley RE, Lee GH, Zhang Y, Fei H, Kim S, Lallone R, Ranganathan S. **Leptin levels in human and rodent: measurement of plasma leptin and ob RNA in obese and weight reduced subjects**. *Nature Medicine* 1(11):1155-1161 (1995).

792 Lammert A, Kiess W, Bottner A, Glasow A, Kratzsch J. **Soluble leptin receptor represents the main leptin binding activity in human blood**. *Biochemistry and Biophysics Research Communications* 283(4):982-988 (2001).

793 Huang L, Wang Z, Li C. **Modulation of circulating leptin levels by its soluble receptor.** *Journal of Biological Chemistry* 276:6343-6349 (2001).

794 Wadden TA, Considine RV, Foster GD, Anderson DA, Sarwer DB, Caro JS. **Short and long-term changes in serum leptin dieting obese women: effects of caloric restriction and weight loss.** *Journal of Clinical Endocrinology and Metabolism* 83(1):214-218 (1998).

795 Rissanen P, Makimattila S, Vehmas T, Taavitsainen M, Rissanen A. **Effect of weight loss and regional fat distribution on plasma leptin concentration in obese women**. *International Journal of Obstetrics and Related Metabolic Disorders* 23(6):645-649 (1999).

796 Bougoulia M, Tzotzas T, Efthymiou H, Koliakos G, Konstantinidis T, Triantos A, Krassas GE. **Leptin concentrations during oral glucose tolerance test (GTT) in obese and normal weight women**. *International Journal of Obstetrics and Related Metabolic Disorders* 23(6):625-628 (1999).

797 Mueller WM, Gregoire FM, Stanhope KL, Mobbs CV, Mizuno TM, Warden CH, Stern JS, Havel PJ. **Evidence that glucose metabolism regulates leptin secretion from cultured rat adipocytes**. *Endocrinology* 139(2):551-558 (1998).

798 Gavrilova O, Barr V, Marcus-Samuels B, Reitman M. **Hyperleptinemia of pregnancy associated with the appearance of a circulating form of the leptin receptor**. *Journal of Biological Chemistry* 272:30546-30551 (1997).

799 Hassink SG, de Lancey E, Sheslow DV, Smith-Kirwin SM, O'Connor DM, Considine RV, Opentanova I, Dostal K, Spear ML, Leef K, Ash M, Spitzer AR, Funanage VL. **Placental leptin: an important new growth factor in intrauterine and neonatal development.** *Pediatrics* 100(1):E1 (1997).

800 Studzinski S, Puzio I, Tatara M**. Leptin and its role at the time around birth**. *Zootechnica* 225(43):5-14 (2001).

801 Zabielski R, Wolinski J. **Role of colostrum and milk leptin in the development of the gastrointestinal tract**. *Zootechnica* 225(43):15-20 (2001).

802 Cohen P, Miyazaki M, Socci ND, Hagge-Greenberg A, Liedtke W, Soukas AA, Sharma R, Hudgins LC, Ntambi JM, Friedman JM. **Role for stearyol-CoA desaturase-1 in leptin-mediated weight loss**. Science 297(5579):240-243 (2002).

803 Heymsfield SB, Greenburg AS, Fujioka K, Dixon RM, Kushner R, Hunt T, Lubina JA, Patane J, Self B, Hunt P, McCamish M. **Recombinant leptin for weight loss in obese and lean adults**. *JAMA* 282(16):1568-1575 (1999).

804 Fruhbeck G, Diez-Caballero A, Salvador J, Alvarez-Cienfuegos J. **Chronobiology of recombinant leptin therapy**. *JAMA* 283(12):1567-1568 (2002).

805 Sinha MK, Caro JF. **Clinical Aspects of Leptin**. *Vitamins and Hormones* 54:1-30 (1998).

806 Tsang SH. **Obesity: from the mouse house to the ambulatory care clinic**. *P&S Medical Review* 5(1) (1998).

Appendix D Notes

Can Colostrum Assist AIDS Patients?

807 Nowa and McMichael. **How HIV defeats the immune system.** *Scientific American* Aug:58-65 (1995).

808 Harmsen MC, Swart PJ, Bethune M, Pauwels R, DeClercq E, The TH, Meijer DK. **Antiviral effects of plasma and milk proteins: lactoferrin shows potent activity against both human immunodeficiency virus and human cytomegalovirus replication *in vitro*.** *Journal of Infectious Diseases* 172(2):380-388 (1995).

809 Stephan W, Dichtelmuller H, Lissner R. **Antibodies from colostrum in oral immunotherapy.** *Journal of Clinical Biochemistry* 28(1):19-23 (1990).

810 Richie DJ, Becker ES. **Update on the Management of Intestinal Cryptosporidiosis in AIDS.** *Annals of Pharmacotherapy* 28(6):767-778 (1994).

811 Rump JA, Aarndt R, Arnold A, Bendick C, Dichtelmuller H, Franke M, Helm EB, Jager H, Kampmann B, Kolb P. **Treatment of diarrhea in human immunodeficiency virus-infected patients with immunoglobulins from bovine colostrum.** *Clinical Investigation* 70(7):588-594 (1992).

812 Ungar BL, Ward DJ, Fayer R, Quinn CA. **Cessation of cryptosporidium-associated diarrhea in AIDS patients after treatment with hyperimmune bovine colostrum.** *Gastroenterology* 98(2):486-489 (1990).

813 Bogstedt AK, Johansen K, Hatta H, Kim M, Casswall T, Svensson L, Hammarstrom L. **Passive immunity against diarrhea.** *Acta Paediatrica* 85(2):125-128 (1996).

814 Plettenberg A, Stoehr A, Stellbrink HJ, Albrecht H, Meigel W. **A preparation from bovine colostrum in the treatment of HIV-positive patients with chronic diarrhea.** *Clinical Investigation* 71(1):42-45 (1993).

815 Bricker DS. **Colostrum: implications for accelerated recovery in damaged muscles and cartilage, prevention of some pathogenic disease.** *The American Chiropractor* Nov. 1991:4-5.